AF411172

Marine Anti-Inflammatory and Antioxidant Agents 2.0

Editors

Donatella Degl'Innocenti
Marzia Vasarri

MDPI • Basel • Beijing • Wuhan • Barcelona • Belgrade • Manchester • Tokyo • Cluj • Tianjin

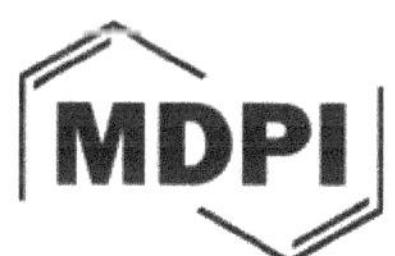

Editors
Donatella Degl'Innocenti
Università degli Studi di
Firenze
Italy

Marzia Vasarri
Università degli Studi di
Firenze
Italy

Editorial Office
MDPI
St. Alban-Anlage 66
4052 Basel, Switzerland

This is a reprint of articles from the Special Issue published online in the open access journal *Marine Drugs* (ISSN 1660-3397) (available at: https://www.mdpi.com/journal/marinedrugs/special_issues/Anti_inflammatoryAntioxidantAgents2).

For citation purposes, cite each article independently as indicated on the article page online and as indicated below:

LastName, A.A.; LastName, B.B.; LastName, C.C. Article Title. *Journal Name* **Year**, *Volume Number*, Page Range.

ISBN 978-3-0365-6784-6 (Hbk)
ISBN 978-3-0365-6785-3 (PDF)

Contents

About the Editors

Donatella Degl'Innocenti

Prof. Donatella Degl'Innocenti obtained a Ph.D. in Biochemistry, and she has been an Associate Professor of Biochemistry in the Department of Experimental and Clinical Biomedical Sciences "Mario Serio" (University of Florence, Italy) since 2001. During her scientific career, she built national and international scientific collaborations.

She is an active researcher and the leader of her department laboratory (https://www.sbsc.unifi.it/vp-223-gruppo-degl-innocenti.html). She has strong, independent research experience, with an impact in the field, as demonstrated by several publications as a senior author in international, peer-reviewed journals. She is also a member of the Scientific Committee of the Interuniversity Center of Marine Biology and Applied Ecology (CIBM) of Livorno (Italy).

In recent years, she has focused her research on the health role of natural and marine compounds. She studied the amyloid aggregation process and potential inhibitory mechanisms of natural compounds and the extract of Mediterranean red seaweed.

Prof. Degl'Innocenti has also studied the biological properties of extracts obtained from the leaves of the *Posidonia oceanica* (L.) Delile marine plant, focusing on these extracts' role in pathophysiological cellular processes, such as inflammation and oxidative stress, as well as on cancer cell migration and protein glycation processes.

Marzia Vasarri

Dr. Marzia Vasarri is a Post-Doc fellow at the Department of Experimental and Clinical Biomedical Sciences "Mario Serio" (University of Florence, Italy). She obtained a Bachelor's degree in Biotechnology in 2014 and a Master's degree in Medical and Pharmaceutical Biotechnology in 2016. During her studies, she acquired technical-scientific skills in biochemistry and molecular biology.

Her research focuses on the bioactive properties of natural products, with particular reference to products of marine origin. Much of her research targets the marine plant Posidonia oceanica (L.) Delile has been investigated by Dr. Vasarri for a variety of pathophysiological cellular processes, from inflammation and oxidative stress to cancer cell migration, protein glycation processes, lipid accumulation in hepatic cells, and their potential as an inducer of autophagy.

Her research interests also include the field of neurodegeneration and amyloid aggregation process, and the protective role of natural compounds against amyloid cytotoxicity. She has also conducted research on the biological properties of natural products delivered within nanoformulations that can improve the efficacy and bioavailability of the encapsulated compounds/phytocomplex to exploit their full potential.

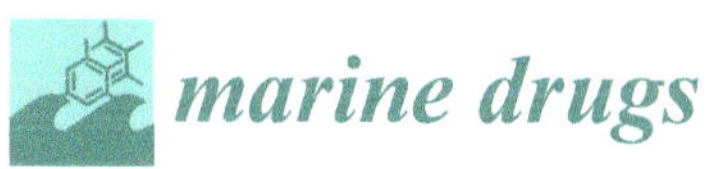

marine drugs

Editorial

News and Updates from 2022 on Antioxidant and Anti-Inflammatory Properties of Marine Products

Marzia Vasarri * and Donatella Degl'Innocenti

Department of Experimental and Clinical Biomedical Sciences, University of Florence, Viale Morgagni 50, 50134 Florence, Italy
* Correspondence: marzia.vasarri@unifi.it

Citation: Vasarri, M.; Degl'Innocenti, D. News and Updates from 2022 on Antioxidant and Anti-Inflammatory Properties of Marine Products. *Mar. Drugs* **2023**, *21*, 26. https://doi.org/10.3390/md21010026

Received: 22 December 2022
Accepted: 27 December 2022
Published: 29 December 2022

Inflammation and oxidative stress are often the common denominators of most modern chronic diseases and disorders, resulting in serious problems for health care systems. The problems associated with the long-term use of conventional therapies have prompted research into new safe, effective, and natural anti-inflammatory and antioxidant agents. In this context, the scientific community is focusing its attention on the rich biodiversity of the marine environment as a molecular source of a variety of bioactive compounds.

This Special Issue of *Marine Drugs*, "Marine Anti-inflammatory and Antioxidant Agents 2.0", brings together six original research papers, two clinical studies, and two comprehensive reviews of natural marine anti-inflammatory and/or antioxidant agents. The natural compounds discussed were sourced from a variety of marine organisms, including oysters, seaweeds, marine plants, deep-sea fungi, Chondrichthyes, and echinoderms. The collected scientific works introduce new perspectives on the applicability of marine products for human health and in biotechnology.

Among all marine organisms, seaweeds have been used since ancient times for their many health benefits, which are mainly due to their bioactive compounds. Therefore, research on the biological properties of seaweed-derived compounds has made considerable progress in various fields of applications possible. In this regard, El-Beltagi et al. (2022) collected information on the composition and beneficial properties of seaweeds [1]. This review described seaweeds as an alternative source of synthetic substances to improve consumer well-being through their incorporation into novel foods or functional medicines.

Research by Roach et al. (2022) also demonstrated valuable health and pharmacological properties of seaweed-derived compounds [2]. Two clinical studies were conducted in humans after ingestion of a single sulfated polysaccharide from the green alga *Ulva* sp. 84, "xylorhamnoglucuronan" (SXRG84). Study 1 found a reduction in non-HDL (high-density lipoprotein) cholesterol and the atherogenic index in all participants, in the insulin levels in overweight adult participants fed 2 g/day of SXRG84, and in the C-reactive protein levels in overweight participants fed 4 g/day of SXRG84. Study 2 described an unchanged lipid level between the groups and lowered plasma concentrations of pro-inflammatory cytokines (IFN-γ, IL-1β, TNF-α, and IL-10) at 12 weeks after SXRG84 treatment. The two studies did not show consistent effects on the gut microbiome, although a change in microbiota composition and abundance following treatment was observed in Study 1. Given the beneficial effects of SXRG84 on inflammatory markers in overweight subjects, the authors suggested the potential use of SXRG84-based supplements to reduce the inflammatory response related to metabolic disorders.

Beside seaweeds, many other marine organisms are sources of polysaccharides. Chondroitin sulfate (CS), an anionic glycosaminoglycan derived from animal cartilage, is widely used in various biopharmaceutical applications. This Special Issue presents a theoretical study on the use of CS derived from shark cartilage as a stabilizing agent of selenium nanoparticles (SeNPs) [3]. Selenium (Se) is an essential micronutrient for human health due to its antioxidant properties, but the narrow margin between beneficial and harmful doses limits its practices in food and medicine. Furthermore, the advantages of using SeNPs as drug carriers are limited by stability issues. Chen et al. (2022) prepared selenium-chondroitin sulfate (SeCS) via a redox reaction of sodium selenite and ascorbic acid, using shark CS as a template. SeCS possessed good storage stability and had higher antioxidant activity than SeNPs and CS [3]. Therefore, the authors proposed the application of SeCS in the prevention and mitigation of oxidative stress-related diseases.

Marine bioactive natural products also include peptides and proteins. The broad spectrum of the bioactivity of these biomolecules makes them potentially valuable nutraceuticals and medicines.

A huge body of literature indicates that the human health benefits of protein hydrolysates can, in part, be attributed to their free-amino-acid-rich and peptide-rich properties. Wang et al. (2022) described how free-amino-acid-rich protein hydrolysates obtained from oysters (*Crassostrea hongkongensis*) had an ameliorative effect of on cadmium (Cd)-induced acute liver injury in mice [4]. As a result of the treatment with oyster protein hydrolysates (OPs), liver function profiles were improved, whereas hemorrhages, lymphocyte accumulation, and inflammatory cell infiltration around the central veins were reduced. Supplementation with OPs reduced malondialdehyde formation and restored the activity of antioxidant enzymes (SOD, CAT, and GPH-Px) in the liver of Cd-exposed mice. OPs blocked inflammatory responses (IL-1β, IL-6, and TNF-α) by inhibiting the expression of inflammation-related proteins (MIP-2 and COX-2) and suppressed hepatocyte apoptosis (Bax, caspase-3, and Blc-2) by regulating ERK/NF-κB- and PI3K/AKT-related signaling pathways in Cd-exposed mice.

Among marine organisms, microalgae represent another rich source of proteins and peptides. *Chlorella vulgaris* is a green microalga used as a source of proteins in aquatic feed to improve growth performance, oxidative status, and immune response in several fish species. The study by Reis et al. (2022) evaluated the effects of short-term supplementation with a 2% *C. vulgaris* biomass and two 0.1% *C. vulgaris* soluble peptide-enriched extracts on immune defenses, oxidative stress, and the inflammatory response of gilthead seabream (*Sparus aurata*) after an inflammatory insult [5]. The *C. vulgaris* peptide-enriched extract had a dual modulatory effect at both the blood and gut levels. In particular, the peptide-enriched extract drives the proliferation of circulating neutrophils in resting gilthead seabream, and, following an inflammatory insult, it can protect the gut from stress.

Carotenoids are among the most common pigments found in the marine environment, and commercially appealing applications are possible due to their many biological properties. Astaxanthin (ATX) is a lipid-soluble carotenoid found in most marine organisms that has documented pharmacological effects, including neuroprotection and antioxidant activity. The study published by Park et al. in 2022 found that the once-daily administration of ATX (100 mg/kg) significantly reduced the death of hippocampal pyramidal cells in gerbils undergoing transient ischemia, as well as DNA damage and lipid peroxidation in the forebrain pyramidal cells [6]. Furthermore, ATX treatment increased the expression of the antioxidant enzyme superoxide dismutase. Therefore, the authors suggested that ATX, due to its antioxidant and neuroprotective properties, can be used as a potential dietary supplement to prevent the progression of severe ischemic brain injury.

The marine environment is also an excellent source of phenolic compounds. Marine-derived phenols exhibit a wide range of biological effects through their uniqueness and structural complexity. The study by Morresi et al. (2022) showed that polyphenol-rich *Posidonia oceanica* leaf hydroalcoholic extract (POE) can reduce glucose transport by lowering GLUT2 levels, promote intestinal barrier integrity by modulating levels of Zonulin-1, and have a protective antioxidant effect against glucose-induced damage in human intestinal Caco-2 cells [7]. This was the first study investigating the behavior of a complex pool of POE phenolic compounds on differentiated Caco-2 cells as a model of the intestinal barrier. Therefore, the authors suggested that the phytocomplex of *Posidonia oceanica* may prevent gut cell dysfunction during the development of inflammation-related diseases associated with oxidative stress.

Furthermore, Vodouhè et al. (2022) demonstrated that the daily consumption of 500 mg of polyphenol-rich brown seaweed (*Ascophyllum nodosum* and *Fucus vesiculosus*) capsules combined with a low-calorie diet had no impact on body weight and blood sugar in overweight prediabetic subjects [8]. Instead, the intake of polyphenol-rich capsules showed a beneficial impact on insulin secretion, heart rate, and inflammatory response. Considering these data, the authors suggested that the early effect of brown seaweed extract on the inflammatory response might be associated with marginal changes in metabolic parameters related to the prevention of type 2 diabetes.

Looking for new bioactive compounds from marine natural products, Anh et al. (2022) isolated and identified three nitrogen-containing secondary metabolites from the ethyl acetate extract of the marine fungus *Aspergillus unguis* IV17-109 [9]. In particular, two new compounds, variotin B (1) and coniosulfide E (2), were identified together with a known compound, unguisin A (3). Compounds 1 and 2 were preliminarily tested for their anti-inflammatory activity by evaluating their inhibitory effect on the lipopolysaccharide-induced production of inflammatory mediators (including NO, IL-6, and iNOS) in RAW 264.7 murine macrophages. Interesting results were obtained for compound 1, which showed moderate anti-inflammatory activity.

In recent decades, many studies have focused on the anti-inflammatory effects of compounds from echinoderms. In this context, Ghelani et al. (2022) collected research articles published between 2010 and 2022 on the anti-inflammatory properties of sea cucumbers, sea urchins, and starfish [10]. In this review, the structures, bioactivity, and molecular mechanisms of these compounds were summarized. In addition, the potential applications of these compounds in the pharmaceutical industry for drug development against chronic inflammation were highlighted.

In conclusion, the studies compiled in this Special Issue confirm that marine organisms are an excellent source of biologically active molecules with antioxidant and anti-inflammatory properties, and that studies of these marine products can contribute to the discovery of new drugs and the scientific validation of their use.

Acknowledgments: Authors and reviewers alike are greatly appreciated for their hard work and the quality of the submitted articles.

Conflicts of Interest: The authors declare no conflict of interest.

References

1. El-Beltagi, H.S.; Mohamed, A.A.; Mohamed, H.I.; Ramadan, K.M.A.; Barqawi, A.A.; Mansour, A.T. Phytochemical and Potential Properties of Seaweeds and Their Recent Applications: A Review. *Mar. Drugs* **2022**, *20*, 342. [CrossRef] [PubMed]
2. Roach, L.A.; Meyer, B.J.; Fitton, J.H.; Winberg, P. Improved Plasma Lipids, Anti-Inflammatory Activity, and Microbiome Shifts in Overweight Participants: Two Clinical Studies on Oral Supplementation with Algal Sulfated Polysaccharide. *Mar. Drugs* **2022**, *20*, 500. [CrossRef] [PubMed]
3. Chen, J.; Chen, X.; Li, J.; Luo, B.; Fan, T.; Li, R.; Liu, X.; Song, B.; Jia, X.; Zhong, S. Preparation and Characterization of Nano-Selenium Decorated by Chondroitin Sulfate Derived from Shark Cartilage and Investigation on Its Antioxidant Activity. *Mar. Drugs* **2022**, *20*, 172. [CrossRef] [PubMed]
4. Wang, J.; Fang, Z.; Li, Y.; Sun, L.; Liu, Y.; Deng, Q.; Zhong, S. Ameliorative Effects of Oyster Protein Hydrolysates on Cadmium-Induced Hepatic Injury in Mice. *Mar. Drugs* **2022**, *20*, 758. [CrossRef] [PubMed]
5. Reis, B.; Ramos-Pinto, L.; Cunha, S.A.; Pintado, M.; da Silva, J.L.; Dias, J.; Conceição, L.; Matos, E.; Costas, B. *Chlorella vulgaris* Extracts as Modulators of the Health Status and the Inflammatory Response of Gilthead Seabream Juveniles (*Sparus aurata*). *Mar. Drugs* **2022**, *20*, 407. [CrossRef] [PubMed]
6. Park, J.H.; Lee, T.-K.; Kim, D.W.; Ahn, J.H.; Lee, C.-H.; Kim, J.-D.; Shin, M.C.; Cho, J.H.; Lee, J.-C.; Won, M.-H.; et al. Astaxanthin Confers a Significant Attenuation of Hippocampal Neuronal Loss Induced by Severe Ischemia-Reperfusion Injury in Gerbils by Reducing Oxidative Stress. *Mar. Drugs* **2022**, *20*, 267. [CrossRef] [PubMed]
7. Morresi, C.; Vasarri, M.; Bellachioma, L.; Ferretti, G.; Degl'Innocenti, D., Bacchetti, T. Glucose Uptake and Oxidative Stress in Caco-2 Cells: Health Benefits from *Posidonia oceanica* (L.) Delile. *Mar. Drugs* **2022**, *20*, 457. [CrossRef] [PubMed]
8. Vodouhè, M.; Marois, J.; Guay, V.; Leblanc, N.; Weisnagel, S.J.; Bilodeau, J.-F.; Jacques, H. Marginal Impact of Brown Seaweed *Ascophyllum nodosum* and *Fucus vesiculosus* Extract on Metabolic and Inflammatory Response in Overweight and Obese Prediabetic Subjects. *Mar. Drugs* **2022**, *20*, 174. [CrossRef] [PubMed]

9. Anh, C.V.; Yoon, Y.D.; Kang, J.S.; Lee, H.-S.; Heo, C.-S.; Shin, H.J. Nitrogen-Containing Secondary Metabolites from a Deep-Sea Fungus Aspergillus unguis and Their Anti-Inflammatory Activity. *Mar. Drugs* **2022**, *20*, 217. [CrossRef] [PubMed]
10. Ghelani, H.; Khursheed, M.; Adrian, T.E.; Jan, R.K. Anti-Inflammatory Effects of Compounds from Echinoderms. *Mar. Drugs* **2022**, *20*, 693. [CrossRef] [PubMed]

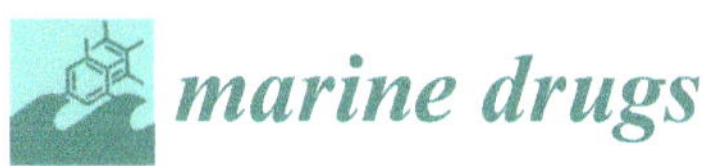

Article

Ameliorative Effects of Oyster Protein Hydrolysates on Cadmium-Induced Hepatic Injury in Mice

Jingwen Wang [1,2,3,4,†], Zhijia Fang [1,2,3,4,*,†], Yongbin Li [1,2,3,4], Lijun Sun [1,2,3,4], Ying Liu [1,2,3,4], Qi Deng [1,2,3,4] and Saiyi Zhong [1,2,3,4,*]

[1] College of Food Science and Technology, Guangdong Ocean University, Zhanjiang 524088, China
[2] Guangdong Provincial Key Laboratory of Aquatic Product Processing and Safety, Zhanjiang 524088, China
[3] Guangdong Provincial Engineering Technology Research Center of Marine Food, Zhanjiang 524088, China
[4] Key Laboratory of Advanced Processing of Aquatic Products of Guangdong Higher Education Institution, Zhanjiang 524088, China
* Correspondence: fangzj@gdou.edu.cn (Z.F.); zsylxc@126.com (S.Z.); Tel./Fax: +86-759-2396027 (Z.F.)
† These authors contributed equally to this work.

Abstract: Cadmium (Cd) is a widespread environmental toxicant that can cause severe hepatic injury. Oyster protein hydrolysates (OPs) have potential effects on preventing liver disease. In this study, thirty mice were randomly divided into five groups: the control, Cd, Cd + ethylenediaminetetraacetic acid (EDTA, 100 mg/kg), and low/high dose of OPs-treatment groups (100 mg/kg or 300 mg/kg). After continuous administration for 7 days, the ameliorative effect of OPs on Cd-induced acute hepatic injury in Cd-exposed mice was assessed. The results showed that OPs significantly improved the liver function profiles (serum ALT, AST, LDH, and ALP) in Cd-exposed mice. Histopathological analysis showed that OPs decreased apoptotic bodies, hemorrhage, lymphocyte accumulation, and inflammatory cell infiltration around central veins. OPs significantly retained the activities of SOD, CAT, and GSH-Px, and decreased the elevated hepatic MDA content in Cd-exposed mice. In addition, OPs exhibited a reductive effect on the inflammatory responses (IL-1β, IL-6, and TNF-α) and inhibitory effects on the expression of inflammation-related proteins (MIP-2 and COX-2) and the ERK/NF-κB signaling pathway. OPs suppressed the development of hepatocyte apoptosis (Bax, caspase-3, and Blc-2) and the activation of the PI3K/AKT signaling pathway in Cd-exposed mice. In conclusion, OPs ameliorated the Cd-induced hepatic injury by inhibiting oxidative damage and inflammatory responses, as well as the development of hepatocyte apoptosis via regulating the ERK/NF-κB and PI3K/AKT-related signaling pathways.

Keywords: cadmium; oyster protein hydrolysate; hepatic injury; oxidative stress; inflammatory response; hepatocyte apoptosis

Citation: Wang, J.; Fang, Z.; Li, Y.; Sun, L.; Liu, Y.; Deng, Q.; Zhong, S. Ameliorative Effects of Oyster Protein Hydrolysates on Cadmium-Induced Hepatic Injury in Mice. *Mar. Drugs* **2022**, *20*, 758. https://doi.org/10.3390/md20120758

Academic Editors: Donatella Degl'Innocenti and Marzia Vasarri

Received: 7 October 2022
Accepted: 28 November 2022
Published: 30 November 2022

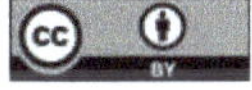

1. Introduction

Cadmium (Cd) is a widespread environmental toxicant that poses a serious threat to human health [1]. Due to its high solubility in water, Cd can easily enter the human body through the food chain from polluted soils and water [2]. Cd exposure will cause metabolic dysfunction and eventually lead to irreversible damage to multiple organs [3,4]. About 50–70% of the absorbed heavy metal accumulates in the kidney and liver [5]. Acute Cd exposure primarily results in liver accumulation and hepatic injury [6]. The liver has been considered one of the main target organs of Cd [7]. Recent research has shown that acute Cd exposure leads to severe hepatic injury, accompanied by oxidative damage, inflammation, and apoptosis [8]. Therefore, reducing oxidative damage, ameliorating inflammatory response, and preventing the development of hepatocyte apoptosis may be practical strategies for the treatment of Cd-induced hepatic injury.

Protein hydrolysates from oysters (*Crassostrea hongkongensis*) have multiple health benefits, including anti-oxidation [9], anti-inflammatory [10], anti-apoptosis [11], anti-cancer, and other properties [12]. In previous studies, oyster-derived hydrolysates have been shown to be protective against D-galactosamine(D-GalN)-induced hepatic injury [13]. The peptides (SCAP1, SCAP3, and SCAP7) produced from oyster protein hydrolysis (OPs) present strong antioxidant and anti-cancer properties [14]. In addition, OPs are considered to be a safe and effective dietetic treatment for alcoholic liver disease by declining ethanol-induced oxidative stress and inflammation [15]. In addition, oyster ferritin was found to efficiently reduce the damage of heavy metals in mice [16]. The evidence suggests that OPs might be a potential candidate for ameliorating Cd-induced hepatic injury. Therefore, this study aimed to investigate the ameliorative effect of OPs on hepatic oxidative damage, inflammation, and apoptosis in Cd-exposed mice.

2. Results

2.1. Sequence Analysis of the Main Peptides of OPs

As shown in Figure 1, the peaks of OPs were mostly in the range of 300 to 900 m/z. Overall, 177 peptides, with molecular weights ranging from 550.250 to 1387.697 Da, and an intensity ranging from 3,857,400 to 171,200,000, were identified from the OPs. The peptide fingerprinting of 40 characteristic peptides in OPs was analyzed using liquid chromatography–tandem mass spectrometry (LC-MS/MS). The scores for evaluating the matches between the theoretical and experimental mass spectrums were obtained by comparing the UniProt database; 20 peptide sequences with higher scores are listed in Table 1. Of interest, they contain a higher percentage of hydrophobic amino acids, such as proline (P, 37/180 residues in 20 peptides), valine (V, 14/180), and alanine (A, 8/180). Specific amino acid motifs, such as PVX, was repeated six times, and PxxP was repeated eight times, X being either a glycine, serine, or a proline residue, x being either an alanine, glycine, valine, threonine, asparagine, leucine, glutamic acid, aspartic acid, or an arginine, can be recognized. Hydrophobic amino acids proline or proline-rich peptides were reported to possess good anti-Cd, anti-oxidation, and anti-inflammatory properties [17–22].

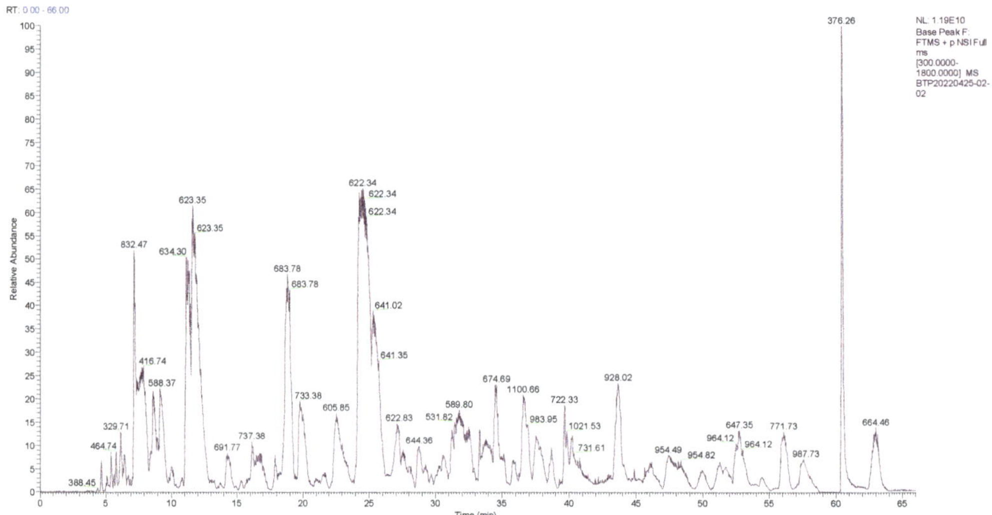

Figure 1. Total ion chromatogram of peptides from oyster enzymatic hydrolysates (OPs).

Table 1. Main peptide sequences of OPs.

Rank	Peptide Sequence	Length	Molecular Mass (Da)	Observed Mass (*m/z*)	Peak Area	Relative Peak Area (%)	Scores
1	GEPGPEGPAGPIGPR	15	1387.697	694.350	18,567,000	0.15	614.6
2	YEETRGVLK	9	1094.584	547.795	9,895,900	0.08	494.2
3	GPTGPVGPL	9	794.441	794.437	3,857,400	0.03	477.2
4	GPSGEPGPE	9	826.358	826.354	12,054,000	0.10	468.7
5	DIERPTYT	8	994.484	497.745	18,359,000	0.15	461.4
6	ENPVPVPS	8	838.431	838.427	6,999,200	0.06	453.3
7	TEAPLNPK	8	869.473	869.471	9,380,400	0.08	451.1
8	TPEEFIPR	8	988.510	494.758	12,323,000	0.10	437.8
9	AGFAGDDAPR	10	976.448	488.727	171,200,000	1.39	430.9
10	TPTYGDL	7	766.362	766.359	46,716,000	0.38	428.1
11	PDVPAGDVDKGK	12	1197.611	399.874	14,901,000	0.12	425.1
12	GPIGGPL	7	610.356	610.354	5,358,100	0.04	423.7
13	SPVGVGA	7	586.320	586.318	13,332,000	0.11	411.4
14	YTPVAYPV	8	586.320	586.318	4,007,500	0.03	388.5
15	LTPSGLPY	8	647.342	647.342	14,591,000	0.12	386.7
16	STPFEGF	7	571.308	571.308	13,332,000	0.11	384.4
17	VSDTVVEPYN	10	550.250	550.250	27,505,000	0.22	383.3
18	DIERPTYTN	9	909.420	909.420	8,461,100	0.07	383.2
19	QGETGDRGPFG	11	879.456	440.231	34,716,000	0.28	383.0
20	PRPPTQVGGS	10	995.525	498.266	38,429,000	0.31	382.8

2.2. Composition of Amino Acid in OPs

According to the data from the automatic analyzer, the content of total amino acids in OPs was 33.73 g/100 g (Table 2). The content of essential amino acids in OPs was 11.82 g/100 g and accounted for 35.04% of the total amino acids. The content of hydrophobic amino acids was 12.76 g/100 g and accounted for 37.83% of the total amino acids. OPs were rich in Glutamic acid (Glu, 4.33 g/100 g), Aspartic acid (Asp, 3.36 g/100 g), Alanine (Ala, 2.63 g/100 g), Proline (Pro, 2.61 g/100 g), and Lysine (Lys, 2.61 g/100 g).

Table 2. Composition and content of amino acids in OPs.

Amino Acids	Contents (g/100 g)	Amino Acids	Contents (g/100 g)
Alanine (Ala) [#]	2.63	Leucine (Leu) [*#]	2.02
Cystine (Cys)	0.40	Methionine (Met) [*#]	0.65
Aspartic acid (Asp)	3.36	Proline (Pro) [#]	2.61
Glutamic acid (Glu)	4.33	Arginine (Arg)	1.71
Phenylalanine (Phe) [*#]	0.72	Serine (Ser)	1.83
Glycine (Gly)	2.92	Threonine (Thr) [*]	1.69
Histidine (His)	0.50	Valine (Val) [*#]	1.81
Isoleucine (Ile) [*#]	1.40	Tyrosine (Tyr)	1.62
Lysine (Lys) [*]	2.61	Tryptophan (Trp) [*#]	0.92
Total amino acids	33.73		
Essential amino acid	11.82		
Hydrophobic amino acids	12.76		

Note: * Essential amino acids. # Hydrophobic amino acids.

2.3. Contents of Free Amino Acids in OPs

Table 3 shows the free amino acid content and composition of OPs. The contents of total free amino acids in OPs were 15.80 g/100 g, indicating OPs contained abundant free amino acids. Among these free amino acids, Pro (2.49 g/100 g), Glu (2.12 g/100 g), Tyr (1.51 g/100 g), Lys (1.43 g/100 g), Gly (1.38 g/100 g), and Val (0.91 g/100 g) were highly detected in OPs. The essential free amino acids accounted for 33.73% of the free total amino acids, and free hydrophobic amino acids accounted for 38.86%.

Table 3. Contents of free amino acids in OPs.

Free Amino Acids	Contents (g/100 g)	Free Amino Acids	Contents (g/100 g)
Ala [#]	0.59	Met [*#]	0.36
Cys	ND	Asn	0.26
Asp	0.37	Pro [#]	2.49
Glu	2.12	Gln	0.85
Phe [*#]	0.18	Arg	0.53
Gly	1.38	Ser	0.29
His	0.08	Thr [*]	0.84
Ile [*#]	0.59	Val [*#]	0.91
Lys [*]	1.43	Trp [*#]	0.52
Leu [*#]	0.50	Tyr	1.51
Total free amino acids	15.80		
Essential free amino acid	5.33		
Hydrophobic free amino acids	6.14		

Note: * Essential free amino acids. # Hydrophobic free amino acids; ND: not detected.

2.4. Effects of OPs on Hepatic Dysfunction in Cd-Exposed Mice

Compared with the control group, the Cd-exposed mice group showed the highest levels of serum alanine transaminase (ALT), aspartate aminotransferase (AST), alkaline phosphatase (ALP), and lactate dehydrogenase (LDH) (Figure 2). EDTA therapy is the most widely used for treating patients with acute or chronic Cd disease [23]. Thus, it was used as a positive control in this test. The supplement of OPs significantly decreased the levels of serum ALT, AST, ALP, and LDH ($p < 0.01$). The effects of OPs were met even better than that of the positive agent EDTA treatment. OPs exhibited a good ameliorative effect on hepatic dysfunction in Cd-exposed mice.

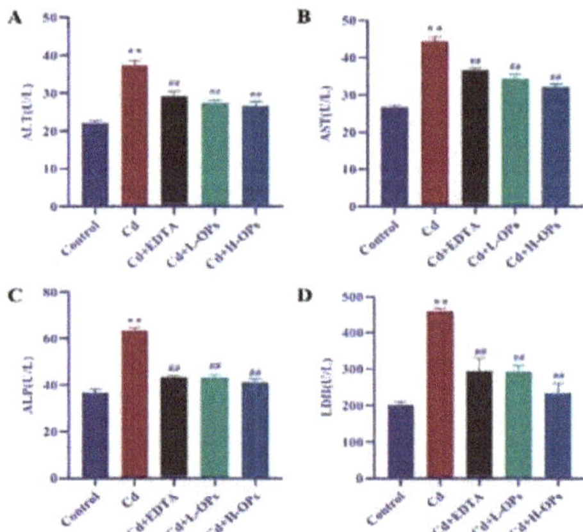

Figure 2. Effect of OPs on the liver function profiles in mice (**A**) ALT: Alanine aminotransferase; (**B**) AST: Aspartate aminotransferase; (**C**) ALP: Alkaline phosphatase; (**D**) LDH: Lactate dehydrogenase; Control: Intraperitoneal injection of 0.9% NaCl (saline) once daily; Cd: Mice were injected intraperitoneally with $CdCl_2$ 5 mg/kg daily; EDTA: Mice were injected with $CdCl_2$ (5 mg/kg) intraperitoneally after 1 hour of oral administration with EDTA (100 mg/kg) daily; Cd+L-OPs: Mice were injected with $CdCl_2$ (5 mg/kg) intra-peritoneally after 1 hour of oral administration with a low dose of OPs (100 mg/kg) daily. Mice were injected with $CdCl_2$ (5 mg/kg) intra-peritoneally after 1 h of oral administration with a high dose of OPs (300 mg/kg) daily. The data were expressed as mean ± SEM, $n = 6$ in each group. Compared with the control group, ** $p < 0.01$; compared with the Cd group, ## $p < 0.01$.

2.5. Effect of OPs on Hepatic Injury in Cd-Exposed Mice

The organ weight coefficient is commonly used to evaluate the toxic effect [24]. The liver weight coefficient of the mice in the Cd-exposed group was significantly higher than that of the mice in the control group ($p < 0.01$). The OPs markedly lowered the liver coefficients in Cd-exposed mice ($p < 0.01$). Histopathological sections of the liver stained with H&E are shown in Figure 3B. Compared with the control group, the mice in the Cd group showed obvious pathological changes in liver tissue, including apoptotic bodies, hemorrhage, lymphocyte accumulation, and inflammatory cell infiltration around the central vein. In the OPs and EDTA-treated groups, liver tissue retained its normal appearance and had fewer apoptotic bodies. OPs showed a protective effect on liver tissue against Cd.

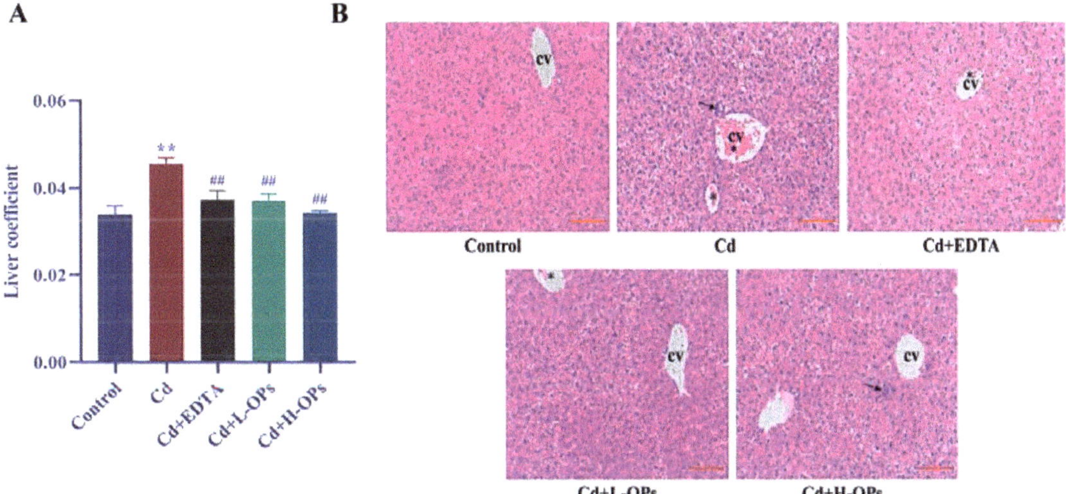

Figure 3. Effects of OPs on liver coefficient and hepatic injury in Cd-exposed mice. (**A**) Liver coefficient = liver weight(g)/mouse weight(g); (**B**) Histopathology with H&E staining ($200\times$) of the liver in mice after treatment for 7 days; CV: Central veins; Arrow: lymphocyte accumulation in the parenchyma; asterisk (*): hemorrhage. Bar = 100 μm. The data were expressed as mean ± SEM, $n = 6$ in each group. Compared with the control group, ** $p < 0.01$; compared with the Cd group, ## $p < 0.01$.

2.6. Effect of OPs on Hepatic Oxidative Indexes in Cd-Exposed Mice

An increased MDA level is an important indicator of oxidative stress. The Cd-exposed mice group showed the highest levels of hepatic MDA, while the OPs treatment significantly lowered the level of MDA ($p < 0.01$, Figure 4A). More importantly, the effects of OPs were better than that of EDTA. OPs markedly inhibited lipid peroxidation (MDA as an indicator) and MDA production in Cd-exposed mice. As shown in Figure 4B–D, antioxidant markers such as SOD, CAT, and GSH-Px were significantly reduced in the Cd-exposed mice group compared to the control group. OPs retained higher activity of antioxidant enzymes in Cd-exposed mice. OPs exhibited a strong reductive effect on Cd-induced oxidative stress in the liver.

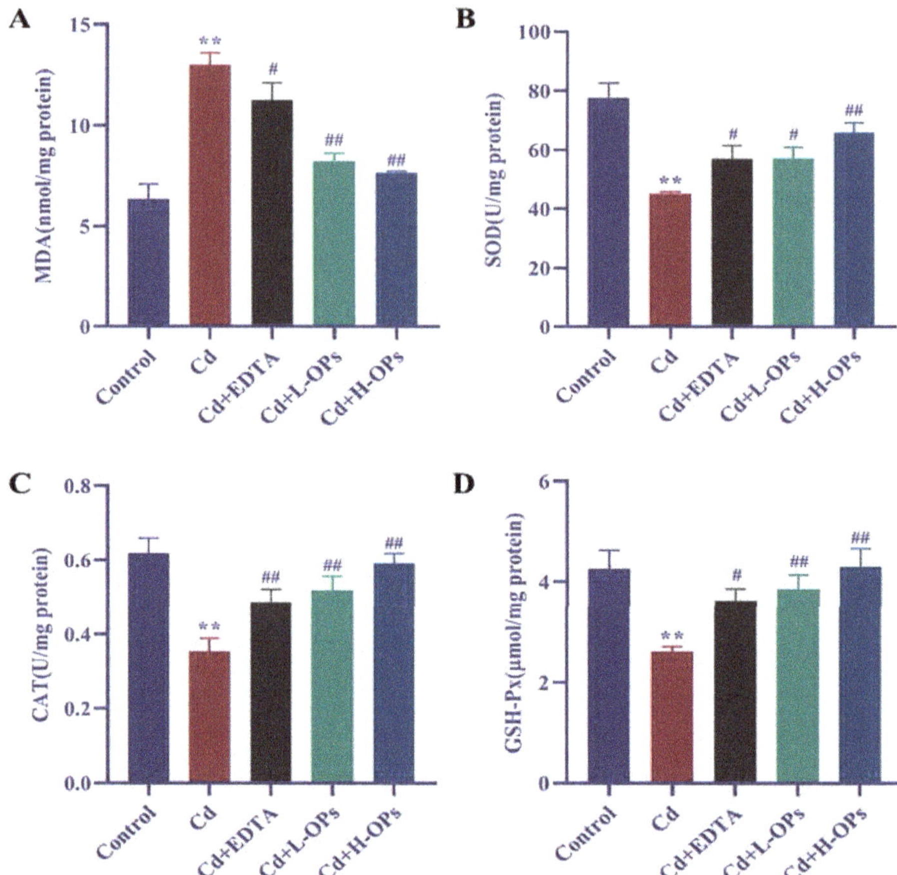

Figure 4. Effects of OPs on MDA level, SOD, CAT, and GSH-Px activities in Cd-induced mice. (**A**) Malondialdehyde (MDA); (**B**) Superoxide dismutase (SOD); (**C**) Catalase (CAT); (**D**) Glutathione peroxidase (GSH-Px). The data were expressed as mean $\pm$ SEM, n = 6 in each group. Compared with the control group, ** $p < 0.01$; compared with the Cd group, [#] $p < 0.05$, [##] $p < 0.01$.

2.7. Effect of OPs on The Hepatic Inflammatory Response (IL-1β, IL-6, TNF-α) in Cd-Exposed Mice

Interleukin IL-1β and IL-6 are two stimulators of the hepatic synthesis of acute-phase proteins in the inflammatory response to stress and important biological markers of hepatic inflammation [25,26]. TNF-α is an important biological marker in substantial hepatic tissue damage [27]. As shown in Figure 5A–C, the mice in the Cd-exposed group have the highest level of hepatic inflammatory cytokines (IL-1β, IL-6, and TNF-α) ($p < 0.01$). OPs significantly attenuated Cd-induced the high level of hepatic IL-1β, IL-6, and TNF-α ($p < 0.01$ and $p < 0.05$, respectively). The results from quantitative reverse-transcription PCR analysis (qRT-PCR) manifested that OPs inhibited the expression of hepatic IL-1β, IL-6, and TNF-α in Cd-exposed mice ($p < 0.01$). These results revealed that the protection of OPs against Cd was associated with its attenuation of the Cd-induced hepatic inflammation in Cd-exposed mice.

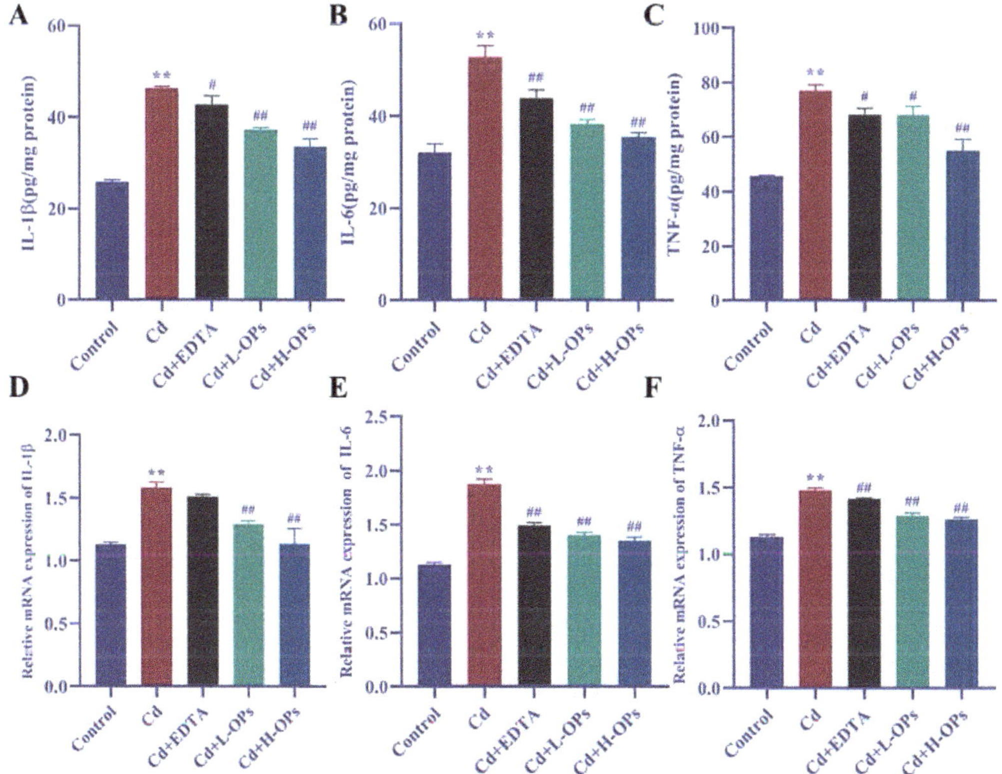

Figure 5. Effect of OPs on inflammatory factor levels and mRNA expression on hepatic in Cd-exposed mice. (**A**) IL-1β level; (**B**) IL-6 level; (**C**) TNF-α level; (**D–F**) Hepatic mRNA expression levels of IL-1β, IL-6, and TNF-α in different groups. These data are expressed as the mean ± SEM, $n = 6$ in each group. Compared with the control group, ** $p < 0.01$; compared with the Cd group, # $p < 0.05$, ## $p < 0.01$.

2.8. Effect of OPs on The Expression of Hepatic COX-2, MIP-2, NF-κB, and p-ERK in Cd-Exposed Mice

COX-2 is a key enzyme in initiating hepatic inflammatory reactions [28]. Meanwhile, macrophage inflammatory protein (MIP)-2 is a potent neutrophil attractant and activator, contributing to the pathogenesis of inflammatory diseases [29]. MIP-2 and COX-2 would be elevated in Cd-induced inflammation [30]. As shown in Figure 6A, enhanced COX-2 and MIP-2 staining were observed around the central vein of hepatocytes in the Cd-exposed group. OPs treatment noticeably reduced the hepatic COX-2 and MIP-2 levels.

In the process of Cd-induced inflammation, the extracellular signal-regulated kinase (ERK) signal pathway would be activated, and the nuclear factor-κB (NF-κB) subsequently was up-regulated [31]. Western blotting assays illustrated that the expression of NF-κB and p-ERK were highly induced in the Cd-exposed group. However, the OPs treatment effectively dampened the expression of NF-κB and p-ERK ($p < 0.01$; Figure 6B,C). The above results implied that OPs might alleviate hepatic inflammation by inhibiting the expression of inflammatory activators (COX-2 and MIP-2) and related inflammatory pathways (NF-κB and ERK).

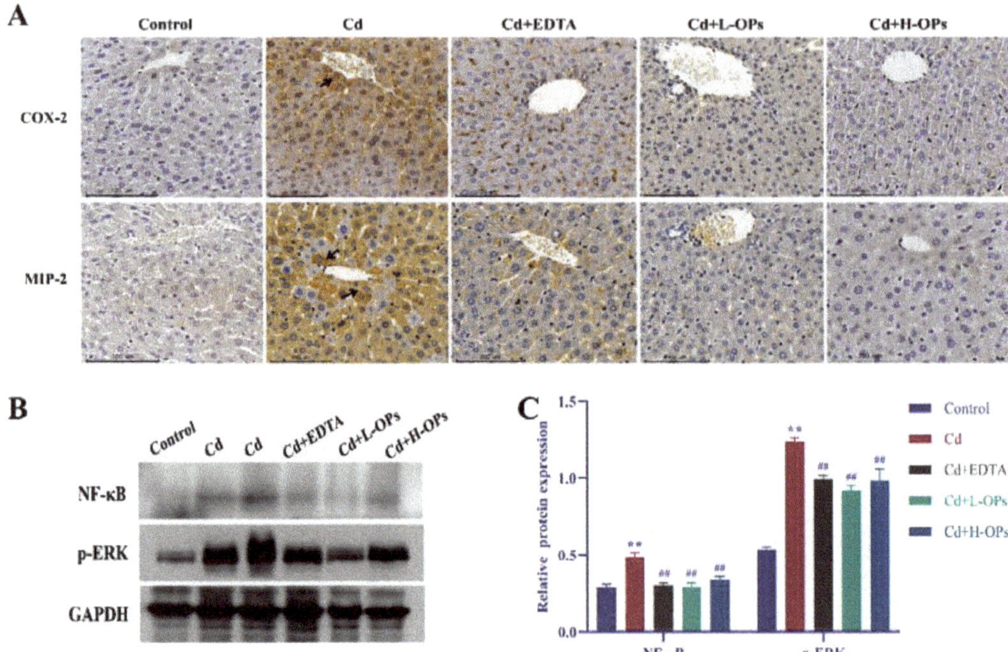

Figure 6. Effect of OPs on the expression of COX-2, MIP-2, NF-κB, and p-ERK in the liver. (**A**) The expression of COX-2 and MIP-2 in the liver by Immunohistochemical (IHC) Staining; (**B**) Western blot analysis of NF-κB and p-ERK proteins, Cd was sampled in 10 µL and 20 µL volumes, respectively; (**C**) Quantitative densitometric analysis of NF-κB and p-ERK proteins. These Data are expressed as the mean ± SEM, $n = 6$ in each group. Compared with the control group, ** $p < 0.01$; compared with the Cd group, ## $p < 0.01$.

2.9. Effect of OPs on Hepatic Apoptosis in Cd-Exposed Mice

Apoptosis-related mitochondrial Bcl2-associated X protein (Bax) and Caspase-3 are two important pro-apoptotic factors. Under the stimulation of oxidative stress caused by Cd, the hepatic Bax increased, then the downstream Caspase-3 was up-regulated, and eventually, apoptosis occurred [32]. Anti-apoptotic Bcl-2 plays a central regulatory role in apoptosis [33]. Accordingly, we examined the effect of OPs on Cd-induced hepatic apoptosis by measuring the levels of pro-apoptotic factors (Bax and caspase-3) and anti-apoptotic factor Bcl-2 in Cd-exposed mice. As shown in Figure 7A–C, Cd significantly decreased the levels of anti-apoptotic Bcl-2 but increased the levels of pro-apoptotic factors (Bax and caspase-3) ($p < 0.01$). On the contrary, OPs treatment significantly increased Bcl-2 while decreasing Bax and caspase-3 levels in Cd-exposed mice ($p < 0.01$). The qRT-PCR results showed that OPs significantly induced the expression of Bcl-2 while suppressing the expression of Bax and caspase-3 in Cd-exposed mice ($p < 0.01$). OPs exhibited a strong anti-apoptotic effect on Cd-induced apoptosis in mice.

Cd can regulate the PI3K/AKT signaling pathway to induce apoptosis [34,35]. Additionally, PI3K/AKT signaling pathway also plays a crucial role in the regulation of inflammatory protein expressions (COX-2 and MIP-2) [36]. Western blotting assays demonstrated that Cd exposure led to the elevation of the expression of PI3K and p-AKT, accompanied by the imbalance of pro-/anti-apoptotic proteins (Bax, caspase-3 and Bcl-2) ($p < 0.05$). By contrast, the OPs treatment inhibited the activation of the PI3K/AKT signaling pathway and restored the balance of pro-/anti-apoptotic proteins in Cd-exposed mice. The results implied that OPs might alleviate hepatic apoptosis by restoring the balance of pro-

/anti-apoptotic proteins via inhibiting the PI3K/AKT signaling pathway in Cd-exposed mice.

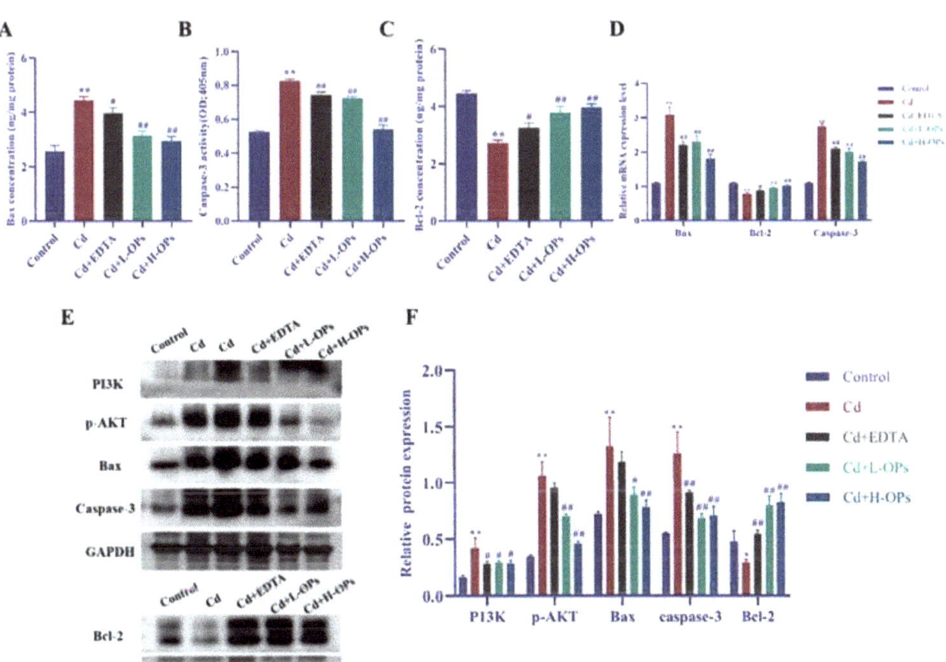

Figure 7. Effect of OPs on apoptotic marker levels and mRNA expression of Cd-induced mice in the liver. (**A**) Bax concentration; (**B**) Caspase-3 activity; (**C**) Bcl-2 concentration; (**D**) Relative mRNA expression levels of Bax, caspase-3 and Bcl-2; (**E**) Western blot analysis of PI3k, p-AKT, Bax, caspase-3 and Bcl-2 protein expression, Cd was sampled in 10 μL and 20 μL volumes, respectively; (**F**) The quantitative densitometric analysis of PI3k, p-AKT, Bax, caspase-3 and Bcl-2. These Data are expressed as the mean ± SEM, $n = 6$ in each group. Compared with the control group, * $p < 0.05$, ** $p < 0.01$; compared with the Cd group, # $p < 0.05$, ## $p < 0.01$.

3. Discussion

As one of the main target organs of Cd, acute hepatic injury was observed in Cd-exposed mice. Fortunately, the OPs treatment clearly ameliorated the Cd-induced hepatic injury in this study. In particular, oxidative damage, inflammation, and cell apoptosis, as crucial triggers and contributors to the development of Cd-induced hepatic injury [30,34,35,37], were improved after OPs application in Cd-exposed mice.

Extensive literature indicates that the health benefits of protein hydrolysates may be partly attributed to their rich in free amino acids and peptides [38,39]. Extracts rich in free amino acids can be used in pharmaceutical applications [40]. A recent study found that free amino acids were related to the antioxidant property of protein hydrolysates of mackerel [38]. The protein hydrolysates with higher contents of free amino acids exhibited better antioxidant properties [41] and metal-chelating ability [42]. In the present study, a high level of free amino acids (15.8%) was detected in OPs. According to a previous report, the royal jelly hydrolysates with 8.389% of free amino acids had a stronger antioxidant activity than those of royal jelly with 0.572% of free amino acids [43]. A similar study also found the anchovy sprat hydrolysates with higher contents of free amino acids (16.28–27.53%) exhibited stronger ferrous-chelating activity and radical-scavenging activity compared to those with lower contents of free amino acids (9.05%) [44]. These data indicated that OPs were rich in free amino acids, which may contribute to the potential health benefits of OPs against Cd toxicity.

Serum ALT and AST are leaked from damaged hepatocytes [45,46]. Cd intoxication led to a significant elevation in the levels of ALT and AST [47]. In the present study, significant improvements were observed in the hepatic injury and dysfunction biomarkers (serum AST, ALT, ALP, and LDH) in Cd-exposed mice after the OPs treatment. Compared to the Cd group, OPs significantly decreased hepatic dysfunction biomarkers in a dose-dependent manner. This result is in line with an earlier report, in which oyster protein hydrolysate could reduce hepatic dysfunction biomarkers (serum AST, ALT, and ALP) and inflammatory response in alcoholic liver disease mice [48]. Likewise, Shi, Sun [49] reported that *ganoderma lucidum* peptides have an alleviative effect on D-GalN-induced hepatocellular injury via reversing AST and ALT levels in the liver. Moreover, Mumtaz, Ali [50] found that elevated level of LDH, AST, and ALT in the Cd-exposed batch was improved by ascorbic acid. Early evidence indicates that hepatic injury and cirrhosis usually lead to metabolic disturbances of amino acids [51]. The bioactive properties of protein hydrolysates mainly depend on free amino acids and peptides [38,39,52]. The present study showed that OPs are rich in hydrophobic free amino acids (i.e., Pro) and proline-rich peptides. Among these amino acids, Pro plays a beneficial role in plants under changing environments, including Cd stress [53]. Exogenous Pro could increase antioxidant enzyme activities and confer tolerance to cadmium stress in cultured tobacco cells [22]. Pro has shown tissue-protective effects against D-galactosamine-induced hepatic injury [54]. Dietary Pro could effectively decrease AST and ALT levels of shrimp under NH3 stress [55]. The derivatives of Pro, N-acetyl-seryl-aspartyl-lysyl-proline, were found to attenuate bile duct ligation-induced liver fibrosis by restoring hepatic dysfunction (serum AST and ALT) in mice [56]. Pro and proline-rich proteins are often implicated in stress tolerance in plants [57–59]. Salivary proline-rich proteins possess good antioxidant properties [60]. Hypothalamic proline-rich polypeptides were found to protect brain neurons in aluminum neurotoxicosis [61]. These data support the idea that OPs could ameliorate hepatic injury and improve hepatic dysfunction in Cd-exposed mice.

Oxidative stress is often implicated in the induction of multi-organ injury under Cd exposure [62]. Lipid peroxidation is a major consequence of Cd-induced oxidative stress [63]. The consequences of the peroxidative of membrane lipids have been considered in relation to the tissue aspects of liver injury, and these peroxidative reactions play a critical role in the pathogenesis of acute liver necrosis [64]. According to a previous report, the liver, kidneys, and heart were most susceptible to Cd-induced oxidative stress in mice [65]. Some amino acid derivatives, such as N-Acetylcysteine, showed ameliorative effects on cisplatin-induced multiple organ toxicity in rats [66–68]. Betulinic acid was found to alleviate the kidney and liver damage induced by Cd [69]. In this study, Cd exposure induced serious hepatic toxicity and oxidative stress, which were significantly improved after the OPs supplement. These data suggest that amelioration of hepatic oxidative injury may be the key to the treatment of Cd toxicity by OPs in mice.

Oxidative stress plays a crucial role in Cd-induced hepatic toxicity [70]. The development of liver injury usually involves the lipid peroxidation of hepatic cell membranes in Cd-exposed mice [71]. According to a recent report, Cd-induced hepatic injury is tightly coupled with enhanced lipid peroxidation (MDA) and the significant depletion of antioxidants (CAT and SOD) [72]. In this study, the OPs supplement clearly reduced the formation of MDA and significantly restored the activity of antioxidant enzymes (SOD, CAT, and GPH-Px) in the liver of the Cd-exposed mice. OPs displayed a strong antioxidant activity, which might also be attributed to their abundance of hydrophobic amino acids. Commonly, protein hydrolysates with higher content of hydrophobic amino acids possess better antioxidant properties due to their more effective interaction with lipid-soluble free radicals and the prevention of lipid peroxidation [17,73–75]. Thus, this evidence clearly indicated that OPs possess good antioxidant properties to delay hepatic oxidative injury via retaining hepatic antioxidant enzymes and preventing MDA production in Cd-exposed mice.

Hepatic histopathological damage in Cd-exposed mice is characterized by apoptotic bodies, hemorrhage, lymphocyte accumulation, and inflammatory cell infiltration in liver tissue. Increasing evidence demonstrates that hepatic injury and fibrosis are accompanied by the elevation of the inflammatory response [76]. As well known, TNF-α and IL-6 are two key inflammatory mediators of tissue injury-induced inflammatory response [77]. IL-1β and IL-6 are two stimulators of the hepatic synthesis of acute-phase proteins in the inflammatory response to stress [25,26]. Cd exposure will trigger an acute inflammatory response in mice [78]. The present study showed that hepatic apoptotic cells in Cd-exposed mice were significantly minimized, and histopathological appearance was obviously improved after OPs treatment. In addition, the Cd-triggered inflammatory responses (IL-1β, IL-6, and TNF-α) were significantly inhibited, as expected. This result is consistent with the findings in an earlier report, in which peptides from oyster soft tissue hydrolysates selectively repressed TNF-α, IL-1β, and IL-6 [79]. To go even further, we found that as important activators and regulators of inflammatory responses, MIP-2 [29], COX-2 [28], NF-κB, and the ERK signal pathway [80], were significantly stimulated in Cd-exposed mice. The results are in agreement with a previous study, in which Cd activated the ERK signal pathway, then subsequently up-regulated TNF-α, COX-2, IL-1β, IL-6, and NF-κB in swine [31]. Likewise, Huang, Xia [30] reported that Cd exposure led to an increase in MIP-2 and COX-2. Actually, ROS production could activate MAPK signaling to induce inflammation and skin aging by promoting the phosphorylation of ERK [32]. Peng, Chen [81] also found that the up-regulated ERK phosphorylation in ultraviolet B-exposed mice was significantly inhibited by the application of oyster protein hydrolysates. A recent study found that seahorse protein hydrolysates could significantly inhibit p-ERK levels in ethanol-exposed cells. [82]. In this study, Western blotting assays showed that OPs significantly decreased the levels of p-ERK and NF-κB proteins, as well as the MIP-2 and COX-2 in Cd-exposed mice. Therefore, the ameliorative effect of OPs in Cd-caused liver injury may be related to its anti-inflammation properties via suppressing the production of inflammatory mediators and inhibiting the inflammatory response associated with NF-κB and the ERK signal pathway.

In addition to inflammatory responses, hepatic injury is also accompanied by the development of apoptosis in Cd-exposed mice. Reducing Cd-induced apoptosis is also considered to be one of the feasible ways to prevent Cd-induced hepatic injury [69]. In the process, the NF-κB inflammation pathway indirectly activated the apoptosis-related factors Bcl-2, Bax, and Caspase-3 [31]. The present study revealed that the OPs supplement strongly up-regulated the expression of the anti-apoptotic factor Bcl-2 while significantly down-regulated the expression of the pro-apoptotic factors (caspase-3 and Bax), eventually restoring the balance of pro-/anti-apoptotic proteins in Cd-exposed mice. Moreover, the PI3K/AKT pathway is an important signaling pathway associated with apoptosis [83]. Actually, Cd selectively induces MIP-2 and COX-2 through the activation of the PI3K/AKT [30]. A previous study showed that curcumin alleviated lipopolysaccharide-induced hepatic injury and apoptosis via inhibiting the PI3K/AKT and NF-κB pathways [84]. MiR-130a alleviated neuronal apoptosis and changes in the expression of Bcl-2/Bax and caspase-3 in cerebral infarction rats through the PI3K/AKT signaling pathway [85]. In the present study, we found that the OPs supplement significantly inhibited the expression of PI3K and p-AKT proteins. These results are in agreement with an earlier report, in which Selenomethionine ameliorated Cd-induced hepatocyte apoptosis by suppressing the PI3K/AKT pathway [86]. Therefore, we may conclude that OPs possess the ability to ameliorate hepatocyte apoptosis, possibly by restoring the balance of pro-/anti-apoptotic proteins via suppressing the PI3K/AKT pathway in Cd-exposed mice.

In conclusion, from our study, we found that OPs could effectively ameliorate Cd-induced hepatic injury through their antioxidative and anti-inflammatory properties. In addition, OPs displayed an important role in restoring the balance between pro-apoptotic and anti-apoptotic proteins by suppressing the activation of the PI3K/AKT pathway, contributing to the development of hepatocyte apoptosis in Cd-exposed mice (Figure 8). These results may provide a new insight for a better understanding of the ameliorative function of OPs to Cd toxicity and provide a theoretical basis for the use of OPs to prevent or treat Cd-induced hepatic injury.

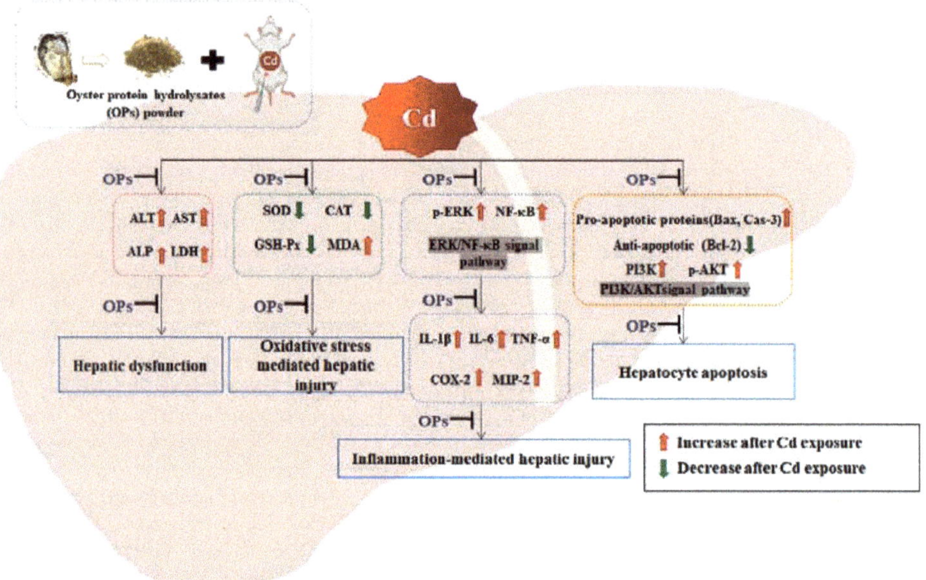

Figure 8. Schematic representation of OPs improved mechanisms of cadmium-induced oxidative stress, inflammation, and apoptosis in mice.

4. Materials and Methods

4.1. Chemical and Materials

Cadmium chloride ($CdCl_2$) was purchased from West Long Chemical (Shantou, Guangdong, China). Fresh oysters (*Crassostrea hongkongensis*) were purchased from the local market in Zhanjiang, China. The kits for measurement of ALT (C009-2-1), AST (C010-2-1), ALP (A059-2-2), and LDH (A020-2-2) were offered by Nanjing Jiancheng Bioengineering Institute (Nanjing, China). The kits used to measure the levels of SOD (BC0170), GSH-Px (BC1195), CAT (BC0205), and MDA (BC0025) were purchased from Solarbio Science & Technology (Beijing, China), and the other chemicals were purchased from Sangon Biotech (Shanghai, China) unless specifically noted otherwise.

4.2. Animals and Experimental Design

Thirty Specific-Pathogen-Free (SPF) mice (Kunming mice, 25–35 g) were obtained from Changsha Tianqin Biotechnology Co., Ltd. (Changsha, China), and the animals were maintained at the Guangdong Ocean University Animal Centre under light (12 h of light and dark) and temperature (~25 °C). The animals were given a standard laboratory diet and water. The experiment was approved by the Animal Ethics Committee of Guangdong Ocean University (No.: GDOU-LAE-2020-009). The animals were randomly divided into 5 groups ($n = 6$). Control group: Intraperitoneal injection of 0.9% NaCl (saline) once daily. Cd-exposed group: the mice were injected intraperitoneally with $CdCl_2$ 5 mg/kg daily [87]. EDTA-treated group (positive control): the mice were injected with $CdCl_2$ (5 mg/kg) intraperitoneally after 1 h of oral administration with EDTA (100 mg/kg) daily. The low dose of OPs(L-OPs)-treated group: the mice were injected with $CdCl_2$ (5 mg/kg) intraperitoneally after 1 h of oral administration with OPs (100 mg/kg) daily. High dose of

OPs (H-OPs)-treated group: the mice were injected with $CdCl_2$ (5 mg/kg) intraperitoneally after 1 h of oral administration with OPs (300 mg/kg) daily. It has been shown that ethylenediaminetetraacetic acid (EDTA) can alleviate cadmium toxicity by enhancing antioxidant enzyme activity and inhibiting inflammatory responses [88]. Therefore, it can be used as a positive control. The doses of EDTA and OPs were determined based on previous studies [89,90]. After 7 days, the mice were executed by cervical dislocation, and the liver was stored at −80 °C for further analysis.

4.3. Preparation of OPs

OPs were prepared by enzymatic hydrolysis from the oyster (*Crassostrea hongkongensis*) meat as described previously [81,90]. Hong Kong oyster meat (~3 kg) was homogenized in distilled water (1:3 (w/w) at 8000 rpm for 5 min. Homogenized oysters were hydrolysed using neutral protease (2×10^5 U/g, Pangbo Biotech, Nanning, China) at a protease/substrate ratio of 2.0% (w/v) (pH 7.0). The neutral protease was incubated for 4 h at 50 °C and then inactivated at 100 °C for 15 min. The hydrolysate was centrifuged at 15,000 rpm for 20 min at 4 °C to obtain the supernatant. The supernatant was collected and ultrafiltered using a membrane bioreactor system with a molecular mass cut-off value of 3 kDa to collect the fractions (<3 kDa). The samples were collected and freeze-dried for further analysis.

4.4. Peptide Sequence Analysis Based on LC-MS/MS

The peptide sequence analysis used an Easy-nLC 1200 system coupled to a Q-Exactive quadrupole-Orbitrap mass spectrometry (Thermo Fisher Scientific, San Jose, CA, USA). One µL of the samples was injected with an autosampler into an Acclaim Pep Map RPLC C18 column (150 µm i.d. × 150 mm, C18, particle size: 1.9 µm, pore size: 100 Å, Dr. Maisch GmbH, Darmstadt, Hessen, Germany) with mobile phase A: 0.1% formic acid in water; B: 0.1% formic acid in the water, 80% acetonitrile. The flow rate was 600 nL/min, and the LC linear gradient ranged from 4% to 40% for 55 minutes and 10 minutes at 95% mobile phase B. Finally, the molecular mass, sequence, peak area (with respect to base peak), and relative peak area (peak area/total peak area) of the peptides were identified and calculated as previously described [81,91]. The conditions of the mass spectrometer were as follows: Resolution: 70,000, AGC target: 3e6, NCE/stepped NCE: 28. The samples were analyzed with a full-scan MS mode in the range of 100–1500 m/z to obtain the total ion chromatogram. The raw MS files were analyzed and searched against the target protein database based on the species of the samples using Byonic.

4.5. LC-MS/MS Analysis of Free Amino Acids

The amino acid composition and content of the OPs were measured, as previously described, with little modification [92]. The OPs samples were accurately weighed to 50 mg and mixed with 600 µL of a water–methanol solution (1:1, v/v) with 10% formic acid in a 2 mL tube. Then, 100 mg of glass beads were added to the mixed samples and vortexed for 30 s. The samples were transferred to a high-throughput tissue grinding machine (MB-96, Mcibi, Jiaxing, Zhejiang, China) and vibrated at 60 Hz for 2 min. The tube was centrifuged at 12,000 rpm for 5 min at 4 °C. Ten µL of supernatant was transferred to a new tube containing 490 µL of the water–methanol solution (1:1, v/v) with 10% formic acid and then vortexed for 30 s. Then, 100 µL of the diluted samples were mixed with 100 µL of 100 µg/L double isotope internal standard (Trp-d3, D87103, Medical Isotopes, USA) and vortexed for 30 s. The mixed samples were filtered through a 0.22 µm hydrophilic PTFE filter and transferred into a labeled vial, and subsequently analyzed via LC–MS/MS.

Five µL of the samples were injected into an ACQUITY UPLC BEH C18 column (2.1 × 100 mm, 1.7 µm, Waters, Milford, MD, USA) with mobile phase A: 10% water -methanol solution with 0.1% formic acid; B: 50% water-methanol solution with 0.1% formic acid. The flow rate: 300 µL/min in 8.5 min, then kept 300–400 µL/min for 4 min. The gradient elution programs: 0~6.5 min, 10~30% B; 6.5~7 min, 30~100% B; 7~8 min, 100% B; 8~8.5 min, 100~10% B; 8.5~12.5 min, 10% B.

Mass spectrometric analysis was performed using an AB SCIEX AB4000 Mass Spectrometer (AB SCIEX, Framingham, MD, USA) equipped with an electrospray ionization (ESI) source using the following parameters: capillary voltage: 5500 V, temperature of the turbo heaters: 500 °C, nebulizer gas (GS1): 50 psi, auxiliary gas (GS2): 50 psi, and curtain gas (CUR): 30 psi, Collision Gas: 6 psi. All of the amino acids were detected in the multiple reaction monitoring mode (MRM).

4.6. Analysis of Amino Acid Composition

According to the previous method with a slight modification [81]. Approximately 30 mg of the sample and 10 mL of 6 mol/L HCl were added to a hydrolysis tube containing phenol. After the tube was vacuumed, the mixture was washed with nitrogen and hydrolyzed at 110 °C for 22 h. After cooling to room temperature, the filtrate is filtered and spun dry under reduced pressure in a centrifuge tube. The 0.02 mol/L HCl solution was added to a dried centrifuge tube and dissolved, and the solution was transferred to the upper sample bottle and determined using an amino acid analyzer (L-8900, Hitachi, Tokyo, Japan). Then, the contents of amino acids in the sample could be determined according to the peak area in comparison with the standard. The content of tryptophan in OP was determined after hydrolysis with 6 mol/L of NaOH instead of HCl.

4.7. Histopathology Examination

The liver samples were fixed in 4% paraformaldehyde for 24 hours and embedded in paraffin. The embedded liver tissue was sectioned into 5 μm sections and fixed on slides, stained with hematoxylin and eosin (H&E) and observed under a BX 53 Olympus microscope according to the method described [93].

4.8. Analysis of Liver Function

The blood samples were collected as previously described [94,95]. Blood samples were gained by removing the eyeballs of mice. Blood was then centrifuged at 4000 rpm for 30 min at 4 °C. The samples were incubated in an electro-thermostatic water bath at 37 °C for 30 min. The serum was collected and subjected to the examination of the activities of alanine transaminase (ALT), aspartate aminotransferase (AST) activities, the activities of lactate dehydrogenase (LDH), and alkaline phosphatase (ALP) with respective commercial kits. The determination of AST, ALT, LDH, and ALP was performed by the instruction of the kits (Nanjing Jianchen Bioengineering Institute, Nanjing, China).

4.9. Measurement of MDA, SOD, CAT and GSH-Px Activities

The changes in hepatic oxidative stress were monitored as previously described [65]. The liver homogenate was centrifuged to obtain the supernatant at 3500 rpm for 10 min at 4 °C, and the superoxide dismutase (SOD), catalase (CAT), glutathione peroxidase (GSH-Px) activity, and malondialdehyde (MDA) levels were measured according to the manufacturer's instructions.

4.10. Measurement of IL-1β, IL-6 and TNF-α in Hepatic Tissue by ELISA Kits

The concentrations of IL-1β (MM-0905M1), IL-6 (MM-1011M1), and TNF-α (MM-0679M1) were measured using an ELISA kit (MeiMian, Yancheng, Jiangsu, China) according to the manufacturer's instructions.

4.11. Immunohistochemistry Analysis

MIP-2 and COX-2 expressions in hepatic tissue were evaluated by immunohistochemistry staining as previously described [96]. The prepared hepatic sections were recovered, and the endogenous peroxidase in tissues was inactivated with 0.1% hydrogen peroxide containing methanol for 15 min. Then, the sections were incubated with a rabbit polyclonal MIP-2 and COX-2 antibody at 4 °C overnight. Subsequently, the sections were washed with PBS and incubated with rabbit anti-mouse (1:1000) secondary antibody at room temperature for 30 min. The sections were rinsed with PBS 3 times and stained with diaminobenzidine (DAB). Additionally, they were evaluated under an optical microscope (Olympus Optical Co., Ltd., Tokyo, Japan).

4.12. Measurement of Bax, Caspase-3 and Bcl-2 in Hepatic Tissue

The levels of pro-apoptotic-related protein Bax (MM-1143H2) and anti-apoptotic-related protein Bcl-2 (MM-0306M2) were performed using an ELISA kit (MeiMian, Yancheng, Jiangsu, China) according to the manufacturer's instructions. Caspase-3 activity was measured using a kit (C1115) purchased from Beyotime Biotechnology (Shanghai, China).

4.13. Quantitative Reverse-Transcription PCR (qRT-PCR) Analyses

The total RNA from each sample was isolated using the Trizol reagent (Sango Shanghai, China), and the first strand cDNA was synthesized using the StarScript II First-strand cDNA Synthesis Mix With gDNA Remover (Genstar) according to the manufacturer's instructions. Quantitative reverse-transcription PCR (qRT-PCR) was conducted to determine the mRNA levels of the IL-1β, IL-6, TNF-α, Bax, Caspase-3, and Bcl-2 (the primer sequences are shown in Table 4), the GAPDH gene was used as an internal control [8,30,97]. Real-time PCR reactions were performed on a CFX Real-time system (CFX96, Bio-Rad, Hercules, CA, USA). All of the samples were analyzed in triplicate, and the $2^{-\Delta\Delta Ct}$ method was used to analyze gene expression levels.

Table 4. Primer sequences for qRT-PCR analyses.

Gene Name	Forward Primer (5′–3′)	Reverse Primer (5′–3′)
IL-1β	GACTTCACCATGGAACCCGT	GGAGACTGCCCATTCTCGAC
IL-6	GGCCCTTGCTTTCTCTTCG	ATAATAAAGTTTTGATTATGT
TNF-α	AGCCCTGGTATGAGCCCATGTA	CCGGACTCCGTGATGTCTAAGT
Bax	CTGAGCTGACCTTGGAGC	GACTCCAGCCACAAGAGATG
Caspase-3	GAGCTTGGAACGGTACGCTA	CCGTACCAGAGCGAGATGAC
Bcl-2	GACAGAAGATCATGCCGTCC	GGTACCAATGGCACTTCAAG
GAPDH	TCACCACCATGGAGAAGGC	GCTAAGCAGTTGGTGGTGCA

4.14. Western Blotting Analyses

The hepatic tissues were lysed with RIPA lysis buffer (Servicebio technology, Wuhan, China), supplemented with protease inhibitor (Servicebio), and homogenized with an ultrasonic processor. According to the manufacturer's instructions, the total protein of the liver tissue was extracted with a commercial kit (Servicebio technology, Wuhan, China). Then, the concentration of the protein was measured with a BCA kit (Beyotime technology, Shanghai, China). Then, the proteins were transferred to a polyvinylidene fluoride (PVDF) membrane, followed by blocking with 5% skim milk (0.5% TBST) and sealed for 1 h. Additionally, then, PDVF membranes were incubated with primary antibodies against NF-κB (1:1000), p-ERK (1:1000), PI3K (1:1000), p-AKT (1:1000), Caspase-3 (1:1000), Bcl-2 (1:1000), Bax (1:1000), and GAPDH (1:3000) were incubated overnight at 4 °C. They were washed with TBST at room temperature on a decolorizing shaker three times. After washing, PVDF membranes were incubated with secondary antibodies (1:3000) at room temperature for 2 h. The antibodies were purchased from Proteintech Group, USA. Finally, they were developed and fixed with developing and fixing reagents, and the Alpha software processing system analyzes the optical density values of the target band.

4.15. Statistical Analysis

The data are expressed as the mean ± SE. Data analyses were carried out using JMP Pro 13. The data were analyzed using general descriptive statistics. One-way analysis of variance (ANOVA) at 95%. $p < 0.05$ was considered statistically significant.

Author Contributions: Conceptualization, J.W. and Y.L. (Ying Liu); methodology, J.W.; validation, L.S., Y.L. (Ying Liu), S.Z. and Q.D.; formal analysis, S.Z. and Y.L. (Yongbin Li); investigation, Z.F. and Q.D.; resources, Z.F.; data curation, J.W., Y.L. (Ying Liu) and Z.F.; writing—original draft preparation, J.W.; writing—review and editing, Z.F.; visualization, L.S., Y.L. (Yongbin Li), S.Z. and Q.D.; funding acquisition, Z.F. All authors have read and agreed to the published version of the manuscript.

Funding: This research was funded by the National Natural Science Foundation of China (No. 32172215 and 31701706). The Program for Scientific Research Start-up Funds of the Guangdong Ocean University (No. R17102), Characteristic Innovation Project of Guangdong Province (No. 2018KTSCX089) and Guangdong Basic and Applied Basic Research Foundation (No. 2019A1515010809, 2021A1515012443). The Innovative Team Program of High Education of Guangdong Province (2021KCXTD021).

Data Availability Statement: The data presented in this study are available on request from the corresponding author.

Conflicts of Interest: The authors declare no conflict of interest.

References

1. Jaishankar, M.; Tseten, T.; Anbalagan, N.; Mathew, B.B.; Beeregowda, K.N. Toxicity, mechanism and health effects of some heavy metals. *Interdiscip. Toxicol.* **2014**, *7*, 60–72. [CrossRef] [PubMed]
2. Jomova, K.; Valko, M. Advances in metal-induced oxidative stress and human disease. *Toxicology* **2011**, *283*, 65–87. [CrossRef] [PubMed]
3. Abdeen, A.; Abou-Zaid, O.A.; Abdel-Maksoud, H.A.; Aboubakr, M.; Abdelkader, A.; Abdelnaby, A.; Abo-Ahmed, A.I.; El-Mleeh, A.; Mostafa, O.; Abdel-Daim, M.; et al. Cadmium overload modulates piroxicam-regulated oxidative damage and apoptotic pathways. *Env. Sci. Pollut. Res. Int.* **2019**, *26*, 25167–25177. [CrossRef] [PubMed]
4. Zhang, J.; Wang, Y.; Fu, L.; Wang, B.; Ji, Y.L.; Wang, H.; Xu, D.X. Chronic cadmium exposure induced hepatic cellular stress and inflammation in aged female mice. *J. Appl. Toxicol.* **2019**, *39*, 498–509. [CrossRef] [PubMed]
5. Nawrot, T.S.; Staessen, J.A.; Roels, H.A.; Munters, E.; Cuypers, A.; Richart, T.; Ruttens, A.; Smeets, K.; Clijsters, H.; Vangronsveld, J. Cadmium exposure in the population: From health risks to strategies of prevention. *BioMetals* **2010**, *23*, 769–782. [CrossRef]
6. Arroyo, V.; Flores, K.; Ortiz, L.; Gómez-Quiroz, L.; Gutiérrez-Ruiz, M. Liver and Cadmium Toxicity. *J. Drug Metab. Toxicol.* **2012**, *5*, 1–7.
7. Andjelkovic, M.; Buha Djordjevic, A.; Antonijevic, E.; Antonijevic, B.; Stanic, M.; Kotur-Stevuljevic, J.; Spasojevic-Kalimanovska, V.; Jovanovic, M.; Boricic, N.; Wallace, D.; et al. Toxic Effect of Acute Cadmium and Lead Exposure in Rat Blood, Liver, and Kidney. *Int. J. Env. Res. Public Health* **2019**, *16*, 274. [CrossRef]
8. Almeer, R.S.; Alarifi, S.; Alkahtani, S.; Ibrahim, S.R.; Ali, D.; Moneim, A. The potential hepatoprotective effect of royal jelly against cadmium chloride-induced hepatotoxicity in mice is mediated by suppression of oxidative stress and upregulation of Nrf2 expression. *Biomed. Pharm.* **2018**, *106*, 1490–1498. [CrossRef]
9. Miao, J.; Liao, W.; Kang, M.; Jia, Y.; Wang, Q.; Duan, S.; Xiao, S.; Cao, Y.; Ji, H. Anti-fatigue and anti-oxidant activities of oyster (*Ostrea rivularis*) hydrolysate prepared by compound protease. *Food Funct.* **2018**, *9*, 6577–6585. [CrossRef]
10. Chalamaiah, M.; Yu, W.; Wu, J. Immunomodulatory and anticancer protein hydrolysates (peptides) from food proteins: A review. *Food Chem.* **2018**, *245*, 205–222. [CrossRef]
11. Fuda, H.; Watanabe, M.; Hui, S.P.; Joko, S.; Okabe, H.; Jin, S.; Takeda, S.; Miki, E.; Watanabe, T.; Chiba, H. Anti-apoptotic effects of novel phenolic antioxidant isolated from the Pacific oyster (*Crassostrea gigas*) on cultured human hepatocytes under oxidative stress. *Food Chem.* **2015**, *176*, 226–233. [CrossRef] [PubMed]
12. Umayaparvathi, S.; Arumugam, M.; Meenakshi, S.; Dräger, G.; Kirschning, A.; Balasubramanian, T. Purification and Characterization of Antioxidant Peptides from Oyster (*Saccostrea cucullata*) Hydrolysate and the Anticancer Activity of Hydrolysate on Human Colon Cancer Cell Lines. *Int. J. Pept. Res. Ther.* **2013**, *20*, 231–243. [CrossRef]
13. Siregar, A.S.; Nyiramana, M.M.; Kim, E.J.; Cho, S.B.; Woo, M.S.; Lee, D.K.; Hong, S.G.; Han, J.; Kang, S.S.; Kim, D.R.; et al. Oyster-Derived Tyr-Ala (YA) Peptide Prevents Lipopolysaccharide/D-Galactosamine-Induced Acute Liver Failure by Suppressing Inflammatory, Apoptotic, Ferroptotic, and Pyroptotic Signals. *Mar. Drugs* **2021**, *19*, 614. [CrossRef] [PubMed]
14. Umayaparvathi, S.; Meenakshi, S.; Vimalraj, V.; Arumugam, M.; Sivagami, G.; Balasubramanian, T. Antioxidant activity and anticancer effect of bioactive peptide from enzymatic hydrolysate of oyster (*Saccostrea cucullata*). *Biomed. Prev. Nutr.* **2014**, *4*, 343–353. [CrossRef]
15. Zhang, C.; Li, X.; Jing, X.; Zhang, B.; Zhang, Q.; Niu, Q.; Wang, J.; Tian, Z. Protective effects of oyster extract against hepatic tissue injury in alcoholic liver diseases. *J. Ocean Univ. China* **2014**, *13*, 262–270. [CrossRef]
16. Li, H.; Xia, X.; Zang, J.; Tan, X.; Wang, Z.; Xu, X.; Du, M. Oyster (*Crassostrea gigas*) ferritin can efficiently reduce the damage of Pb^{2+} in vivo by electrostatic attraction. *Int. J. Biol. Macromol.* **2022**, *210*, 365–376. [CrossRef]
17. Harnedy, P.A.; FitzGerald, R.J. Bioactive peptides from marine processing waste and shellfish: A review. *J. Funct. Foods* **2012**, *4*, 6–24. [CrossRef]

18. Rakesh, K.P.; Suhas, R.; Gowda, D.C. Anti-inflammatory and Antioxidant Peptide-Conjugates: Modulation of Activity by Charged and Hydrophobic Residues. *In. J. Pept. Res. Ther.* **2019**, *25*, 227–234. [CrossRef]

19. Mahmood, S.; Wahid, A.; Azeem, M.; Zafar, S.; Bashir, R.; Sharif, O.; Ali, S. Tyrosine or lysine priming modulated phenolic metabolism and improved cadmium stress tolerance in mung bean (*Vigna radiata* L.). *S. Afr. J. Bot.* **2022**, *149*, 397–406. [CrossRef]

20. Zemanová, V.; Pavlík, M.; Pavlíková, D.; Tlustoš, P. The significance of methionine, histidine and tryptophan in plant responses and adaptation to cadmium stress. *Plant Soil Environ.* **2014**, *60*, 426–432. [CrossRef]

21. Domínguez-Solís, J.R.; López-Martín, M.C.; Ager, F.J.; Ynsa, M.D.; Romero, L.C.; Gotor, C. Increased cysteine availability is essential for cadmium tolerance and accumulation in *Arabidopsis thaliana*. *Plant Biotechnol. J.* **2004**, *2*, 469–476. [CrossRef] [PubMed]

22. Islam, M.M.; Hoque, M.A.; Okuma, E.; Banu, M.N.A.; Shimoishi, Y.; Nakamura, Y.; Murata, Y. Exogenous proline and glycinebetaine increase antioxidant enzyme activities and confer tolerance to cadmium stress in cultured tobacco cells. *J. Plant Physiol.* **2009**, *166*, 1587–1597. [CrossRef] [PubMed]

23. Born, T.; Kontoghiorghe, C.N.; Spyrou, A.; Kolnagou, A.; Kontoghiorghes, G.J. EDTA chelation reappraisal following new clinical trials and regular use in millions of patients: Review of preliminary findings and risk/benefit assessment. *Toxicol. Mech. Methods* **2013**, *23*, 11–17. [CrossRef] [PubMed]

24. Michael, B.; Yano, B.; Sellers, R.S.; Perry, R.; Morton, D.; Roome, N.; Johnson, J.K.; Schafer, K. Evaluation of Organ Weights for Rodent and Non-Rodent Toxicity Studies: A Review of Regulatory Guidelines and a Survey of Current Practices. *Toxicol. Pathol.* **2007**, *35*, 742–750. [CrossRef]

25. Arranz, J.; Soriano, A.; Garcia, I.; García, I.; Concepción, M.T.; Navarro, J.; Arteaga, A.; Filella, X.; Bravo, P.; Barrera, M.; et al. Effect of proinflammatory cytokines (IL-6, TNF-α, IL-1β) on hemodynamic performance during orthotopic liver transplantation. *Transpl. P.* **2003**, *35*, 1884–1887. [CrossRef]

26. Arras, D.S.; John, S.R. IL-6 pathway in the liver: From physiopathology to therapy. *J. Hepatol.* **2016**, *64*, 1403–1415. [CrossRef]

27. Schwabe, R.F.; Brenner, D.A. Mechanisms of Liver Injury. I. TNF-α-induced liver injury: Role of IKK, JNK, and ROS pathways. *Am. J. Physiol. Gastr. L.* **2006**, *290*, G583–G589. [CrossRef]

28. Yu, J.; Ip, E.; dela Peña, A.; Hou, J.Y.; Sesha, J.; Pera, N.; Hall, P.; Kirsch, R.; Leclercq, I.; Farrell, G.C. COX-2 induction in mice with experimental nutritional steatohepatitis: Role as pro-inflammatory mediator. *Hepatology* **2006**, *43*, 826–836. [CrossRef]

29. Zhao, Y.; Huang, S.; Liu, J.; Wu, X.; Zhou, S.; Dai, K.; Kou, Y. Mitophagy Contributes to the Pathogenesis of Inflammatory Diseases. *Inflammation* **2018**, *41*, 1590–1600. [CrossRef]

30. Huang, Y.-Y.; Xia, M.-Z.; Wang, H.; Liu, X.-J.; Hu, Y.-F.; Chen, Y.-H.; Zhang, C.; Xu, D.-X. Cadmium Selectively Induces MIP-2 and COX-2 Through PTEN-Mediated Akt Activation in RAW264.7 Cells. *Toxicol. Sci.* **2014**, *138*, 310–321. [CrossRef]

31. Zhang, Y.; Li, Y.; Zhang, J.; Qi, X.; Cui, Y.; Yin, K.; Lin, H. Cadmium induced inflammation and apoptosis of porcine epididymis via activating RAF1/MEK/ERK and NF-κB pathways. *Toxicol. Appl. Pharmacol.* **2021**, *415*, 115449. [CrossRef] [PubMed]

32. Habeebu, S.S.M.; Liu, J.; Klaassen, C.D. Cadmium-Induced Apoptosis in Mouse Liver. *Toxicol. Appl. Pharm.* **1998**, *149*, 203–209. [CrossRef] [PubMed]

33. Thomadaki, H.; Scorilas, A. BCL2 Family of Apoptosis-Related Genes: Functions and Clinical Implications in Cancer. *Crit. Rev. Clin. Lab. Sci.* **2006**, *43*, 1–67. [CrossRef] [PubMed]

34. Yiming, L.; Yanfei, H.; Hang, Y.; Yimei, C.; Guangliang, S.; Shu, L. Cadmium induces apoptosis of pig lymph nodes by regulating the PI3K/AKT/HIF-1α pathway. *Toxicology* **2021**, *451*, 152694. [CrossRef] [PubMed]

35. Cui, W.; Zhou, S.; Wang, Y.; Shi, X.; Liu, H. Cadmium exposure activates the PI3K/AKT signaling pathway through miRNA-21, induces an increase in M1 polarization of macrophages, and leads to fibrosis of pig liver tissue. *Ecotoxicol. Environ. Saf.* **2021**, *228*, 113015. [CrossRef] [PubMed]

36. Rodríguez Barbero, A.; Dorado, F.; Velasco, S.; Pandiella, A.; Banas, B.; López Novoa, J.M. TGF-β1 induces COX-2 expression and PGE2 synthesis through MAPK and PI3K pathways in human mesangial cells. *Kidney Int.* **2006**, *70*, 901–909. [CrossRef]

37. Matović, V.; Buha, A.; Đukić-Ćosić, D.; Bulat, Z. Insight into the oxidative stress induced by lead and/or cadmium in blood, liver and kidneys. *Food Chem. Toxicol.* **2015**, *78*, 130–140. [CrossRef]

38. Wu, H.-C.; Chen, H.-M.; Shiau, C.-Y. Free amino acids and peptides as related to antioxidant properties in protein hydrolysates of mackerel (*Scomber austriasicus*). *Food Res. Int.* **2003**, *36*, 949–957. [CrossRef]

39. Nasri, M. Chapter Four—Protein Hydrolysates and Biopeptides: Production, Biological Activities, and Applications in Foods and Health Benefits. A Review. In *Advances in Food and Nutrition Research*; Toldrá, F., Ed.; Academic Press: Cambridge, MA, USA, 2017; pp. 109–159.

40. Ghaly, A.E.; Vv, R.; Brooks, M.S.-L.; Budge, S.M.; Dave, D. Fish Processing Wastes as a Potential Source of Proteins, Amino Acidsand Oils: A Critical Review. *J. Microb. Biochem. Technol.* **2013**, *2*, 107–129.

41. Yang, B.; Yang, H.; Li, J.; Li, Z.; Jiang, Y. Amino acid composition, molecular weight distribution and antioxidant activity of protein hydrolysates of soy sauce lees. *Food Chem.* **2011**, *124*, 551–555. [CrossRef]

42. Rania, J.H.; Hassan, H.M.M.; Afify, A.S. Evaluation of Antioxidant and Metal Chelating Activities of Protein Hydrolysates Produced from Leather Waste by Alkaline and Enzymatic Hydrolysis. *Res. J. Pharm. Biol. Chem. Sci.* **2016**, *7*, 910–919.

43. Gu, H.; Song, I.B.; Han, H.-J.; Lee, N.-Y.; Cha, J.-Y.; Son, Y.-K.; Kwon, J. Antioxidant Activity of Royal Jelly Hydrolysates Obtained by Enzymatic Treatment. *Korean J. Food Sci. Anim. Resour.* **2018**, *38*, 135–142. [PubMed]

44. Ovissipour, M.; Rasco, B.; Shiroodi, S.G.; Modanlow, M.; Gholami, S.; Nemati, M. Antioxidant activity of protein hydrolysates from whole anchovy sprat (*Clupeonella engrauliformis*) prepared using endogenous enzymes and commercial proteases. *J. Sci. Food Agric.* **2013**, *93*, 1718–1726. [CrossRef] [PubMed]

45. DeRosa, G.; Swick, R.W. Metabolic implications of the distribution of the alanine aminotransferase isoenzymes. *J. Biol. Chem.* **1975**, *250*, 7961–7967. [CrossRef]

46. Fernando, S.; Wijewickrama, A.; Gomes, L.; Punchihewa, C.T.; Madusanka, S.D.; Dissanayake, H.; Jeewandara, C.; Peiris, H.; Ogg, G.S.; Malavige, G.N. Patterns and causes of liver involvement in acute dengue infection. *BMC Infect. Dis.* **2016**, *16*, 319. [CrossRef]

47. Noor, K.K.; Ijaz, M.U.; Ehsan, N.; Tahir, A.; Yeni, D.K.; Neamul Kabir Zihad, S.M.; Uddin, S.J.; Ashraf, A.; Simal-Gandara, J. Hepatoprotective role of vitexin against cadmium-induced liver damage in male rats: A biochemical, inflammatory, apoptotic and histopathological investigation. *Biomed. Pharmacother.* **2022**, *150*, 112934. [CrossRef]

48. Wang, K.; Shi, J.; Gao, S.; Hong, H.; Tan, Y.; Luo, Y. Oyster protein hydrolysates alleviated chronic alcohol-induced liver injury in mice by regulating hepatic lipid metabolism and inflammation response. *Food Res. Int.* **2022**, *160*, 111647. [CrossRef]

49. Shi, Y.; Sun, J.; He, H.; Guo, H.; Zhang, S. Hepatoprotective effects of Ganoderma lucidum peptides against d-galactosamine-induced liver injury in mice. *J. Ethnopharmacol.* **2008**, *117*, 415–419. [CrossRef]

50. Mumtaz, S.; Ali, S.; Khan, R.; Andleeb, S.; Ulhaq, M.; Khan, M.A.; Shakir, H.A. The protective role of ascorbic acid in the hepatotoxicity of cadmium and mercury in rabbits. *Environ. Sci. Pollut. R.* **2019**, *26*, 14087–14096. [CrossRef]

51. Holeček, M.; Mráz, J.; Tilšer, I. Plasma amino acids in four models of experimental liver injury in rats. *Amino Acids* **1996**, *10*, 229–241. [CrossRef]

52. Ryu, B.; Shin, K.-H.; Kim, S.-K. Muscle Protein Hydrolysates and Amino Acid Composition in Fish. *Mar. Drugs* **2021**, *19*, 377. [CrossRef] [PubMed]

53. Hayat, S.; Hayat, Q.; Alyemeni, M.N.; Wani, A.S.; Pichtel, J.; Ahmad, A. Role of proline under changing environments. *Plant Signal. Behav.* **2012**, *7*, 1456–1466. [CrossRef] [PubMed]

54. Obayashi, Y.; Arisaka, H.; Yoshida, S.; Mori, M.; Takahashi, M. Proline protects liver from d-galactosamine hepatitis by activating the IL-6/STAT3 survival signaling pathway. *Amino Acids* **2012**, *43*, 2371–2380. [CrossRef] [PubMed]

55. Xie, S.-W.; Tian, L.-X.; Li, Y.-M.; Zhou, W.; Zeng, S.-L.; Yang, H.-J.; Liu, Y.-J. Effect of proline supplementation on anti-oxidative capacity, immune response and stress tolerance of juvenile Pacific white shrimp, *Litopenaeus vannamei*. *Aquaculture* **2015**, *448*, 105–111. [CrossRef]

56. Zhang, L.; Xu, L.; Chen, Y.; Ni, Q.I.; Zhou, M.; Qu, C.; Zhang, Y. Antifibrotic effect of N-acetyl-seryl-aspartyl-lysyl-proline on bile duct ligation induced liver fibrosis in rats. *World J. Gastroenterol.* **2012**, *18*, 5283–5288.

57. Gujjar, R.; Pathak, A.D.; Karkute, S.; Supaibulwattana, K. Multifunctional proline rich proteins and their role in regulating cellular proline content in plants under stress. *Biol. Plant.* **2019**, *63*, 448–454. [CrossRef]

58. Yao Chai, T.; Didierjean, L.; Burkard, G.; Genot, G. Expression of a green tissue-specific 11 kDa proline-rich protein gene in bean in response to heavy metals. *Plant Sci.* **1998**, *133*, 47–56. [CrossRef]

59. Kavi Kishor, P.B.; Sreenivasulu, N. Is proline accumulation per se correlated with stress tolerance or is proline homeostasis a more critical issue? *Plant Cell Environ.* **2014**, *37*, 300–311. [CrossRef]

60. Komatsu, T.; Kobayashi, K.; Morimoto, Y.; Helmerhorst, E.; Oppenheim, F.; Chang-Il Lee, M. Direct evaluation of the antioxidant properties of salivary proline-rich proteins. *J. Clin. Biochem. Nutr.* **2020**, *67*, 131–136. [CrossRef]

61. Galoyan, A.A.; Shakhlamov, V.A.; Aghajanov, M.I.; Vahradyan, H.G. Hypothalamic Proline-Rich Polypeptide Protects Brain Neurons in Aluminum Neurotoxicosis. *Neurochem. Res.* **2004**, *29*, 1349–1357. [CrossRef]

62. Das, S.C.; Al-Naemi, H.A. Cadmium Toxicity: Oxidative Stress, Inflammation and Tissue Injury. *Occup. Dis. Environ. Med.* **2019**, *7*, 144–163. [CrossRef]

63. Valko, M.; Rhodes, C.J.; Moncol, J.; Izakovic, M.; Mazur, M. Free radicals, metals and antioxidants in oxidative stress-induced cancer. *Chem. Biol. Interact.* **2006**, *160*, 1–40. [CrossRef] [PubMed]

64. Poli, G.; Albano, E.; Dianzani, M.U. The role of lipid peroxidation in liver damage. *Chem. Phys. Lipids* **1987**, *45*, 117–142. [CrossRef] [PubMed]

65. Wang, J.; Zhang, Y.; Fang, Z.; Sun, L.; Wang, Y.; Liu, Y.; Xu, D.; Nie, F.; Gooneratne, R. Oleic Acid Alleviates Cadmium-Induced Oxidative Damage in Rat by Its Radicals Scavenging Activity. *Biol. Trace Elem. Res.* **2019**, *190*, 95–100. [CrossRef] [PubMed]

66. Elsayed, A.; Elkomy, A.; Elkammar, R.; Youssef, G.; Abdelhiee, E.Y.; Abdo, W.; Fadl, S.E.; Soliman, A.; Aboubakr, M. Synergistic protective effects of lycopene and N-acetylcysteine against cisplatin-induced hepatorenal toxicity in rats. *Sci. Rep.* **2021**, *11*, 13979. [CrossRef] [PubMed]

67. Elsayed, A.; Elkomy, A.; Alkafafy, M.; Elkammar, R.; Fadl, S.E.; Abdelhiee, E.Y.; Abdeen, A.; Youssef, G.; Shaheen, H.; Soliman, A.; et al. Ameliorating Effect of Lycopene and N-Acetylcysteine against Cisplatin-Induced Cardiac Injury in Rats. *Pak. Vet. J.* **2022**, *42*, 107–111.

68. Elsayed, A.; Elkomy, A.; Alkafafy, M.; Elkammar, R.; El-Shafey, A.; Soliman, A.; Aboubakr, M. Testicular toxicity of cisplatin in rats: Ameliorative effect of lycopene and N-acetylcysteine. *Environ. Sci. Pollut. R.* **2022**, *29*, 24077–24084. [CrossRef]

69. Fan, R.; Hu, P.-C.; Wang, Y.; Lin, H.-Y.; Su, K.; Feng, X.-S.; Wei, L.; Yang, F. Betulinic acid protects mice from cadmium chloride-induced toxicity by inhibiting cadmium-induced apoptosis in kidney and liver. *Toxicol. Lett.* **2018**, *299*, 56–66. [CrossRef]

70. Shaikh, Z.A.; Vu, T.T.; Zaman, K. Oxidative Stress as a Mechanism of Chronic Cadmium-Induced Hepatotoxicity and Renal Toxicity and Protection by Antioxidants. *Toxicol. Appl. Pharmacol.* **1999**, *154*, 256–263. [CrossRef]

71. Jemai, H.; Messaoudi, I.; Chaouch, A.; Kerkeni, A. Protective effect of zinc supplementation on blood antioxidant defense system in rats exposed to cadmium. *J. Trace Elem. Med. Biol.* **2007**, *21*, 269–273. [CrossRef]
72. Jemai, H.; Mahmoudi, A.; Feryeni, A.; Fki, I.; Bouallagui, Z.; Choura, S.; Chamkha, M.; Sayadi, S. Hepatoprotective Effect of Oleuropein-Rich Extract from Olive Leaves against Cadmium-Induced Toxicity in Mice. *Biomed. Res. Int.* **2020**, *2020*, 4398924. [CrossRef]
73. Li, Y.; Yu, J. Research Progress in Structure-Activity Relationship of Bioactive Peptides. *J. Med. Food* **2014**, *18*, 147–156. [CrossRef] [PubMed]
74. Zhu, L.; Chen, J.; Tang, X.; Xiong, Y.L. Reducing, Radical Scavenging, and Chelation Properties of in Vitro Digests of Alcalase-Treated Zein Hydrolysate. *J. Agric. Food Chem.* **2008**, *56*, 2714–2721. [CrossRef] [PubMed]
75. Zou, T.-B.; He, T.-P.; Li, H.-B.; Tang, H.-W.; Xia, E.-Q. The Structure-Activity Relationship of the Antioxidant Peptides from Natural Proteins. *Molecules* **2016**, *21*, 72. [CrossRef]
76. Wree, A.; Holtmann, T.M.; Inzaugarat, M.E.; Feldstein, A.E. Novel Drivers of the Inflammatory Response in Liver Injury and Fibrosis. *Semin. Liver Dis.* **2019**, *39*, 275–282. [CrossRef] [PubMed]
77. Diao, L.; Li, N.; Brayman, T.G.; Hotz, K.J.; Lai, Y. Regulation of MRP2/ABCC2 and BSEP/ABCB11 Expression in Sandwich Cultured Human and Rat Hepatocytes Exposed to Inflammatory Cytokines TNF-α, IL-6, and IL-1β. *J. Biol. Chem.* **2010**, *285*, 31185–31192. [CrossRef]
78. Zhao, Z.; Hyun, J.S.; Satsu, H.; Kakuta, S.; Shimizu, M. Oral exposure to cadmium chloride triggers an acute inflammatory response in the intestines of mice, initiated by the over-expression of tissue macrophage inflammatory protein-2 mRNA. *Toxicol. Lett.* **2006**, *164*, 144–154. [CrossRef]
79. Qian, B.; Zhao, X.; Yang, Y.; Tian, C. Antioxidant and anti-inflammatory peptide fraction from oyster soft tissue by enzymatic hydrolysis. *Food Sci. Nutr.* **2020**, *8*, 3947–3956. [CrossRef]
80. Li, S.; Sun, W.; Zhang, K.; Zhu, J.; Jia, X.; Guo, X.; Zhao, Q.; Tang, C.; Yin, J.; Zhang, J. Selenium deficiency induces spleen pathological changes in pigs by decreasing selenoprotein expression, evoking oxidative stress, and activating inflammation and apoptosis. *J. Anim. Sci. Biotechno.* **2021**, *12*, 65. [CrossRef]
81. Peng, Z.; Chen, B.; Zheng, Q.; Zhu, G.; Cao, W.; Qin, X.; Zhang, C. Ameliorative Effects of Peptides from the Oyster (*Crassostrea hongkongensis*) Protein Hydrolysates against UVB-Induced Skin Photodamage in Mice. *Mar. Drugs* **2020**, *18*, 288. [CrossRef]
82. Qian, Z.-J.; Chen, M.-F.; Chen, J.; Zhang, Y.; Zhou, C.; Hong, P.; Yang, P. Intracellular ethanol-mediated oxidation and apoptosis in HepG2/CYP2E1 cells impaired by two active peptides from seahorse (*Hippocampus kuda* bleeler) protein hydrolysates via the Nrf2/HO-1 and akt pathways. *Food Sci. Nutr.* **2021**, *9*, 1584–1602. [CrossRef] [PubMed]
83. Li, Y.; Lu, L.; Luo, N.; Wang, Y.Q.; Gao, H.M. Inhibition of PI3K/AKt/mTOR signaling pathway protects against d-galactosamine/lipopolysaccharide-induced acute liver failure by chaperone-mediated autophagy in rats. *Biomed Pharm.* **2017**, *92*, 544–553. [CrossRef] [PubMed]
84. Zhong, W.; Qian, K.; Xiong, J.; Ma, K.; Wang, A.; Zou, Y. Curcumin alleviates lipopolysaccharide induced sepsis and liver failure by suppression of oxidative stress-related inflammation via PI3K/AKT and NF-kappaB related signaling. *Biomed. Pharm.* **2016**, *83*, 302–313. [CrossRef] [PubMed]
85. Wang, Y.; Gu, J.; Hu, L.; Kong, L.; Wang, T.; Di, M.; Li, C.; Gui, S. miR-130a alleviates neuronal apoptosis and changes in expression of Bcl-2/Bax and caspase-3 in cerebral infarction rats through PTEN/PI3K/Akt signaling pathway. *Exp. Med.* **2020**, *19*, 2119–2126. [CrossRef] [PubMed]
86. Xiong, X.; Zhang, Y.; Xing, H.; Xu, S. Ameliorative Effect of Selenomethionine on Cadmium-Induced Hepatocyte Apoptosis via Regulating PI3K/AKT Pathway in Chickens. *Biol. Trace Elem. Res.* **2020**, *195*, 559–568. [CrossRef] [PubMed]
87. Augustine, N.; Ani, C.; Eze, W.; Ugwudike, P.; Anyaeji, P.; Ude, V.C.; Agu, F.U.; Nworgu, C.; Ikwuka, D.; Ugwuishi, E.; et al. The effect of aqueous extract of zest of citrus sinensis (AEZCs) on cadmium chloride induced liver toxicity in wistar rats. *Afr. J. Biochem. R.* **2020**, *14*, 5–17. [CrossRef]
88. Najeeb, U.; Jilani, G.; Ali, S.; Sarwar, M.; Xu, L.; Zhou, W. Insights into cadmium induced physiological and ultra-structural disorders in *Juncus effusus* L. and its remediation through exogenous citric acid. *J. Hazard. Mater.* **2011**, *186*, 565–574. [CrossRef]
89. El-Naggar, S.A.; El-Said, K.S.; Elwan, M.; Mobasher, M.; Mansour, F.; Elbakry, M.; Kabil, D.I. Toxicity of bean cooking media containing EDTA in mice. *Toxicol. Ind. Health* **2020**, *36*, 436–445. [CrossRef]
90. Zhang, X.; Peng, Z.; Zheng, H.; Zhang, C.; Lin, H.; Qin, X. The Potential Protective Effect and Possible Mechanism of Peptides from Oyster (*Crassostrea hongkongensis*) Hydrolysate on Triptolide-Induced Testis Injury in Male Mice. *Mar. Drugs* **2021**, *19*, 566. [CrossRef]
91. Jansen, R.; Lachatre, G.; Marquet, P. LC-MS/MS systematic toxicological analysis: Comparison of MS/MS spectra obtained with different instruments and settings. *Clin. Biochem.* **2005**, *38*, 362–372. [CrossRef]
92. Łozowicka, B.; Kaczyński, P.; Iwaniuk, P. Analysis of 22 free amino acids in honey from Eastern Europe and Central Asia using LC-MS/MS technique without derivatization step. *J. Food Compos. Anal.* **2021**, *98*, 103837. [CrossRef]
93. He, S.; Zhuo, L.; Cao, Y.; Liu, G.; Zhao, H.; Song, R.; Liu, Z. Effect of cadmium on osteoclast differentiation during bone injury in female mice. *Environ. Toxicol.* **2020**, *35*, 487–494. [CrossRef] [PubMed]
94. Zhu, Y.; Chen, X.; Rao, X.; Zheng, C.; Peng, X. Saikosaponin a ameliorates lipopolysaccharide and d-galactosamine-induced liver injury via activating LXRα. *Int. Immunopharmacol.* **2019**, *72*, 131–137. [CrossRef]

95. Yang, P.; Xu, F.; Li, H.-F.; Wang, Y.; Li, F.-C.; Shang, M.-Y.; Liu, G.-X.; Wang, X.; Cai, S.-Q. Detection of 191 Taxifolin Metabolites and Their Distribution in Rats Using HPLC-ESI-IT-TOF-MSn. *Molecules* **2016**, *21*, 1209. [CrossRef] [PubMed]
96. Fornetti, J.; Jindal, S.; Middleton, K.; Borges, V.; Schedin, P. Physiological COX-2 Expression in Breast Epithelium Associates with COX-2 Levels in Ductal Carcinoma in Situ and Invasive Breast Cancer in Young Women. *Am. J. Pathol.* **2014**, *184*, 1220–1229. [CrossRef]
97. He, Q.; Luo, Y.; Xie, Z. Sulforaphane ameliorates cadmium induced hepatotoxicity through the up-regulation of /Nrf2/ARE pathway and the inactivation of NF-κB. *J. Funct. Foods* **2021**, *77*, 104297. [CrossRef]

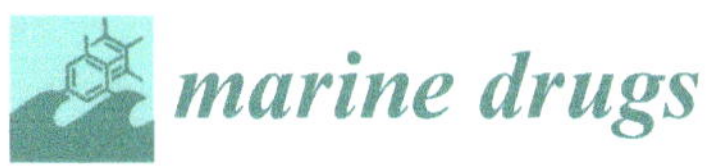

marine drugs

Article

Improved Plasma Lipids, Anti-Inflammatory Activity, and Microbiome Shifts in Overweight Participants: Two Clinical Studies on Oral Supplementation with Algal Sulfated Polysaccharide

Lauren A. Roach [1,*], Barbara J. Meyer [1,*], J. Helen Fitton [2] and Pia Winberg [3,*]

[1] Molecular Horizons, Illawarra Health and Medical Research Institute, School of Medical, Indigenous and Health Sciences, University of Wollongong, Wollongong, NSW 2522, Australia
[2] RDadvisor, Hobart, TAS 7006, Australia; drfitton@rdadvisor.com
[3] Venus Shell Systems Pty Ltd., Nowra, NSW 2540, Australia
* Correspondence: lroach@uow.edu.au (L.A.R.); bmeyer@uow.edu.au (B.J.M.); pia@venusshellsystems.com.au (P.W.)

Abstract: Seaweed polysaccharides in the diet may influence both inflammation and the gut microbiome. Here we describe two clinical studies with an *Ulva* sp. 84-derived sulfated polysaccharide—"xylorhamnoglucuronan" (SXRG84)—on metabolic markers, inflammation, and gut flora composition. The first study was a double-blind, randomized placebo-controlled trial with placebo, and either 2 g/day or 4 g/day of SXRG84 daily for six weeks in 64 overweight or obese participants (median age 55 years, median body mass index (BMI) 29 kg/m^2). The second study was a randomized double-blind placebo-controlled crossover trial with 64 participants (median BMI 29 kg/m^2, average age 52) on placebo for six weeks and then 2 g/day of SXRG84 treatment for six weeks, or vice versa. In Study 1, the 2 g/day dose exhibited a significant reduction in non-HDL (high-density lipoprotein) cholesterol (-10% or -0.37 mmol/L, $p = 0.02$) and in the atherogenic index (-50%, $p = 0.05$), and two-hour insulin (-12% or -4.83 mU/L) showed trends for reduction in overweight participants. CRP (C-reactive protein) was significantly reduced (-27% or -0.78 mg/L, $p = 0.03$) with the 4 g/day dose in overweight participants. Significant gut flora shifts included increases in *Bifidobacteria*, *Akkermansia*, *Pseudobutyrivibrio*, and *Clostridium* and a decrease in *Bilophila*. In Study 2, no significant differences in lipid measures were observed, but inflammatory cytokines were improved. At twelve weeks after the SXRG84 treatment, plasma cytokine concentrations were significantly lower than at six weeks post placebo for IFN-γ (3.4 vs. 7.3 pg/mL), IL-1β (16.2 vs. 23.2 pg/mL), TNF-α (9.3 vs. 12.6 pg/mL), and IL-10 (1.6 vs. 2.1 pg/mL) ($p < 0.05$). Gut microbiota abundance and composition did not significantly differ between groups ($p > 0.05$). Together, the studies illustrate improvements in plasma lipids and an anti-inflammatory effect of dietary SXRG84 that is participant specific.

Keywords: seaweed; metabolic syndrome; prediabetes; sulfated polysaccharide; anti-inflammation; cholesterol; Ulva; microbiome

Citation: Roach, L.A.; Meyer, B.J.; Fitton, J.H.; Winberg, P. Improved Plasma Lipids, Anti-Inflammatory Activity, and Microbiome Shifts in Overweight Participants: Two Clinical Studies on Oral Supplementation with Algal Sulfated Polysaccharide. *Mar. Drugs* **2022**, 20, 500. https://doi.org/10.3390/md20080500

Academic Editors: Donatella Degl'Innocenti and Marzia Vasarri

Received: 6 July 2022
Accepted: 29 July 2022
Published: 2 August 2022

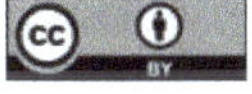

1. Introduction

Maintaining a healthy gut microbiome and a noninflammatory state is key to avoiding metabolic syndrome. In the studies described here, we sought to understand how the gut microbiome is affected by ingesting a type of ulvan from the green seaweed *Ulva* sp. 84, and the effects it has on plasma lipids and inflammation markers. The ulvan is referred to as SXRG84.

The gut microbiome is a complex system of microbes necessary for digestion and homeostasis [1]. A dysregulated microbiome may lead to inflammation and gut permeability. The chronic low-grade inflammation that accompanies metabolic disorder [2] may also give rise to comorbidities such as cardiovascular disease [3], depression [4], and neuropathy [5]. Inflammatory biomarkers, such as interleukin-6 (IL-6) and high-sensitivity C-reactive protein (hsCRP) independently predict future cardiovascular events with a magnitude of effect comparable to that of low-density lipoprotein cholesterol (LDL-C). Treatments for atherosclerosis may require both inflammation inhibition and additional cholesterol reduction [6]. Gut florae respond directly and indirectly to dietary and intestinal glycans, and the microbiome is important to digestive enzyme activity, synthesis of vitamins, interaction with the immune system, interaction with pathogens, and control of inflammatory activity across the gut–blood barrier [7]. Consequently, glycans and the gut florae they support have a lifetime role on the status of the metabolic and immune system.

Seaweeds contain large amounts of resistant dietary glycan. These include the alginates, laminarin and fucoidan (from brown seaweeds), carrageenan and agar (from red seaweeds) and "ulvans"—a diverse group of high-rhamnose-content polysaccharides from green seaweeds. This has recently been well reviewed by Shannon et al. [8]. Seaweed glycans are highly diverse [9,10]. The specificity of bacterial enzymes to dietary glucans implies that each seaweed mucopolysaccharide will have distinct effects on the composition of the microbiome and its metabolic function [11]. Consequently, a response to dietary glycans will also be specific, reflecting individual microbiome profiles, although commonalities related to the microbiome and gut processes are predicted.

Whole *Ulva* sp. seaweeds have been shown to influence gut metabolic processes [12]. There is low toxicity in purified ulvans [13], with doses of up to 600 mg/kg of body weight over six months shown to be well tolerated in rats. *Ulva* sp. and ulvans show effective lipid-lowering qualities. More recent research has shown a consistency in these findings and a diversity in similar metabolic disease related effects from diverse algae [14,15].

In previous studies, brown seaweeds and their components have been shown to exert beneficial effects on allergy and inflammation [16]. The brown seaweed extract fucoidan restored gut lysozyme levels in athletes [17], but fucoidan did not affect metabolic markers in obese nondiabetic subjects [18]. Green seaweeds, including the Ulvacean species similar to the one used in this study, contain a class of polysaccharides known as "ulvans". These heterodisperse sulfated polymers are quite diverse, but generally contain rhamnose, xylose, galactose, and uronic acid. They exhibit lipid-lowering activity [13], protective effects in irritable bowel syndrome (IBD) models [19], and antioxidant and antihyperlipidemic effects [20–22]. A hyperlipidemic rat model showed reductions in non-HDL-cholesterol and increases in HDL-cholesterol and a corresponding improvement in the atherogenic index (log (triglycerides/HDL-cholesterol)) [21]. At 300 mg/kg body weight, hypolipidemic effects were observed in a dose-dependent manner in high-fat-fed mice—an effect comparable to the drug simvastatin [23]. These studies were conducted primarily in animal models and human studies are warranted.

This research presents two consecutive clinical trials investigating the effects of a specific type of ulvan, sulfated xylorhamnoglucuronan, or "SXRG-84", on the metabolic disease markers, the microbiota, and inflammation.

The aim of Study 1 was to investigate the effects of "SXRG84" on plasma lipid levels, glucose, and insulin levels in overweight and obese individuals and assess the impact on the gut microbiota. The primary outcome measures were changes in plasma lipid levels. Secondary outcomes were carbohydrate metabolism, gut microbiota, inflammation, and oxidative stress. It was hypothesized that SXRG84 would have a favorable effect on plasma lipid levels, measures of carbohydrate metabolism, inflammation, and oxidative stress and would result in shifts in the gut microbiota when compared to the placebo group.

The second study (Study 2) was powered on the change in non-HDL-C observed in Study 1, using a randomized placebo-controlled crossover design. The primary objective was to confirm the Study 1 findings that SXRG84 would reduce non-HDL cholesterol in overweight participants. Secondary objectives were to examine the effects of the SXRG84 on further metabolic, inflammatory, and gut microbiota measures.

In this paper, we describe two studies that recruited participants who had a high BMI, and therefore, who had the potential for being metabolically challenged. The BMIs extended from 24 to 40, implying a range of metabolic flexibility. Metabolic flexibility is basically defined as being able to switch between utilizing glucose and lipids as a source of energy during fasting and fed states, as well as during exercise and resting, in order to maintain energy homeostasis [24]. A recent systematic review has shown that metabolic flexibility to glucose and insulin stimulation is inversely associated with the total amount of adipose tissue, waist circumference, and visceral adipose tissue [25]. This suggests that as the weight of a person increases, the metabolic flexibility decreases. Therefore, an additional aim of the first study is to compare metabolic markers across people that were overweight versus those that were obese on the various metabolic outcome measures as the potential to respond to treatments would be affected by metabolic flexibility.

2. Results

2.1. Participants Study 1

Sixty-five participants in Study 1 were randomly assigned to the three blinded treatment groups. This assignment resulted in 21 participants being assigned to the placebo group, 21 participants to the 2 g dose of extract group, and 23 participants to the 4 g dose of extract group. One participant who was assigned to the 4 g dose of extract group withdrew consent due to reasons unrelated to the study (Figure S1 during the trial and so 64 participants completed the trial. Study participants had a median age of 55 years and a median BMI of 29 kg/m^2. There were more female ($n = 40$) than male ($n = 24$) participants recruited, but the distribution of gender was not significantly different between the treatment groups ($p = 0.26$) so the population was analyzed as one. There were no significant differences at baseline between the three treatment gro ups for any of the outcome measures (Table 1).

Table 1. Baseline demographics across treatment groups in Study 1.

	Placebo $n = 21$	2 g SXRG84/day $n = 21$	4 g SXRG84/day $n = 22$	*p*-Value
Gender, F, n (%)	16 (76)	11 (52)	13 (59)	0.259
Age (years)	55.0 (47.0, 60.5)	54.0 (51.0, 57.5)	54.0 (46.8, 63.3)	0.788
BMI (kg/m^2)	29.0 (26.0, 36.0)	29.0 (27.5, 31.0)	30.0 (26.8, 33.3)	0.625
Plasma Lipids				
Total Cholesterol (mmol/L)	5.21 (4.75, 5.96)	5.05 (4.48, 5.60)	5.46 (5.06, 6.07)	0.254
Triglyceride (mmol/L) [1]	1.07 (0.75, 1.56)	1.08 (0.76, 1.56)	1.10 (0.76, 1.82)	0.685
HDL (mmol/L) [1]	1.52 (1.34, 2.13)	1.34 (1.20, 1.84)	1.43 (1.14, 1.93)	0.397
Cholesterol/HDL (mmol/L) [1]	3.10 (2.55, 3.95)	3.60 (2.60, 4.10)	3.70 (2.85, 4.83)	0.265
LDL (mmol/L)	3.10 (2.35, 3.90)	3.00 (2.40, 3.45)	3.35 (2.78, 3.88)	0.412
Non-HDL (mmol/L)	3.45 (2.76, 4.35)	3.55 (3.01, 3.96)	3.84 (3.01, 4.46)	0.335
Atherogenic Index of Plasma (Log TG/HDL)	−0.16 (−0.34, 0.02)	−0.14 (−0.36, 0.12)	−0.12 (−0.32, 0.15)	0.539
Inflammation				
CRP (mg/L) *	2 (1, 4)	2 (1, 3)	3 (2, 4)	0.273
Carbohydrate Metabolism				
Fasting Glucose * (mmol/L)	5.00 (4.80, 5.15)	5.10 (4.75, 5.40)	5.15 (4.80, 5.73)	0.417
HOMA IR [1]	2.10 (1.20, 3.09)	1.93 (1.25, 3.14)	2.11 (1.63, 4.39)	0.401
Glucose After 75 g Glucose load and 2 h [1] (mmol/L)	4.60 (3.55, 5.70)	5.50 (4.35, 6.50)	4.75 (4.15, 6.30)	0.110
C-Peptide [1] (nmol/L)	0.87 (0.53, 1.16)	0.75 (0.59, 0.98)	0.81 (0.66, 1.31)	0.492
Fasting Insulin [1] (mU/L)	9.30 (5.30, 14.75)	8.40 (5.60, 13.75)	9.20 (7.20, 17.78)	0.448
Insulin After 75 g Glucose load and 2 h [1,§] (mU/L)	29.40 (14.70, 68.50)	29.40 (20.60, 63.60)	36.30 (30.80, 129.20)	0.275

Data presented as median, 25th, and 75th percentile. SXRG84—sulfated xylorhamnogalactouronan, BMI—body mass index, HDL—high-density lipoprotein, LDL—low-density lipoprotein, TG—triglyceride, CRP—C-reactive protein, HOMA IR—Homeostatic model assessment for insulin resistance. [1] Log-transformed variable, * Nonparametric Kruskal–Wallis test; [§] $n = 19$ for 2-h insulin due to missing data (Placebo = 6, 2 g = 6 and 4 g = 7).

There were no significant changes post intervention between the three treatment groups. However, given the differences in metabolic flexibility between overweight and obese participants, a secondary data analysis was conducted comparing overweight and obese participants. The baseline characteristics of overweight and obese participants only are shown in Table 2. As expected, there were significant differences between overweight and obese participants; notably an 18% increase in BMI, a 67% increase in CRP, a 47% increase in HOMA, a 36% increase in C-peptide, a 49% increase in fasting insulin, and a trend towards a 47% increase ($p = 0.07$) in insulin following a two-hour OGTT in the obese participants compared to the overweight participants.

Table 2. Comparison of overweight and obese participants at baseline in Study 1.

	Overweight $n = 30$	Obese $n = 30$	p-Value
Sex F, n (%)	18 (60%)	19 (63%)	0.791
Age *	55 (49, 59)	55 (50, 63)	0.819
BMI [1] (kg/m^2)	28 (26, 29)	33 (31, 38)	0.0001
Lipids			
Total Cholesterol (mmol/L)	5.5 (4.9, 6.2)	5.1 (4.5, 5.7)	0.061
Triglyceride [1] (mmol/L)	1.1 (0.7, 1.5)	1.2 (1.0, 1.7)	0.343
HDL [1] (mmol/L)	1.5 (1.3, 2.0)	1.4 (1.2, 1.7)	0.130
Chol/HDL [1] (mmol/L)	3.7 (2.6, 4.5)	3.6 (3.0, 4.2)	0.874
LDL (mmol/L)	3.3 (2.7, 4.1)	2.8 (2.3, 3.5)	0.115
Non-HDL (mmol/L)	3.9 (3.2, 4.7)	3.6 (3.0, 4.0)	0.210
Atherogenic Index of Plasma (Log TG/HDL)	-0.14 (-0.40, 0.11)	-0.04 (-0.26, 0.12)	0.207
CRP (mg/L) *	1 (1, 2)	3 (2, 4)	0.0001
U-Creatinine [1] (mmol/L)	6.3 (4.4, 8.1)	7.9 (6.0, 12.2)	0.041
U-Creatinine Excretion (mmol/d)	11.5 (8.9, 14.8)	12.2 (9.7, 18.1)	0.154
Urine Sodium Excretion (mmol/day)	104 (77, 142)	115 (87, 133)	0.586
Urine Potassium Excretion (mmol/day)	73 (60, 83)	75 (57, 88)	0.641
Na/K [2]	1.5 (1.1, 1.9)	1.5 (1.3, 2.0)	0.749
Fasting Glucose * (mmol/L)	5.0 (4.7, 5.2)	5.3 (5.0, 5.8)	0.099
HOMA [1]	1.7 (1.1, 2.1)	3.2 (2.0, 5.1)	0.0001
Glucose After 75 g Glucose load and 2 h [1]	4.7 (4.0, 5.6)	5.4 (4.2, 6.5)	0.098
C-Peptide [1] (nmol/L)	0.7 (0.5, 0.8)	1.1 (0.9, 1.4)	0.0001
Fasting Insulin [1] (mU/L)	7.5 (5.1, 9.6)	14.8 (9.1, 18.1)	0.0001
Insulin After 75 g Glucose load and 2 h [1] (mU/L) [§]	29.9 (24.7, 42.0)	56.5 (30.8, 129.2)	0.073

Median (25th and 75th percentile). [1] *t*-test on log10-transformed data. [2] *t*-test on square root-transformed data. * nonparametric Wilcoxon signed-rank test used for nonparametric data. [§] $n = 10$ overweight and 7 obese for 2-h insulin levels due to missing data.

However, the baseline parameters between the three treatment groups (placebo, 2 g, and 4 g) did not differ in either the overweight participants or the obese participants (Table 3).

2.1.1. Plasma Lipids Study 1

Given the difference in metabolic flexibility between participants who are overweight and obese, a secondary analysis was conducted for the change scores calculated per treatment group for both overweight and obese groups. The overweight participants had a mean baseline total cholesterol of 5.5 mmol/L (all groups) and there was a significant decrease in non-HDL cholesterol (-10%) in the 2 g dose group ($p = 0.02$) and a trend toward a reduction in the atherogenic index (-50%) in the 2 g dose group ($p = 0.05$) (Figure 1) determined by ANOVA. There were no significant effects in the obese group who started the trial with a slightly lower baseline mean total cholesterol of 5.1 mmol/L (all groups).

Table 3. Baseline for overweight and obese participants per treatment group in Study 1.

Overweight	Placebo $n = 11$	2 g SXRG84/day $n = 10$	4 g SXRG84/day $n = 9$	*p*-Value
Baseline Total Cholesterol (mmol/L)	5.56 (4.76, 6.33)	5.15 (4.79, 5.90)	5.59 (5.28, 6.35)	0.485
Baseline LDL Cholesterol (mmol/L)	3.10 (2.40, 4.20)	3.00 (2.50, 3.65)	3.50 (3.30, 4.10)	0.347
Baseline Non-HDL Cholesterol (mmol/L)	3.41 (2.75, 4.89)	3.89 (3.19, 4.20)	4.08 (3.65, 4.82)	0.463
Baseline Triglycerides (mmol/L) [1]	1.02 (0.62, 1.09)	1.32 (0.79, 2.10)	1.37 (0.66, 1.65)	0.288
Baseline Atherogenic Index of Plasma (Log TG/HDL)	−0.29 (−0.52, -0.10)	−0.06 (−0.37, 0.25)	−0.08 (−0.50, 0.16)	0.269
Baseline C-Reactive Protein (mg/L) *	1 (1, 2)	1 (1, 2)	2 (1, 5)	0.117
Baseline Fasting Glucose (mmol/L) *	5.00 (4.60, 5.10)	5.00 (4.68, 5.30)	4.90 (4.75, 5.15)	0.902
Baseline Glucose after 75 g Glucose Load and 2 h (mmol/L) [1]	4.10 (3.50, 5.00)	5.50 (4.13, 6.65)	4.70 (4.20, 5.25)	0.062
Baseline Insulin 2-h Response to OGTT (mU/L) [§]	28.30 (15.20, 30.40)	27.90 (11.50, 64.10)	36.10 (30.95, 53.48)	0.531
Baseline HOMA IR [1]	1.30 (0.86, 2.10)	1.83 (1.21, 2.42)	1.71 (1.23, 2.11)	0.504
Obese	**Placebo** $n = 9$	**2 g SXRG84/day** $n = 9$	**4 g SXRG84/day** $n = 12$	*p*-Value
Baseline Total Cholesterol (mmol/L) Baseline	4.92 (4.36, 5.82)	4.76 (4.01, 5.73)	5.31 (4.75, 5.92)	0.487
Baseline LDL Cholesterol (mmol/L)	2.80 (2.30, 3.50)	2.60 (2.30, 3.45)	3.00 (2.40, 3.75)	0.646
Baseline Non-HDL Cholesterol (mmol/L)	3.56 (2.85, 4.10)	3.46 (2.82, 3.93)	3.74 (3.23, 4.23)	0.442
Baseline Triglycerides (mmol/L) [1]	1.39 (1.00, 1.71)	1.08 (0.69, 1.56)	1.10 (0.98, 1.95)	0.667
Baseline Atherogenic Index of Plasma (Log TG/HDL)	−0.01 (−0.23, 0.10)	0.00 (−0.32, 0.11)	−0.15 (−0.26, 0.22)	0.871
Baseline C-Reactive Protein (mg/L) *	4 (2, 10)	2 (2, 6)	3 (2, 4)	0.628
Baseline Fasting Glucose (mmol/L) baseline *	5.00 (4.80, 5.95)	5.30 (5.00, 5.60)	5.65 (5.15, 6.28)	0.237
Baseline Glucose After 75 g Glucose Load and 2 h (mmol/L) baseline [1]	5.40 (4.20, 6.50)	5.50 (4.35, 6.80)	5.30 (3.83, 7.05)	0.772
Baseline Insulin 2-h Response to OGTT (mU/L) [‡]	80.45 (56.50, 104.40)	27.20 (23.60, 30.80)	129.2 (30.8, 220.5)	0.379
Baseline HOMA IR [1]	3.11 (2.52, 4.49)	2.73 (1.34, 3.93)	3.89 (2.16, 7.87)	0.266

Data presented as median, 25th and 75th percentile. SXRG—sulfated xylorhamnoglucuronan, HDL—high-density lipoprotein, LDL—low-density lipoprotein, TG—triglyceride, CRP—C-reactive protein, OGTT—oral glucose tolerance test. [1] Log-transformed variable. * Nonparametric Kruskal–Wallis test. [§] $n = 9$ for overweight 2-h insulin due to missing data (Placebo = 3, 2 g = 3, and 4 g = 3). [‡] $n = 7$ for obese 2-h insulin due to missing data (Placebo = 2, 2 g = 2, and 4 g = 3).

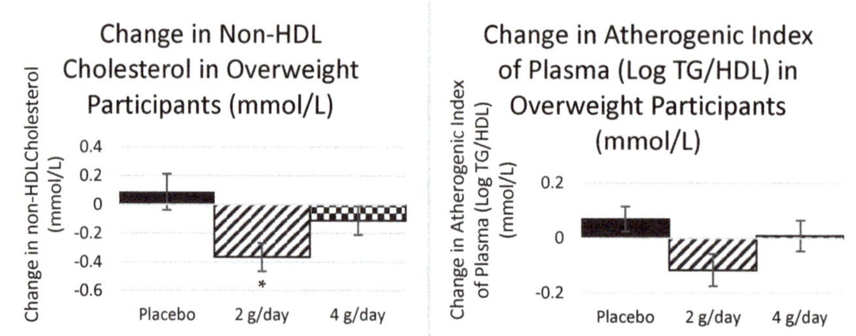

Figure 1. The mean change in non-HDL cholesterol and the atherogenic index of plasma after six weeks of treatment for each of the placebo and active treatments in the overweight participants. $n = 30$ (Placebo = 11, 2 g = 10, and 4 g = 9). Standard error bars shown. * Significant at $p < 0.05$.

2.1.2. Inflammatory Markers Study 1

There was a significant reduction in CRP (-27%) in the 4 g dose in the overweight participants ($p = 0.03$) and a trend towards a reduction in CRP (-27%) in the 2 g dose in the obese participants ($p = 0.06$), as determined by a Kruskal–Wallis test (Figure 2). The obese group started at a considerably higher inflammation status than the overweight group.

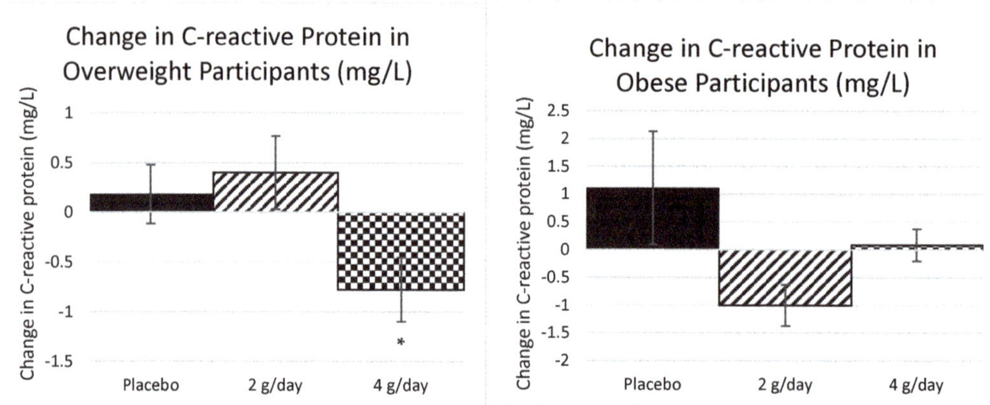

Figure 2. The mean change in CRP after 6 weeks of each of the three treatments for overweight $n = 30$ (Placebo = 11, 2 g = 10, and 4 g = 9) and obese participants $n = 30$ (Placebo = 9, 2 g = 9, and 4 g = 12), separately. Standard error bars shown. * Significant at $p < 0.05$.

2.1.3. Carbohydrate Metabolism Study 1

There were no consistent changes in fasting glucose, fasting insulin, C-peptide, HOMA, or two-hour glucose response to the OGTT across the three treatment groups for either the overweight ($p = 0.17, 0.34, 0.49, 0.15$, and 0.86, respectively) or the obese groups ($p = 0.86$, $0.14, 0.14, 0.22$, and 0.28, respectively) (ANOVA for fasting glucose and two-hour glucose; Kruskal–Wallis for remaining variables). However, there was a trend towards a reduction to the two-hour insulin response to the OGTT (-12%) in the 4 g dose for the overweight participants only ($p = 0.05$), as determined by a Kruskal–Wallis test (Figure 3).

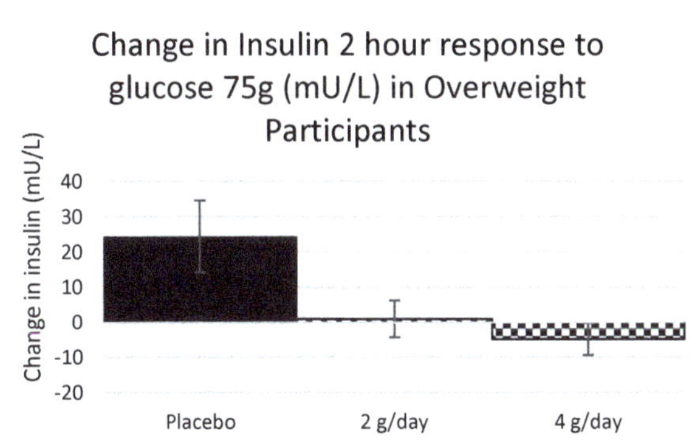

Figure 3. The difference in the 2-h insulin response to the OGTT for overweight participants. N = 9 for overweight 2-h insulin due to missing data (Placebo = 3, 2 g = 3, and 4 g = 3). Standard error bars shown.

2.1.4. Microbiome Results Study 1

There were significant differences ($p < 0.05$) between the pooled active treatments groups (2 g SXRG84/day and 4 g SXRG84/day combined) compared to the placebo group for both overweight and obese participants as separate groups in terms of the most-changed composition and abundance of genera of bacteria from before and after the six-week intervention. This pattern was consistent for both the overweight and the obese participant groups (Figure S3). Below, Figure 4 depicts the change in composition and abundance of genera over a six-week period between the overweight and obese participants on placebo (enclosed circles), which was much smaller compared to those on the active treatment (open circles).

Permutational multivariate analysis is a powerful tool to demonstrate the overall ecological shifts of significance in the treatment and control communities of the microbiome, or the effective changes to the betadiversity. However, translating ecosystem shifts in local diversity compared to the global diversity, or betadiversity, to select species is only complicated by cascading interaction and external effects. Nevertheless, it is of interest to determine which species contributed to the significant change in betadiversity, as experiments can be designed to test cause-and-effect studies over time. Therefore, SIMPER analysis revealed 15 genera that contributed to at least 90% of the differences between placebo and pooled active group changes (Table 4). These 15 genera were examined individually to assess whether there were consistent changes in the two treatment groups compared to the placebo group. Five genera were identified that appeared to demonstrate a treatment effect. The individual genera that increased most in contrast to the placebo group were *Akkermansia, Clostridium, Pseudobutyrivibrio,* and *Bifidobacteria* (mostly *B. longum*) sp. Although not identified in the SIMPER analysis, only one genus seemed to decrease, and this was *Bilophila* sp. (Figure 5)—although the frequency of this change was not large enough to be considered one that contributed to 90% of the variation across treatments.

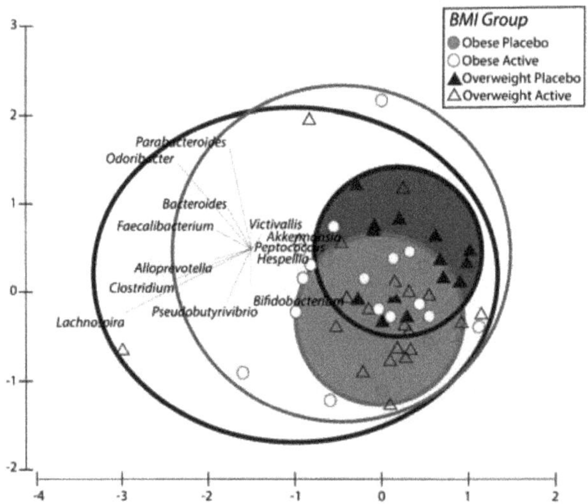

Figure 4. Principle component analysis of the change of composition of genera that was present in each treatment group, including Obese (light) and Overweight (dark) people on active treatments (open shapes) and placebo treatments (closed shapes). Obese Active = Obese participants on active (2 g/SXRG84 or 4 g/SXRG84), Overweight Placebo = Overweight participants on placebo, Overweight Active = Overweight participants on active (2 g/SXRG84 or 4 g/SXRG84), Obese Placebo = Obese participants on placebo.

Table 4. Genera as identified in SIMPER analysis that contributed to the differences between treatment groups. * Indicates potential for treatment effect.

Genera	Contribution%	Cum.%	
Odoribacter	9.32	9.32	Increased across all groups slightly—no treatment effect
* *Akkermansia (muciniphila)*	9.08	18.39	Variable effect in some people.
Lachnospira	9.06	27.46	Significant decrease in placebo—no treatment effect
* *Clostridium*	7.95	35.40	Slight decrease in placebo—limited treatment effect
Parabacteroides	7.84	43.24	Variable trends—no evident treatment effect
Faecalibacterium	7.35	50.60	Random nonsignificant effects
* *Pseudobutyrivibrio*	6.73	57.32	Significant increases in 2 and 4 g treatments but not in placebo.
Catenibacterium	5.17	62.49	Random increase and decrease across groups
* *Bifidobacterium (longum)*	5.05	67.54	Apparent shifts in all groups but much higher in 2 g and 4 g treatments.
Desulfovibrio	5.05	72.59	Random increase and decrease across groups
Bacteroides	4.76	77.35	Decreased in all groups
Victivallis	4.28	81.64	Random increase and decrease across groups
Hespellia	4.11	85.75	Random increase and decrease across groups
Acidaminococcus	3.59	89.34	
Alloprevotella	2.29	91.63	

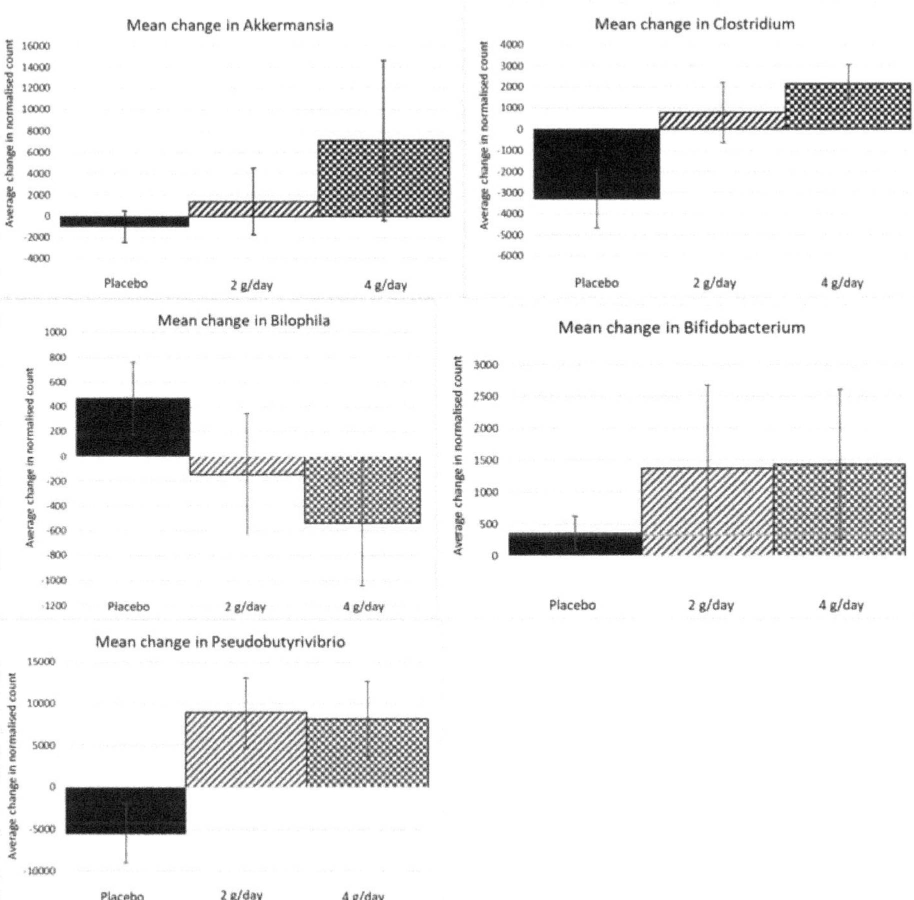

Figure 5. Univariate genera that were identified as those that contributed most to the difference between the active and placebo treatments consistently. Standard error bars are shown.

2.1.5. Dietary Data, Bowel Movements, Urinary F_2-Isoprostanes—Blood Count Results Study 1

Dietary intake and urinary F_2-isoprostanes were included as a tertiary outcome in the study. Dietary intake between the three treatment groups was not significantly different at baseline for total energy (kJ), all macronutrients, sugar (g), and dietary fiber (g) and all three groups had no difference in total diet score. In the 4 g treatment group, there was a trend towards a 10% reduction in saturated fat ($p = 0.06$), as determined by ANOVA, and a trend towards a 33% reduction in added sugar as a percent of total energy after the six-week treatment, as determined by ANOVA ($p = 0.08$, Table S1, Supplementary Material).

There was no significant difference between treatment groups in regard to a change in frequency in bowel movements throughout the trial (results not shown). Safety measures such as full blood-count data (Table S4 and urinary F_2-isoprostanes remained stable throughout the trial, with no significant changes detected between groups ($p > 0.05$) (Table S2).

2.2. Study 2

2.2.1. Participants Study 2

Study two was a double-blind, crossover design with 70 participants randomized to either treatment regime. Each group included both active (2 g SXRG84) and placebo treatments in different orders. Six participants discontinued the intervention for the following reasons: one withdrew consent and provided no reason, one was unable to attend the final appointment due to work commitments, one was unable to attend the final appointment due to medical reasons, one did not want to continue the intervention, one fell pregnant, and one experienced a flare up of gut symptoms but was on the placebo treatment at the time. Therefore, 30 participants (15 female, 15 male) completed the placebo then treatment regime (AB) and 34 (18 female, 16 male) completed the treatment then placebo regime (BA) (Figure S2).

At baseline there were no significant differences between the two groups (placebo then treatment (AB) or treatment then placebo (BA)). There was no significant difference in gender distribution between the two groups with 50–53% female ($p = 0.8142$) in each group (Table 5). Overall, at baseline participants had a median BMI of 29 kg/m^2 and an average age of 52. The proportion of participants meeting the estimated average requirement (EAR) for nutrients remained constant across the three timepoints. The nutrients that were at risk (i.e., less than 50% of the study group met the EAR) were calcium, magnesium, and zinc for males and calcium for females (Table S3).

Table 5. Baseline, post (6 or 12 weeks) and change data after placebo or SXRG treatment (Study 2) for blood pressure and weight.

	AA Baseline to 6 Weeks (Placebo) $n = 30$	AB Baseline to 12 Weeks (Placebo then Active) $n = 30$	BB Baseline to 6 Weeks (Active) $n = 34$	BA Baseline to 12 Weeks (Active then Placebo) $n = 34$	*p*-Value *
Gender, F (%)	15 (50%)	15 (50%)	18 (53%)	18 (53%)	0.814
Age	51.7 ± 15	51.7 ± 15	52.2 ± 11	52.2 ± 11	0.887
BMI (kg/m^2)					
Baseline §	28 (26, 31)	28. (26, 31)	29 (27, 31)	29 (27, 31)	0.101
Post	29 (26, 31)	29 (26, 31)	29 (28, 31)	29 (27, 31)	0.363
Change	0 (0, 1)	0 (0, 0)	0 (0, 0)	0 (−1, 0)	
Waist Circumference (cm)					
Baseline	95 (85, 104)	95 (85, 104)	96 (92, 105)	96 (92, 105)	0.257
Post	97 (85, 106)	99 (87, 107)	100 (93, 106)	99 (92, 107)	0.660
Change	1 (−1, 4)	2 (−1, 5)	3 (−1, 5)	1 (−3, 4)	
Systolic BP (mmHg)					
Baseline §	132 (117, 142)	132 (117, 142)	130 (122, 139)	130 (122, 139)	0.850
Post	127 (114, 141)	122 (114, 139)	129 (119, 135)	125 (114, 136)	0.809
Change	−5.0 (−10.8, 1.8)	−6.0 (−13.5, 1.0)	−4.0 (−14.5, 4.8)	−6.0 (−16.3, 0.5)	
Diastolic BP (mmHg)					
Baseline	82 (71, 89)	82 (71, 89)	83 (75, 94)	83 (75, 94)	0.524
Post	79 (72, 87)	76 (70, 85)	80 (73, 87)	79 (67, 87)	0.653
Change	−1.5 (−8.0, 2.8)	−4.0 (−8.0, 3.0)	−4.0 (−8.0, 4.0)	−3.0 (−10.8, 1.0)	

Data are presented as number and % for gender, mean ± standard deviation or median (25th and 75th percentile). AA = Placebo for 6 weeks; AB = Placebo for 6 weeks then SXRG treatment for 6 weeks; BB = SXRG treatment for 6 weeks; BA = SXRG treatment for 6 weeks then placebo for 6 weeks. Change determined by median post value (6 or 12 weeks) minus median baseline value. * *p*-value at baseline determined by *T*-test on normal or log-transformed (§) data between the two baseline regime groups. *p*-value for post measure determined by ANCOVA using absolute data from 6 weeks (for placebo and active group) and 12 weeks (for placebo then active group and active then placebo group) using baseline data as a covariate.

2.2.2. Biochemical Analysis Study 2

There were no significant differences detected between the four groups for any of the lipid measures, blood pressure and glucose, both fasting glucose, and two-hour response to the OGTT (Table 6).

Table 6. Lipid and glucose baseline, post (6 or 12 weeks) and change data after placebo or SXRG84 treatment (Study 2). Data are presented as median (25th and 75th percentile). AA = Placebo for 6 weeks; AB = Placebo for 6 weeks then SXRG treatment for 6 weeks; BB = SXRG treatment for 6 weeks; BA = SXRG treatment for 6 weeks then placebo for 6 weeks.

	AA Baseline to 6 weeks (Placebo) $n = 30$	AB Baseline to 12 weeks (Placebo then Active) $n = 30$	BB Baseline to 6 weeks (Active) $n = 34$	BA Baseline to 12 weeks (Active then Placebo) $n = 34$	*p*-Value *
Total Cholesterol (mmol/L)					
Baseline	5.2 (4.5, 5.9)	5.2 (4.5, 5.9)	5.2 (4.5, 6.1)	5.2 (4.5, 6.1)	0.697
Post	4.6 (3.9, 5.4)	4.8 (4.2, 5.7)	5.3 (4.2, 5.9)	5.0 (4.4, 5.9)	0.120
Change	−0.3 (−1.0, 0.1)	−0.1 (−0.7, 0.6)	−0.1 (−0.6, 0.4)	−0.3 (−1.0, 0.2)	
HDL Cholesterol (mmol/L)					
Baseline [§]	1.3 (1.0, 1.6)	1.3 (1.0, 1.6)	1.3 (0.9, 1.8)	1.3 (0.9, 1.8)	0.810
Post	1.1 (1.0, 1.7)	1.2 (1.0, 1.7)	1.3 (0.9, 1.9)	1.2 (0.9, 1.6)	0.493
Change	−0.0 (−0.2, 0.1)	−0.1 (−0.3, 0.2)	−0.0 (−0.2, 0.1)	−0.2 (−0.3, 0.1)	
Triglycerides (mmol/L)					
Baseline [§]	1.0 (0.7, 1.2)	1.0 (0.7, 1.2)	1.2 (0.8, 1.8)	1.2 (0.8, 1.8)	0.112
Post	0.8 (0.7, 1.3)	1.1 (0.7, 1.3)	1.0 (0.8, 1.4)	1.0 (0.8, 1.8)	0.663
Change	−0.1 (−0.3, 0.2)	0.0 (−0.2, 0.3)	−0.1 (−0.4, 0.2)	−0.1 (−0.4, 0.1)	
Non-HDL Cholesterol (mmol/L)					
Baseline	3.7 (3.0, 4.5)	3.7 (3.0, 4.5)	4.0 (3.1, 4.4)	4.0 (3.1, 4.4)	0.651
Post	3.4 (2.6, 3.9)	3.6 (2.7, 4.3)	3.8 (3.0, 4.6)	3.7 (3.3, 4.3)	0.086
Change	−0.3 (−0.9, 0.1)	−0.1 (−0.7, 0.6)	0.0 (−0.4, 0.3)	−0.2 (−0.7, 0.4)	
LDL Cholesterol (mmol/L)					
Baseline	3.3 (2.6, 3.9)	3.3 (2.6, 3.9)	3.3 (2.6, 3.9)	3.3 (2.6, 3.9)	0.906
Post	2.9 (2.2, 3.4)	3.2 (2.2, 3.9)	3.4 (2.4, 3.7)	3.2 (2.6, 3.7)	0.103
Change	−0.3 (−0.8, 0.1)	−0.2 (−0.7, 0.5)	−0.1 (−0.5, 0.3)	−0.1 (−0.6, 0.3)	
Fasting Glucose (mmol/L)					
Baseline [¥]	4.5 (4.1, 5.3)	4.5 (4.1, 5.3)	4.9 (4.6, 5.3)	4.9 (4.6, 5.3)	0.071
Post	4.5 (4.1, 5.0)	4.8 (4.1, 5.7)	5.0 (4.2, 5.5)	4.8 (4.3, 5.5)	0.369
Change	−0.1 (−0.4, 0.4)	0.2 (−0.4, 1.0)	−0.0 (−0.5, 0.4)	−0.1 (−0.8, 0.3)	
2-h Glucose Response to OGTT (mmol/L)					
Baseline [¥]	4.9 (4.1, 5.7)	4.9 (4.1, 5.7)	4.8 (4.0, 6.1)	4.8 (4.0, 6.1)	0.844
Post	4.5 (4.2, 5.7)	5.1 (4.3, 5.8)	4.5 (3.8, 5.9)	5.2 (4.0, 6.8)	0.629
Change	0.0 (−0.8, 0.5)	0.0 (−0.5, 0.6)	−0.1 (−1.0, 1.0)	0.1 (−1.1, 1.2)	

Change determined by median post value (6 or 12 weeks) minus median baseline value. * *p*-value at baseline determined by *T*-test on normal, log-transformed ([§]), or Wilcoxon signed rank test ([¥]) between the two baseline regime groups. *p*-value for post measure determined by ANCOVA using absolute data from 6 weeks (for placebo and active group) and 12 weeks (for placebo then active group and active then placebo group) using baseline data as a covariate.

2.2.3. Inflammatory Markers Study 2

Significant differences were detected between the four groups for post intervention inflammatory markers using the corresponding baseline value as a covariate (Tables 7 and 8).

Table 7. Inflammatory markers baseline, post 6 or 12 weeks, and change data after placebo or SXRG (Study 2).

	AA Baseline to 6 Weeks (Placebo) $n = 30$	AB Baseline to 12 Weeks (Placebo then Active) $n = 30$	BB Baseline to 6 Weeks (Active) $n = 34$	BA Baseline to 12 Weeks (Active then Placebo) $n = 34$	*p*-Value [*]
C-Reactive Protein (mg/L)					
Baseline [¥]	0 (0, 4.5)	0 (0, 4.5)	0 (0, 0.6)	0 (0, 0.6)	0.409
Post	0 (0, 6.9)	0.1 (0, 5.1)	0 (0, 4.5)	0 (0, 0.2)	0.240
Change	0 (0, 1.4)	0 (−0.5, 0.6)	0 (0, 3.5)	0 (0, 0)	
IFN-gamma (pg/mL)					
Baseline [¥]	3.2 (1.8, 5.4)	3.2 (1.8, 5.4)	3.4 (1.8, 4.8)	3.4 (1.8, 4.8)	0.877
Post	3.0 (2.2, 5.8) [a]	2.7 (1.9, 4.0) [b]	3.6 (2.0, 4.2) [a,b]	2.3 (1.3, 3.1) [b]	0.014
Change	0.4 (−0.6, 1.6)	−0.4 (−2.2, 0.6)	0.2 (−1.3, 0.8)	−1.0 (−2.0, 0.0)	
IL-1 beta (pg/mL)					
Baseline [‡]	17.5 (9.4, 27.7)	17.5 (9.4, 27.7)	14.7 (9.9, 23.3)	14.7 (9.9, 23.3)	0.547
Post	17.6 (13.0, 25.1) [a]	15.2 (9.9, 21.7) [b]	16.4 (13.3, 21.3) [a,b]	10.6 (8.0, 18.3) [b]	0.005
Change	−0.3 (−3.9, 8.9)	−1.1 (−9.0, 4.6)	1.4 (−5.9, 5.9)	−3.7 (−11.0, 0.8)	
IL-6 (pg/mL)					
Baseline [‡]	11.8 (8.3, 20.8)	11.8 (8.3, 20.8)	12.9 (7.9, 22.3)	12.9 (7.9, 22.3)	0.896
Post	14.8 (10.5, 19.5)	12.0 (9.4, 16.5)	13.8 (9.3, 17.1)	10.3 (7.0, 16.1)	0.226
Change	1.3 ± 8.1	−2.0 ± 7.8	−1.5 ± 8.7	−2.3 ± 8.0	
TNF-alpha (pg/mL)					
Baseline [§]	7.7 (4.0, 12.1)	7.7 (4.0, 12.1)	5.4 (2.9, 10.0)	5.4 (2.9, 10.0)	0.528
Post	8.1 (6.3, 16.9) [a]	8.0 (3.6, 13.1) [b]	8.7 (6.1, 11.6) [a,b]	4.5 (2.8, 10.1) [b]	0.005
Change	1.7 (−1.4, 7.6)	0.3 (−2.0, 3.3)	1.3 (−2.3, 5.0)	−1.2 (−6.2, 2.4)	
IL-10 (pg/mL)					
Baseline [¥]	1.3 (0.8, 2.4)	1.3 (0.8, 2.4)	1.1 (0.7, 2.1)	1.1 (0.7, 2.1)	0.780
Post	1.5 (1.2, 2.5) [a]	1.3 (0.8, 2.2) [b,c]	1.6 (1.2, 2.0) [a,b]	1.0 (0.7, 1.9) [c]	0.009
Change	0.3 (−0.3, 1.1)	0.0 (−0.3, 0.5)	0.1 (−0.4, 0.8)	−0.2 (−0.9, 0.3)	
IL-8 (pg/mL)					
Baseline [§]	5.2 (3.5, 10.1)	5.2 (3.5, 10.1)	4.7 (2.7, 8.5)	4.7 (2.7, 8.5)	0.607
Post	5.7 (3.9, 8.8)	3.9 (3.0, 6.9)	5.2 (4.0, 7.0)	3.9 (1.7, 9.2)	0.254
Change	0.2 (−1.3, 3.0)	−1.1 (−2.8, 0.2)	−0.2 (−2.6, 2.6)	−0.5 (−2.1, 0.9)	

Data are presented as median (25th and 75th percentile). AA = Placebo for 6 weeks; AB = Placebo for 6 weeks then SXRG treatment for 6 weeks; BB = SXRG treatment for 6 weeks; BA = SXRG treatment for 6 weeks then placebo for 6 weeks. Change determined by median post value (6 or 12 weeks) minus median baseline value. * *p*-value at baseline determined by T-test on normal, log-transformed (§), square root-transformed data (‡), or Wilcoxon signed rank test (¥) between the two baseline regime groups. *p*-value for post measure determined by ANCOVA using absolute data from 6 weeks (for placebo and active group) and 12 weeks (for placebo then active group and active then placebo group) using baseline data as a covariate. Values with different superscript letters denotes statistical significance ($p < 0.05$).

There were multiple significant changes in specific inflammatory markers, but not in CRP, bearing in mind that CRP was lower at baseline in Study 2.

Table 8. Significant correlations with baseline measures and gut microbiota genera in Study 2.

Baseline Variable	Genus	Spearman's Correlation Coefficient	*p*-Value
Weight (kg)	*Flavonifractor*	−0.282	0.039
	Intestinibacter	−0.413	0.002
	Megasphaera	0.587	0.001
	Thalassospira	−0.538	0.001
BMI (kg/m²)	*Anaerotruncus*	−0.295	0.027
	Blautia	−0.289	0.028
	Intestinibacter	−0.325	0.016
	Megasphaera	−0.519	0.004
	Ordoribacter	0.290	0.048
	Romboutsia	0.288	0.047
Waist Circumference (cm)	*Anaerotruncus*	−0.360	0.007
	Bifidobacterium	−0.315	0.048
	Flavobacterium	−0.333	0.044
	Flavonifractor	−0.363	0.007
	Intestinibacter	−0.479	0.000
	Megasphaera	0.476	0.009
	Thalassospira	−0.464	0.005
CRP	*Erysipelatoclostridium*	0.297	0.031
	Parasutterella	0.398	0.010
	Subdoligranulum	0.317	0.017
Total Cholesterol	*Megasphaera*	−0.375	0.045
	Mogibacterium	−0.313	0.032
	Parabacteroides	−0.303	0.025
HDL Cholesterol	*Anaerotruncus*	0.318	0.017
	Intestinibacter	0.308	0.024
	Megasphaera	−0.482	0.008
	Thalassospira	0.519	0.001
Triglycerides	*Anaerotruncus*	−0.328	0.014
	Barnesiella	−0.365	0.015
	Corynebacterium	0.373	0.016
	Flavobacterium	−0.362	0.025
	Flavonifractor	−0.315	0.020
	Intestinibacter	−0.433	0.001
	Pseudoflavonifractor	−0.422	0.010
	Sarcina	−0.360	0.006
	Thalassospira	−0.380	0.022
Non-HDL Cholesterol	*Parabacteroides*	−0.330	0.014
LDL Cholesterol	*Collinsella*	−0.272	0.045
	Parabacteroides	−0.325	0.015
Fasting Glucose	*Alloprevotella*	−0.529	0.043
	Bacteroides	0.278	0.034
	Erysipelatoclostridium	0.289	0.036
	Flavonifractor	−0.480	0.000
	Haemophilus	−0.362	0.010
	Intestinibacter	−0.277	0.043
	Megamonas	−0.810	0.015
	Pseudoflavonifractor	−0.504	0.002
	Subdoligranulum	0.280	0.036
	Veillonella	−0.305	0.030
2 h Glucose Post Oral Glucose Tolerance Test	*Haemophilus*	−0.374	0.014
	Intestinibacter	−0.284	0.048

Table 8. *Cont.*

Baseline Variable	Genus	Spearman's Correlation Coefficient	*p*-Value
IFNγ	*Clostridium*	−0.271	0.045
	Granulicatella	0.467	0.012
IL-1β	*Actinomyces*	0.301	0.034
	Clostridium	−0.351	0.008
	Corynebacterium	0.324	0.039
	Granulicatella	0.447	0.015
	Prevotella	0.330	0.028
IL-6	*Adlercreutzia*	0.300	0.048
	Corynebacterium	0.348	0.028
	Granulicatella	0.386	0.042
TNF-α	*Clostridium*	−0.321	0.017
	Granulicatella	0.428	0.023
	Prevotella	0.354	0.018
IL-10	*Clostridium*	−0.321	0.016
	Corynebacterium	0.370	0.017
	Granulicatella	0.428	0.020
	Parabacteroides	−0.280	0.038
	Prevotella	0.361	0.016
	Thalassospira	−0.446	0.006
IL-8	*Adlercreutzia*	0.311	0.042
	Alistipes	0.296	0.035
	Bifidobacterium	0.317	0.049
	Flavonifractor	0.278	0.046
	Granulicatella	0.464	0.015

2.2.4. Gut Flora Results Study 2

A permutational multivariate analysis of variance was used to determine if there were any significant differences in gut microbiota between the two treatment regimens across the three time points, resulting in comparisons between six groups. There were no significant differences between the six groups ($p > 0.05$). A correlation plot was then used to assess the movement of gut microbiota per regime group and time point (Figure 6), on which each data point represented a time point per regime group. After visual inspection of the correlation plot, it was apparent that the two regime groups at baseline varied greatly, with movement occurring at each time point. A SIMPER analysis was conducted to determine whether there were any consistent increases or decreases in genera common to both the active treatments and not the placebo treatment. There were three genera identified that consistently changed in both regimes after the SXRG84 treatment with no effect or an opposing effect in the placebo groups—these were an increase in both *Fusicatenibacter* and *Parabacteroides* and a decrease in *Clostridium*.

There were a number of genera at baseline that significantly correlated with baseline measures of weight, BMI, waist circumference, lipids, glucose, CRP, and cytokines, which are summarized in Table 8. There were also significant correlations between the change of cytokines that were observed in this study (IFNγ, IL-1β, TNF-α, and IL-10) and the change in specific gut genera (below, Table 9).

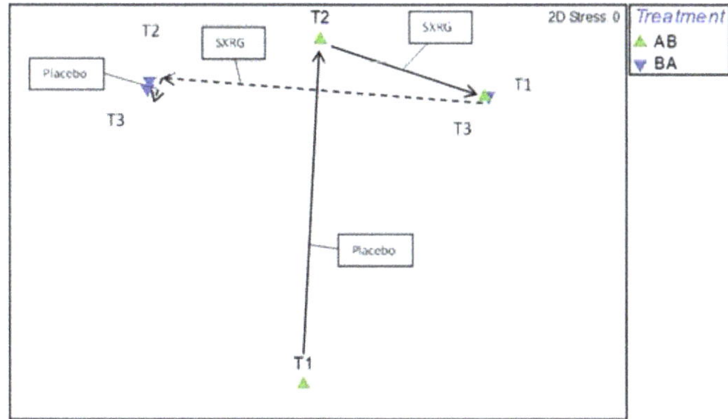

Figure 6. Correlation plot of gut microbiome movement per treatment group. Green triangles are regime AB (starting on placebo then crossing to SXRG84 treatment), blue triangles are regime BA (starting on SXRG84 treatment then crossing to placebo). T1 is baseline measure, T2 is measure from six weeks, and T3 is measure from 12 weeks.

Table 9. Cytokines that significantly changed in Study 2 correlate with a change in specific gut microbiota genera.

Cytokine	Genus	Spearman Correlation Coefficient	*p*-Value
IFN-γ	*Collinsella*	−0.298	0.023
	Oscillibacter	−0.297	0.023
	Romboutsia	−0.278	0.034
IL-1β	*Collinsella*	−0.299	0.023
	Lactobacillus	−0.289	0.028
TNF-α	*Bacteroides*	−0.332	0.011
	Dorea	−0.320	0.014
	Peptococcus	0.270	0.040
IL-10	*Bacteroides*	−0.369	0.004
	Dorea	−0.300	0.022

3. Discussion

This research presents two approaches to clinical studies in humans following the ingestion of a unique ulvan polysaccharide, SXRG-84. The studies explored the intervention effects on metabolic health outcomes wherein the links between lipid markers, inflammation status, and gut microbiota composition were recognized.

The primary outcome measure of Study 1 was plasma lipids, for which a significant 10% reduction in non-HDL cholesterol was observed in overweight participants. Study 2 was then powered to show the reduction in non-HDL cholesterol seen in Study 1, although this was not confirmed with potentially less metabolically challenged participants at baseline.

There was strong agreement between the two studies that dietary SXRG84 effectively reduced inflammatory markers. In the first study, the marker CRP was significantly reduced (−27%) in the 4 g/day dose group. In Study 2, a wider range of proinflammatory cytokines were reduced: IFN-γ (3.4 vs. 7.3 pg/mL), IL-1β (16.2 vs. 23.2 pg/mL), and TNF-α (9.3 vs. 12.6 pg/mL), as well as the anti-inflammatory cytokine IL-10 (1.6 vs. 2.1 pg/mL) ($p < 0.05$). These marked findings indicate a positive effect on metabolic health over a relatively short period of time.

Each study looked at gut microbiomes. There was no consistent effect on the microbiome seen between the two studies, although Study 1 demonstrated a significant change in overall composition and abundance of microbiota in SXRG-84 treatments versus placebo, and some key biota that were important in this shift were identified.

In more detail, Study 1 subgroups (based on BMI) presented changes in lipids, inflammation, and insulin levels and shifts in gut flora. The reduction in non-HDL cholesterol in overweight participants on the 2 g dose also showed a trend to reduction in the atherogenic index (log(triglycerides/HDL-cholesterol)). Although the changes observed in non-HDL cholesterol were much lower than those observed in statin trials [26], this group was not necessarily hypercholesterolemic to begin with. Non-HDL cholesterol is a clinically relevant target as it has strong correlations with atherogenic lipoproteins and is suggested to be a better predictor of CVD events than LDL-cholesterol [6].

Although Study 2 was adequately powered to show a reduction in non-HDL cholesterol, Study 1 findings were not confirmed. One reason for this null finding may be that Study 2 used a different population from Study 1. Whilst the two study populations did not differ in total cholesterol, non-HDL cholesterol, and LDL-cholesterol levels at baseline (Table 10), they differed in regard to CRP, fasting glucose, and HDL-cholesterol at baseline, with participants from Study 1 having significantly higher levels. The higher glucose and CRP indicate a slightly more metabolically challenged group in Study 1, which may have elicited a stronger treatment effect.

Table 10. Comparison of baseline data from Study 1 to Study 2.

	Study 1 $n = 64$	Study 2 $n = 64$	*p*-Value
Gender, F, M (%)	42, (63%)	33, (52%)	0.198
Age (years)	54 ± 10	52 ± 13	0.326
Weight (kg) [§]	85 (74, 101)	84 (76, 95)	0.584
BMI [¥] (kg/m²)	29 (26, 33)	29 (27, 31)	0.471
Total Cholesterol (mmol/L)	5.3 ± 0.9	5.3 ± 1.2	0.750
HDL Cholesterol (mmol/L) [‡]	1.4 (1.2, 2.0)	1.3 (1.0, 1.7)	0.007
Non-HDL Cholesterol (mmol/L) [‡]	3.6 (3.1, 4.1)	3.9 (3.0, 4.4)	0.180
LDL Cholesterol (mmol/L) [‡]	3.0 (2.4, 3.6)	3.3 (2.6, 3.9)	0.143
Triglycerides (mmol/L) [§]	1.1 (0.7, 1.6)	1.1 (0.8, 1.6)	0.898
Fasting Glucose (mmol/L) [¥]	5.1 (4.8, 5.4)	4.8 (4.3, 5.2)	0.004
Glucose 2-h Post OGTT (mmol/L) [¥]	4.7 (4.0, 6.3)	4.8 (4.0, 5.8)	0.837
CRP (mg/L) [¥]	2 (1, 4)	0 (0, 3)	0.000

Data presented as absolute values and (percentage) for female gender; mean ± standard deviation for normally distributed variables or median (25th, 75th percentile) for non-normally distributed variables. BMI—body mass index, OGTT—oral glucose tolerance test. Two groups were compared using an independent samples t-test on normally distributed data, log-transformed data ([§]), square root-transformed data ([‡]), or the Wilcoxon signed rank test ([¥]).

The inconsistency of lipid-lowering effects highlights the need for further research with this extract, with recruitment restricted to hypercholesterolemic participants. Although Study 2 failed to show an improvement in lipid levels, the major finding was the improvements in proinflammatory cytokines after SXRG84 treatment, including IFN-γ, IL-1β, TNF-α, and the generally anti-inflammatory IL-10 [27].

Previous work from animal trials has shown that certain seaweed glycan extracts reduce plasma lipid levels through the action of bile acid sequestering [21,28,29], supported by the increase in bile acids in the feces of these animals following seaweed glycan supplementation [21]. Mechanistically, plasma lipids are lowered as they are required for the synthesis of bile acids; thus, the removal of lipids from the circulation is upregulated [21]. It was of interest that the genus Bilophila was one of the microbiotas that decreased during SXRG-84 treatment in support of this hypothesis [30,31]. Another potential reason for the lipid-lowering effects is via short-chain fatty acid propionate produced by *Bacteroides* and

Akkermansia [32], which both increased in Study 1. Propionate production has been shown to increase up to five times more from L-rhamnose than from other sugars [33] (SXRG84 is rhamnose rich).

In Study 1, there were significant reductions in CRP in overweight participants on 4 g of SXRG84 and a trend towards a reduction in CRP in obese participants. Although CRP is a nonspecific marker of inflammation, it is predictive of coronary heart disease and gastrointestinal diseases [34]. There was a trend towards a reduction in the two-hour insulin response to the OGTT, with no observed changes to glucose levels, suggesting an improvement in insulin sensitivity.

In Study 2, the observed reductions in a suite of inflammatory cytokines (IFN-γ, IL-1β, and TNF-α) may be beneficial as elevated levels are implicated in metabolic and cardiovascular conditions. IFN-γ has been implicated in the development of cardiovascular disease [35]. Additionally, IL-1β and TNF-α levels are chronically raised in metabolic disease [36]. Reducing these proinflammatory cytokines may benefit overweight participants who are otherwise generally healthy but may be at increased risk. IL-10 is generally regarded as an anti-inflammatory cytokine, and it is possible that the reduction indicates a reduced inflammatory pressure [27]. In contrast, probiotic supplementation in ulcerative colitis generally decreases proinflammatory cytokines and raises IL-10 levels.

In Study 1, the change in microbiome species composition over time (six weeks) was significantly different and more variable for participants on SXRG84 versus placebo. The impact of dietary SXRG84 on the gut flora can be summarized as an increasing shift of up to 15 taxa. In Study 1, of the 15 taxa responsible for significant differences in the active groups vs. placebo groups, 25% of the significant shift was explained by a quartet of assumed beneficial or probiotic microbiota, including *Pseudobutyrivibrio*, *Bifidobacteria*, *Akkermansia*, and *Clostridium*. These bacteria are known to respond positively to soluble dietary glycans in the distal colon. *Akkermansia* and *Bifidobacterium*, which are thought to be important for a broad range of health-related processes [37], are regarded as target organisms by researchers in the field of metabolic disease and gut health-related disorders. *Bifidobacterium* has specifically been shown to increase in response to larger molecular polysaccharides, more so than for the recognized fructo-oligosaccharides, including those with rhamnose [38]. There has been a lot of recent work focusing on the beneficial effects of probiotic *Akkermansia* intervention, and it is suggested that there is a strong synergistic relationship between the host and the bacterium in defending the gut lining and reducing leaky gut-triggered inflammation in exchange for increased mucilage production for food [39]. Achieving healthy levels of *Akkermansia* has been identified as a potential probiotic target to decrease inflammation, reduce obesity, and improve insulin sensitivity [39].

Akkermansia seems to have a high specificity, growing only on specific polysaccharides, including amine sugars, in the presence of proteins [40]. This makes sense in the case of this study, which includes amine-polysaccharides. The mechanism for protection by *Akkermansia* is still not fully understood but it is thought to relate to endocannabinoids that modulate glucose metabolism and protect against pathogenic bacteria [37,39]. *Bacteroides* was shown to decrease in all treatment groups at the largest magnitude. It is unclear as to why this occurred in all groups; however, Bacteroides is a dominant genus in the human gut, and has been shown to reflect a more western diet that is high in animal fat and protein [41]. Therefore, a reduction across the study population may suggest improved dietary habits in the participants. This, however, is only supported in the 4 g treatment group in our dietary analysis.

In Study 2, we did not observe a significant difference in gut microbiome composition between the two regimes at each timepoint. We *did* observe a consistent change in certain genera, including an increase in *Fusicatenibacter* and *Parabacteroides* and a decrease in *Clostridium* while on the SXRG84 treatment and not while on the placebo treatment for both regimes. *Parabacteroides* have increased in rats after laminarin supplementation [42], as has the species *Parabacteroides distasonis* [43], which is also a common species in rats fed with alginate. *Parabacteroides distasonis* has been identified as a laminarin fermenter [43].

It is possible, as our work has suggested, that *Parabacteroides* also responds to seaweed polysaccharides from Ulva Sp., which may infer benefits to the host. This is because *Parabacteroides* has been shown to modulate immunity [44] by suppressing the increase in inflammatory cytokines (IFN-γ, IL-12, IL-17, and IL-6) from gut tissue and increasing serum antibodies in a murine model of intestinal inflammation [44]. In Study 1, there was an increase in beneficial species of *clostridium*. In contrast, Study 2 showed a decrease in *Clostridium*. *Clostridium* as a genus, and species of clostridium have had different responses to seaweed extracts. In a murine model, *Clostridium cluster* XIVb and XI decreased in prevalence after laminarin supplementation [42]. Alternatively, both *Clostridium histolyticum* and *Clostridium coccoides* did not respond to ten different low-molecular-weight polysaccharides from either alginate or agar seaweeds when they were inoculated with human feces [45]. In Study 2, *Clostridium* at baseline was negatively correlated with the baseline value of the cytokines that were reduced (IFN-γ, IL-1β, TNF-α, and IL-10), suggesting an overall anti-inflammatory role of *Clostridium*. Further work is needed to determine the effects of SXRG84 extract on *Clostridium* levels across species as the current evidence is contradictory.

Limitations and Future Work

These two studies are the first dietary clinical investigations of an ulvan, and specifically of SXRG84. They indicated a highly consistent anti-inflammatory effect. However, the lipid effects were not replicated in Study 2, possibly because of differences in the study population.

The use of the crossover designs—as in Study 2—in randomized clinical trials are popular because they can reduce bias from confounding variables and allow participants to act as their own control. Crossover trials are appropriate for use where treatment effects are short-lived in chronic conditions [46]. However, crossover trials also have complications, including the possibility of "order effects". In Study 2, there were no consistent effects found for either of the treatment groups or the placebo groups when examining the significant outcomes. As such, we analyzed the data as four groups instead of collapsing them into two treatment groups. The need to analyze four separate groups does undermine the strengths of running a crossover trial. The true baseline at week zero was used as a covariate in all of the metabolic and inflammatory outcome measures in an attempt to reduce any carryover effects. Study 2 did not include a washout period, with the belief that six weeks on the placebo post SXRG84 treatment would not result in any carried over benefits. Furthermore, any improvements seen after six weeks on the SXRG84 treatment should have returned to baseline after the placebo in the second arm. Indeed, the gut microbiota can revert back to their initial state within 48 h of ceasing specific diets [47]. Figure 6 suggests that the gut microbiota shift that was observed in the placebo group following the SXRG84 was minimal, and many shifts observed after six weeks on the SXRG84 reverted back in the subsequent placebo period. For example, Bacteroides decreased following the SXRG84 treatment and then increased again following the placebo. Regardless, not including a washout period can make identifying treatment effects difficult. Future crossover trials examining the gut microbiome should consider a washout period.

Lastly, the multiple comparisons used in this study makes the likelihood of type I errors more common and need to be considered when assessing the results. We did not adjust for multiple comparisons, as this can have the opposite effect and make type II errors more common [48], therefore making it difficult to determine whether any effect exists. Due to the novel nature of this work, we would prefer to present unadjusted p-values to identify potential treatment effects.

In conclusion, Study 1 showed that the dietary inclusion of SXRG84 had a beneficial effect on a number of lipid and inflammation markers and showed a relationship broadly consistent to gut flora shifts in overweight and obese humans. The results of Study 2 failed to confirm the reduction in non-HDL cholesterol from Study 1 but did confirm the anti-inflammatory potential of SXRG84 in overweight adults across a range of specific cytokine markers. These anti-inflammatory effects may exert benefits to the host as inflammatory cytokines are interrelated with metabolic and cardiovascular diseases. Three genera (*Fusicatenibacter*, *Parabacteroides*, and *Clostridium*), which consistently responded whilst on the SXRG84 treatment, were identified, supporting the prebiotic potential of this extract.

Importantly, there were no changes in blood counts or other markers that indicated a compromise in health. The potential for the supplements as a preventative or additional therapy is apparent but requires further investigation. It is evident that effects will also be highly specific to an individual considering their baseline metabolic state as well as gut flora composition.

4. Materials and Methods

4.1. Study 1 Design

This double-blind randomized placebo-controlled parallel design trial was approved by the University of Wollongong Human Research Ethics Committee (approval CT13/002), and prospectively registered with the Australian New Zealand Clinical Trials Registry (ACTRN12615001057572). Sixty-four participants were recruited, with all providing written informed consent. Exclusion criteria were <18 years of age and antibiotic use in the previous two months. Participants with an overweight or obese BMI (>25 kg/m^2) were included in the study, with one participant of a BMI of 22 kg/m^2. Participants were randomly assigned to three treatment groups of externally identical capsules: a placebo group, a 2 g dose of seaweed extract, and a 4 g dose of seaweed extract; participants and investigators were blinded to the treatment allocations. Two treatment doses were chosen to determine if there was a dose effect, as there were no previous data on humans. Randomization to treatment groups was determined using a computer-generated sequence and groups were assigned by someone independent from the study. The trial ran for a six-week period with sampling occurring at baseline and the end of week six. Participants were advised to maintain diet and exercise routines throughout the trial period and to continue to take any medications.

4.2. Study 2 Design

This double-blind placebo-controlled trial was prospectively registered with the Australian New Zealand Clinical Trial Registry (ACTRN12617001010381) and approved by the University of Wollongong Human Research Ethics Committee (approval 2017/101). Participants were enrolled in the study if they were 18 years or over, had an overweight BMI ($25 - <30$ kg/m^2), had not recently consumed antibiotics (previous two months), and were not pregnant.

Participants with an inflammatory skin condition were also included in the study, although this subgroup was analyzed separately (data presented in Roach et al., anticipated publication 2022).

Participants were advised to maintain their usual diet and medication regimes. The sample size was determined using a power calculation with data from Study 1 and an online calculator (https://www.stat.ubc.ca/~rollin/stats/ssize/n2.html, accessed on 7 June 2017). The change in non-HDL cholesterol that was observed in Study 1 (-0.37 mmol/L) was used as the primary outcome, the test was two sided, with a power of 80% and alpha set at 0.05. A sample of ten per group was calculated as being statistically sufficient, with a view to recruit up to 30 per group to allow for participants that may potentially withdraw consent and missing data. Furthermore, 17 per group and 19 per group were required to detect changes in LDL-cholesterol and total cholesterol, respectively. Overweight participants were recruited as they showed the greatest response to the treatment in Study 1. A 2 g dose of SXRG84 was selected, as this dose reduced non-HDL cholesterol in Study 1.

Participants were randomized into two regimes: placebo group for six weeks and then crossed to the treatment group for six weeks (AB) or vice versa (BA) (Figure 7). Therefore, all participants consumed both the treatment and the placebo during the trial, but they were blinded as to when they consumed each treatment. Allocation of the treatment regime and labeling of the study treatments were completed by an individual independent of the study. There was no washout between the first six weeks and then second six weeks of the trial.

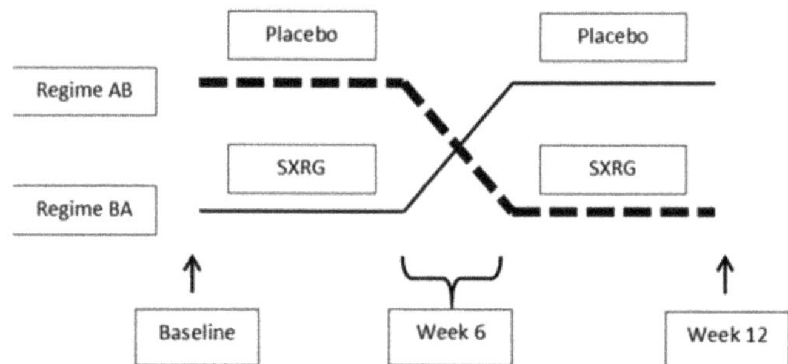

Figure 7. Study Design Regime AB, placebo followed by SXRG84 treatment. Regime BA, SXRG84 treatment followed by placebo.

4.3. Seaweed Extract

Sulfated xylorhamnoglucuronan-rich extract (SXRG84) from Ulva sp. 84 (PhycoDigest®Biobelly) was supplied by Venus Shell Systems Pty. Ltd. SXRG84 is an 80% pure proteoglycan extract containing 42% rhamnose, 20% glucose, and 5% xylose, as well as glucuronic and iduronic acids, and small amounts of galactose, mannose, and arabinose, with >16% sulfation and 15% protein. The molecular weight is above 600 kDa. The extract was approved for use in a clinical setting by the Australian Therapeutic Goods Administration (TGA) Clinical Trial Notification (CTN) (CT2015CTN021221) after assessment by the University of Wollongong Human Research Ethics Committee (approval CT13/002). No adverse events were recorded during the intervention.

For Study 1, dry milled extract was formulated into 2 g and 4 g doses per 8, opaque, 0 cellulosic, vegetarian capsules, with a milled brown rice additive that was also used for the placebo capsules. Milled dark seaweed residue (without glycans) was used in trace amounts (<1%) to make all treatments visually consistent. Six-week supplies of capsules at eight per day were allocated into jars in a three-stage double-blinding system, with the key held until post-data analysis from the clinical intervention. For Study 2, the formulation was the same as described above for Study 1 and the 2 g dose was used.

Participants ingested eight capsules throughout the day and recorded daily compliance, bowel movements, and flatulence. Self-assessment compliance charts were provided at commencement and were collected at the end of the study.

4.4. Blood Analysis

Blood samples were collected after an overnight fast into EDTA tubes and placed on ice immediately for transport to laboratory facilities for spinning separation and were frozen for analysis, as outlined across the two studies below.

Blood Analysis Study 1

Blood samples were collected after an overnight fast into EDTA tubes by qualified phlebotomists from a professional pathology service supplier (Southern Pathology IML). Fasted blood samples were analyzed for total cholesterol, triglycerides, non-HDL cholesterol, LDL-cholesterol, CRP, glucose, C-peptide, and insulin. Samples were analyzed using a Roche Cobas 8000 or Roche Cobas Pro by Southern Pathology IML. Total cholesterol was measured using the cholesterol oxidase/peroxidase method, triglycerides were measured using the lipase/glycerol kinase method, non-HDL and LDL cholesterol were measured using the dextran sulfate/polyethylene glycol modified enzymes method, CRP was measured using a turbidimetric assay, glucose was measured using the hexokinase method, and C-peptide and insulin were measured using an electrochemiluminescence assay.

Further blood-count variables were measured for safety context and are provided in the Supplementary Material (Table S4).

Blood Analysis Study 2

Blood samples were collected after an overnight fast into 10 mL EDTA and 10 mL SST tubes. EDTA tubes were subjected to centrifugation within 30 min of collection for analysis of cytokines.

EDTA plasma was analyzed by Crux Biolab (https://cruxbiolab.com.au/, accessed on 7 June 2017), using an immunoassay high sensitivity Luminex Panel for the following cytokines: IFNγ, IL-1β, IL-6, TNFα, IL-10, and IL-8. Calculated coefficients of variation (CVs) ranged from 9.6−19.3% for inter-assay variation and 0.8−7.3% for intra-assay variation. Limits for detection of the cytokines were as follows: 1.16−4770 pg/mL for IFNγ, 0.21−875 pg/mL for IL-1β, 0.74−3050 pg/mL for IL-6, 0.97−3960 pg/mL for TNFα, 0.20−810 pg/mL for IL-10, and 0.24−985 pg/mL for IL-8.

Serum was analyzed in-house on a Konelab 20XT auto-analyzer. Commercially available kits, reagents, and standards were obtained from Thermo Fisher Scientific Australia Pty. Ltd. and were used to analyze total cholesterol (kit code 981813), HDL-cholesterol (kit code 981823), triglycerides (kit code 981786), glucose hexokinase (kit code 981779), and C-reactive protein (kit code 981934). The first four tests were colorimetric assays, while CRP was an immunoturbidimetric assay. Samples were run in singular; however, for any unusually high or low results, they were analyzed again to confirm the reading. LDL levels were calculated using the Friedwald equation (Friedewald, Levy et al., 1972) [49].

4.5. Oral Glucose Tolerance Test (OGTT) in Both Studies

After the fasted blood sample was collected, participants consumed a glucose drink containing 75 g of glucose. Participants then waited for 2 h and remained rested with minimal activity during this period. Then, after 2 h, another blood sample was taken into an EDTA tube via venipuncture. These samples were analyzed for glucose (Study 1 and 2) and insulin levels (Study 1).

4.6. Study 1 Urine Analysis

Urine was collected by participants for a 24-h period prior to the clinic appointment in large plastic bottles provided to participants. These samples were also analyzed by the NATA-accredited pathology laboratory for creatinine, sodium, and potassium excretion. Samples were analyzed fresh in singular; any abnormal results were flagged and rerun to verify results. Samples were analyzed on a either a Roche Cobas 8000 or a Roche Cobas Pro using the creatininase method for creatinine and the ion-specific electrode-indirect method for potassium and sodium.

From this urine bottle, 1.5 mL was retained and aliquoted in cryovials. These cryovials were stored at −80 °C with no preservative prior to F$_2$ isoprostane assessment using previously described methods [50]. Briefly, urine samples were thawed, acidified to a pH of 3, and internal standard was added. Separation of F$_2$-isoprostanes was achieved by using silica and reverse-phase cartridges and high-performance liquid chromatography. Samples were analyzed in singular, using gas chromatography/electron capture negative-ionization mass spectrometry and the peaks were identified through the comparison of retention times with known standards. The within- and between-assay reproducibility was 6.7% and 3.7%, respectively.

4.7. Gut Flora Analysis

Participants were provided with a gut testing kit by uBiome (https://en.wikipedia.org/wiki/UBiome, (131 kit numbers from November 2015 (Study 1) and 185 kit numbers June 2017 (Study 2)), which sequenced 16S rRNA of the microbiome from fecal swabs.

uBiome provided the sequencing service for registered research groups which provided access to the full suite of 16s RNA raw data sets. Swabs were taken before and after the treatment interventions. Participants were required to swab a fecal sample from toilet paper using the provided swab and place the swab into a provided vial filled with a stabilization liquid. The swab was then swirled in the vial, removed, and discarded. Then, the vial was capped and stored at ambient temperature. Raw data across all taxonomic levels for each participant and time were retrieved.

The raw taxonomic data were downloaded from Ubiome from 122 individual data sets in .json format, converted to .csv using konklone (http://konklone.io/json/, accessed on January to March 2016 for Study 1 and October 2017 to February 2018 for Study 2), and realigned in a single .xlsx database for multivariate analysis. Multivariate analysis was undertaken with PRIMER6+ using multidimensional scaling (MDS) plots to visualize patterns, which were subsequently tested statistically using PERMANOVA. Data were used as untransformed, square root-transformed, and presence/absence data to account for differences in abundance as well as composition. Data were tested using Bray Curtis similarity distance, as these are ecological data of biodiversity with a lot of zeros in the data. Where there were differences in treatment groups, SIMPER analysis was applied to determine which taxonomic group(s) contributed most to this variation. These were then tested in univariate *t*-tests using SPSS (Version 21).

The data were organized for analysis in PRIMER (version 6 with PERMANOVA) and PERMANOVA as per the following Table 11. The level of Genus provided the greatest detail of taxa without losing too much of the quantity, although overall patterns were very similar.

Table 11. Data for analysis in PRIMER and PERMANOVA at each taxonomic level.

	Untransformed	**Square Root**	**Presence/Absence**
Phylum			
Class			
Order	General spread	General spread	none
Family	General spread but similar to Genus		
Genus MOST DATA HIGHEST RESOLUTION	General spread—but most hopeful with just T4 visible	General spread	none
	Select > 10% contribution general spread but similar to above = any change is linked to dominant taxa shifts		
Species	Less pattern than lower taxonomic levels —potentially due to data loss		

In the study, 6.5 million gut flora were quantified across close to 200 genera (Table 12 below). The species level of bacteria from the gut is still a field of research in rapid growth in line with the application of genetic tools, so the quantity of over 200 species is an underestimate and is the reason why only 30% of organisms can be identified at this level. Therefore, data that were analyzed at the genus level were selected as a sensitive level of taxonomy but with adequate resolution of diversity accounting for 86% of the total count, while the species level only accounted for 32% of the total count.

Table 12. Summary of the taxonomic levels of microorganisms represented in the BioBelly gut flora data from 122 samples from 67 participants.

Row Labels	Number Categories	TOTAL Count
superkingdom	3	6,377,013
superphylum	3	1,763,398
phylum	15	6,376,988
class	25	6,376,121
order	34	6,357,174
family	71	6,089,366
genus	191	5,601,385
species	221	2,107,685
species_group	3	444
subclass	8	462,343
no_rank (total)	13	6,518,503

The data were analyzed at the taxonomic level of genus as this accounted for 86% of the total count, while species level only accounted for 32% of the total count.

Data were prepared as the change in number of normalized counts of genera for each participant. The number of genera were reduced based on the genera that contributed to the change to reduce the noise of the multivariate data or the influence of highly abundant species. Data were visually analyzed in untransformed, square root-transformed, and in presence–absence transformations in multidimensional scaling (MDS) and in principal component analysis (PCA) plots in the PRIMER-E software package (Plymouth Marine Laboratories). Permutational multivariate analysis of variance was used to compare the dissimilarities between groups using the PERMANOVA+ for PRIMER software extension. Data were analyzed in transformed and untransformed formats to determine if shifts were predominantly species abundance or composition changes. Analyses were completed using PCA and PERMANOVA models. Further identification of the genera that contributed most to the differences between groups was undertaken using the SIMPER analysis in the PRIMER-E package.

4.8. Dietary Intake

Study 1 participants completed a single 24-h dietary recall at the beginning and end of the six-week trial outlining all foods and beverages consumed within that 24-h period. Study 2 participants completed a single 24-h dietary recall at the beginning and again after six and 12 weeks of the trial, outlining all foods and beverages consumed within that 24-h period. These data were entered into Foodworks software (Version 7.0.3016, Xyris Software, Highgate Hill, Brisbane, Australia) for nutrient analysis.

4.9. Bowel Movements

The number of bowel movements were self-recorded by participants for the six-week (Study 1) and twelve-week (Study 2) trial periods on a calendar sheet. This sheet was also used to record compliance of capsule consumption. Bowel movements were counted by the investigator.

4.10. Statistical Analysis of Biochemical Data

The researchers were blinded for all preliminary analyses. The atherogenic index of plasma was calculated using log(triglycerides/HDL-cholesterol) (Dobiášová and Frohlich 2001) [51]. The insulin-resistance homeostasis model assessment (HOMA) index was calculated as (fasting insulin (mU/L) × fasting glucose (mmol/L))/22.5 (Matthews, Hosker et al., 1985) [52]. The OGTT was assessed by the fasting glucose measure (mmol/L) and the 2-h glucose measure (mmol/L). Participants who withdrew from the study were excluded from the statistical analysis. For those who completed the study, all participant demographics, as well as plasma, urine, and dietary data were expressed as the median (25th and 75th percentile) and were tested for normality using the Shapiro–Wilk test.

Gender across the three treatment groups was compared using a chi-squared test. Baseline, finish, and change data were compared across the three treatment groups using ANOVA for normally distributed data or Kruskal–Wallis for nonparametric data. If a significant difference among the three groups existed, further post hoc tests were applied: Tukey's test for parametric data and Dunn's test for nonparametric data, with statistical significance assessed as $p < 0.05$. JMP Pro was used for plasma and dietary data statistical analyses.

In Study 2, SPSS Version 21 was used for analysis. For all metabolic and inflammatory outcome variables, an ANCOVA was used to test for a treatment effect of the SXRG extract on the six-week and twelve-week outcome measures using four groups. In all analyses, the baseline value was used as the only covariate to control for baseline values. The six-week to twelve-week measures were not analyzed separately due to potential carryover effects; instead, the baseline to twelve weeks was considered, which used the true baseline as a covariate.

The relationship between the different genera and the outcome variables at baseline was assessed using Spearman's correlation. Spearman's correlations were also used to determine whether the change in cytokines was related to the change in any specific gut microbiota genera.

5. Conclusions

Favorable effects on non-HDL cholesterol levels were only seen in the study population, with baseline elevated levels in Study 1. SXRG84 had a beneficial effect on inflammatory markers in overweight and obese participants. The relationship to gut flora shifts is complex, and more work is needed. Importantly, there were no changes in blood counts or other markers that indicated a compromise in health. There is potential for SXRG84 supplements to reduce inflammatory markers connected to metabolic disorders in overweight and obese participants.

Supplementary Materials: The following are available online at https://www.mdpi.com/article/10.3390/md20080500/s1, Figure S1: Flow diagram of study participants in study 1, Figure S2: Participant diagram for study 2, Figure S3: The different genera of bacteria are shown with the change in bacteria in the placebo group in blue and the change in the average active groups shown in yellow, Table S1: Comparison of Dietary Intake between three treatment groups, Table S2: Urinary F_2-Isoprostane levels per treatment group for overweight and obese participants. Study 1, Table S3: Adherance to dietary guidelines for study population at each of the three timepoints, Table S4: blood count data from Study 1, post intervention across the three groups, including change data. Average change in before versus after for each treatment of 2 g, 4 g and placebo groups, and final levels.

Author Contributions: Conceptualization, L.A.R., B.J.M. and P.W.; methodology, L.A.R.; formal analysis, L.A.R.; investigation, P.W. and B.J.M.; resources, B.J.M. and P.W.; data curation, L.A.R.; writing—original draft preparation, L.A.R. and J.H.F.; writing—review and editing, J.H.F., B.J.M., L.A.R. and P.W; supervision, B.J.M.; project administration, L.A.R.; funding acquisition, B.J.M. and P.W. All authors have read and agreed to the published version of the manuscript.

Funding: This research was funded by the University of Wollongong, Science, Medicine and Health Research Partnership Grants (Gut, skin and metabolic health study of seaweed dietary fibers—BioBelly Study 2, 2017).

Institutional Review Board Statement: The study was conducted according to the guidelines of the Declaration of Helsinki and approved by the University of Wollongong Human Research Ethics Committee (approval CT13/002 and approval 2017/101) and registered with the Australian New Zealand Clinical Trials Registry (ACTRN12615001057572 and ACTRN12617001010381).

Informed Consent Statement: Informed consent was obtained from all subjects involved in the study.

Data Availability Statement: Data are not publicly available due to participant confidentiality as defined by ethics committee. De-identified data are available on request from the corresponding author.

Acknowledgments: We would like to acknowledge our participants for taking part in Study 1 and Study 2; Trevor Mori for the F_2 isoprostane analysis; and Nicola Zamai and William Paton for their research assistant support and Eluned Price for assistance with the dietary analysis. We would also like to acknowledge to Dan Harmelin for his guidance.

Conflicts of Interest: P.W. is the CEO of Venus Shell Systems, which provided the extract for this study.

References

1. Dabke, K.; Hendrick, G.; Devkota, S. The gut microbiome and metabolic syndrome. *J. Clin. Investig.* **2019**, *129*, 4050–4057. [CrossRef]
2. McCracken, E.; Monaghan, M.; Sreenivasan, S. Pathophysiology of the metabolic syndrome. *Clin. Dermatol.* **2018**, *36*, 14–20. [CrossRef]
3. Jardon, K.M.; Canfora, E.E.; Coossens, G.H.; Blaak, E.E. Dietary macronutrients and the gut microbiome: A precision nutrition approach to improve cardiometabolic health. *Gut* **2022**, *71*, 1214–1226. [CrossRef]
4. Chan, K.L.; Cathomas, F.; Russo, S.J. Central and Peripheral Inflammation Link Metabolic Syndrome and Major Depressive Disorder. *Physiology (Bethesda)* **2019**, *34*, 123–133. [CrossRef]
5. Zhang, C.; Ward, J.; Dauch, J.R.; Tanzi, R.E.; Cheng, H.T. Cytokine-mediated inflammation mediates painful neuropathy from metabolic syndrome. *PLoS ONE* **2018**, *13*, e0192333. [CrossRef]
6. Ridker, P.M.; MacFadyen, J.G.; Glynn, R.J.; Bradwin, G.; Hasan, A.A. Comparison of interleukin-6, C-reactive protein, and low-density lipoprotein cholesterol as biomarkers of residual risk in contemporary practice: Secondary analyses from the Cardiovascular Inflammation Reduction Trial. *Eur. Heart J.* **2020**, *41*, 2952–2961. [CrossRef]
7. Wong, J.M.; Jenkins, D.J. Carbohydrate digestibility and metabolic effects. *J. Nutr.* **2007**, *137*, 2539S–2546S. [CrossRef]
8. Shannon, E.; Conlon, M.; Hayes, M. Seaweed Components as Potential Modulators of the Gut Microbiota. *Mar. Drugs* **2021**, *19*, 358. [CrossRef] [PubMed]
9. Winberg, P.C.; Fitton, J.H.; Stringer, D.; Karpiniec, S.S.; Gardiner, V.A. Controlling seaweed biology, physiology and metabolic traits in production for commercially relevant bio-actives in glycobiology. *Adv. Bot. Res.* **2013**, *71*, 221–252.
10. Cardoso, M.J.; Costa, R.R.; Mano, J.F. Marine Origin Polysaccharides in Drug Delivery Systems. *Mar. Drugs* **2016**, *14*, 34. [CrossRef] [PubMed]
11. Ndeh, D.; Gilbert, H.J. Biochemistry of complex glycan depolymerisation by the human gut microbiota. *FEMS Microbiol. Rev.* **2018**, *42*, 146–164. [CrossRef]
12. Andrieux, C.; Hibert, A.; Houari, A.-M.; Bensaada, M.; Popot, F.; Szylit, O. *Ulva lactuca* is poorly fermented but alters bacterial metabolism in rats inoculated with human faecal flora from methane and non-methane producers. *J. Sci. Food Agricul.* **1998**, *77*, 25–30. [CrossRef]
13. Qi, H.; Liu, X.; Wang, K.; Liu, D.; Huang, L.; Liu, S.; Zhang, Q. Subchronic toxicity study of ulvan from *Ulva pertusa* (Chlorophyta) in Wistar rats. *Food Chem. Toxicol.* **2013**, *62*, 573–578. [CrossRef]
14. Dvir, I.; Chayoth, R.; Sod-Moriah, U.; Shany, S.; Nyska, A.; Stark, A.H.; Madar, Z.; Arad, S.M. Soluble polysaccharide and biomass of red microalga *Porphyridium* sp. alter intestinal morphology and reduce serum cholesterol in rats. *Br. J. Nutr.* **2000**, *84*, 469–476. [CrossRef]
15. Kumar, S.A.; Magnusson, M.; Ward, L.C.; Paul, N.A.; Brown, L. Seaweed supplements normalise metabolic, cardiovascular and liver responses in high-carbohydrate, high-fat fed rats. *Mar. Drugs* **2015**, *13*, 788–805. [CrossRef]
16. Olsthoorn, S.E.M.; Wang, X.; Tillema, B.; Vanmierlo, T.; Kraan, S.; Leenen, P.J.M.; Mulder, M.T. Brown Seaweed Food Supplementation: Effects on Allergy and Inflammation and Its Consequences. *Nutrients* **2021**, *13*, 2613. [CrossRef]
17. Cox, A.J.; Cripps, A.W.; Taylor, P.A.; Fitton, J.H.; West, N.P. Fucoidan Supplementation Restores Fecal Lysozyme Concentrations in High-Performance Athletes: A Pilot Study. *Mar. Drugs* **2020**, *18*, 412. [CrossRef]
18. Wright, C.M.; Dezuhie, W.; Fitton, J.H.; Stringer, D.N.; Derezifickl, L.R.E.; Peterson, G.M. Effect of a Fucoidan Extract on Insulin Resistance and Cardiometabolic Markers in Obese, Nondiabetic Subjects: A Randomized, Controlled Trial. *J. Altern. Complement. Med.* **2019**, *25*, 346–352. [CrossRef]
19. Li, Y.; Ye, H.; Wang, T.; Wang, P.; Liu, R.; Li, Y.; Tian, Y.; Zhang, J. Characterization of Low Molecular Weight Sulfate Ulva Polysaccharide and its Protective Effect against IBD in Mice. *Mar. Drugs* **2020**, *18*, 499. [CrossRef]
20. Li, B.; Xu, H.; Wang, X.; Wan, Y.; Jiang, N.; Qi, H.; Liu, X. Antioxidant and antihyperlipidemic activities of high sulfate content purified polysaccharide from *Ulva pertusa*. *Int. J. Biol. Macromol.* **2020**, *146*, 756–762. [CrossRef]
21. Pengzhan, Y.; Ning, L.; Xiguang, L.; Gefei, Z.; Quanbin, Z.; Pengcheng, L. Antihyperlipidemic effects of different molecular weight sulfated polysaccharides from *Ulva pertusa* (Chlorophyta). *Pharmacol. Res.* **2003**, *48*, 543–549. [CrossRef]
22. Tas, S.; Celikler, S.; Ziyanok-Ayvalik, S.; Sarandol, E.; Dirican, M. *Ulva rigida* improves carbohydrate metabolism, hyperlipidemia and oxidative stress in streptozotocin induced diabetic rats. *Cell. Biochem. Funct.* **2011**, *29*, 108–113. [CrossRef]
23. Tang, Z.; Cao, H.; Wang, S.; Wen, S.; Qin, S. Hypolipidemic and antioxidant properties of a polysaccharide fraction from *Enteromorpha prolifera*. *Int. J. Biol. Macromol.* **2013**, *58*, 186–189. [CrossRef]

24. Galgani, J.E.; Fernandez-Verdejo, R. Pathophysiological role of metabolic flexibility on metabolic health. *Obes. Rev.* **2021**, *22*, e13131. [CrossRef]
25. Glaves, A.; Díaz-Castro, F.; Farías, J.; Ramírez-Romero, R.; Galgani, J.E.; Fernández-Verdejo, R. Association Between Adipose Tissue Characteristics and Metabolic Flexibility in Humans: A Systematic Review. *Front. Nutr.* **2021**, *8*, 744187. [CrossRef]
26. Ballantyne, C.M.; Bertolami, M.; Hernandez Garcia, H.R.; Nul, D.; Stein, E.A.; Theroux, P.; Weiss, R.; Cain, V.A.; Raichlen, J.S. Achieving LDL cholesterol, non-HDL cholesterol, and apolipoprotein B target levels in high-risk patients: Measuring Effective Reductions in Cholesterol Using Rosuvastatin therapY (MERCURY) II. *Am. Heart J.* **2006**, *151*, 975.e1–975.e9. [CrossRef]
27. Shouval, D.S.; Ouahed, J.; Biswas, A.; Goettel, J.A.; Horwitz, B.H.; Klein, C.; Muise, A.M.; Snapper, S.B. Interleukin 10 receptor signaling: Master regulator of intestinal mucosal homeostasis in mice and humans. *Adv Immunol.* **2014**, *122*, 177–210.
28. Qi, H.; Liu, X.; Zhang, J.; Duan, Y.; Wang, X.; Zhang, Q. Synthesis and antihyperlipidemic activity of acetylated derivative of ulvan from *Ulva pertusa*. *Int. J. Biol. Macromol.* **2012**, *50*, 270–272. [CrossRef]
29. BelHadj, S.; Hentati, O.; Elfeki, A.; Hamden, K. Inhibitory activities of *Ulva lactuca* polysaccharides on digestive enzymes related to diabetes and obesity. *Arch. Physiol. Biochem.* **2013**, *119*, 81–87. [CrossRef]
30. Natividad, J.M.; Lamas, B.; Pham, H.P.; Michel, M.L.; Rainteau, D.; Bridonneau, C.; da Costa, G.; van Hylckama Vlieg, J.; Sovran, B.; Chamignon, C.; et al. *Bilophila wadsworthia* aggravates high fat diet induced metabolic dysfunctions in mice. *Nat. Commun.* **2018**, *9*, 2802. [CrossRef]
31. Devkota, S.; Chang, E.B. Interactions between Diet, Bile Acid Metabolism, Gut Microbiota, and Inflammatory Bowel Diseases. *Dig. Dis.* **2015**, *33*, 351–356. [CrossRef] [PubMed]
32. Rodríguez-Carrio, J.; Salazar, N.; Margolles, A.; González, S.; Gueimonde, M.; de Los Reyes-Gavilán, C.G.; Suárez, A. Free Fatty Acids Profiles Are Related to Gut Microbiota Signatures and Short-Chain Fatty Acids. *Front. Immunol.* **2017**, *8*, 823. [CrossRef] [PubMed]
33. Vogt, J.A.; Pencharz, P.B.; Wolever, T.M. L-Rhamnose increases serum propionate in humans. *Am. J. Clin. Nutr.* **2004**, *80*, 89–94. [CrossRef] [PubMed]
34. Łykowska-Szuber, L.; Rychter, A.M.; Dudek, M.; Ratajczak, A.E.; Szymczak-Tomczak, A.; Zawada, A.; Eder, P.; Lesiak, M.; Dobrowolska, A.; Krela-Kaźmierczak, I. What Links an Increased Cardiovascular Risk and Inflammatory Bowel Disease? A Narrative Review. *Nutrients* **2021**, *13*, 2661. [CrossRef] [PubMed]
35. Elyasi, A.; Voloshyna, I.; Ahmed, S.; Kasselman, L.J.; Behbodikhah, J.; De Leon, J.; Reiss, A.B. The role of interferon-γ in cardiovascular disease: An update. *Inflamm. Res.* **2020**, *69*, 975–988. [CrossRef] [PubMed]
36. Silveira Rossi, J.L.; Barbalho, S.M.; Reverete de Araujo, R.; Bechara, M.D.; Sloan, K.P.; Sloan, L.A. Metabolic syndrome and cardiovascular diseases: Going beyond traditional risk factors. *Diabetes Metab. Res. Rev.* **2021**. [CrossRef] [PubMed]
37. Cani, P.D.; Plovier, H.; Van Hul, M.; Geurts, L.; Delzenne, N.M.; Druart, C.; Everard, A. Endocannabinoids—At the crossroads between the gut microbiota and host metabolism. *Nat. Rev. Endocrinol.* **2016**, *12*, 133–143. [CrossRef]
38. Thomassen, L.V.; Vigsnæs, L.K.; Licht, T.R.; Mikkelsen, J.D.; Meyer, A.S. Maximal release of highly bifidogenic soluble dietary fibers from industrial potato pulp by minimal enzymatic treatment. *Appl. Microbiol. Biotechnol.* **2011**, *90*, 873–884. [CrossRef]
39. Everard, A.; Belzer, C.; Geurts, L.; Ouwerkerk, J.P.; Druart, C.; Bindels, L.B.; Guiot, Y.; Derrien, M.; Muccioli, G.G.; Delzenne, N.M.; et al. Cross-talk between *Akkermansia muciniphila* and intestinal epithelium controls diet-induced obesity. *Proc. Natl. Acad. Sci. USA* **2013**, *110*, 9066–9071. [CrossRef]
40. Derrien, M.; Vaughan, E.E.; Plugge, C.M.; de Vos, W.M. *Akkermansia muciniphila* gen. nov., sp. nov., a human intestinal mucin-degrading bacterium. *Int. J. Syst. Evol. Microbiol.* **2004**, *54*, 1469–1476. [CrossRef]
41. Chen, T.; Long, W.; Zhang, C.; Liu, S.; Zhao, L.; Hamaker, B.R. Fiber-utilizing capacity varies in *Prevotella*- versus *Bacteroides*-dominated gut microbiota. *Sci. Rep.* **2017**, *7*, 2594. [CrossRef]
42. Nguyen, S.G.; Kim, J.; Guevarra, R.B.; Lee, J.H.; Kim, E.; Kim, S.I.; Unno, T. Laminarin favorably modulates gut microbiota in mice fed a high-fat diet. *Food. Funct.* **2016**, *7*, 4193–4201. [CrossRef]
43. An, C.; Kuda, T.; Yazaki, T.; Takahashi, H.; Kimura, B. FLX pyrosequencing analysis of the effects of the brown-algal fermentable polysaccharides alginate and laminaran on rat cecal microbiotas. *Appl. Environ. Microbiol.* **2013**, *79*, 860–866. [CrossRef]
44. Kverka, M.; Zakostelska, Z.; Klimesova, K.; Sokol, D.; Hudcovic, T.; Hrncir, T.; Rossmann, P.; Mrazek, J.; Kopecny, J.; Verdu, E.F.; et al. Oral administration of Parabacteroides distasonis antigens attenuates experimental murine colitis through modulation of immunity and microbiota composition. *Clin. Exp. Immunol.* **2010**, *163*, 250–259. [CrossRef]
45. Ramnani, P.; Chitarrari, R.; Tuohy, K.; Grant, J.; Hotchkiss, S.; Philp, K.; Campbell, R.; Gill, C.; Rowland, I. In vitro fermentation and prebiotic potential of novel low molecular weight polysaccharides derived from agar and alginate seaweeds. *Anaerobe* **2012**, *18*, 1–6. [CrossRef]
46. Mills, E.J.; Chan, A.-W.; Wu, P.; Vail, A.; Guyatt, G.H.; Altman, D.G. Design, analysis, and presentation of crossover trials. *Trials* **2009**, *10*, 27. [CrossRef]
47. David, L.A.; Maurice, C.F.; Carmody, R.N.; Gootenberg, D.B.; Button, J.E.; Wolfe, B.E.; Ling, A.V.; Devlin, A.S.; Varma, Y.; Fischbach, M.A.; et al. Diet rapidly and reproducibly alters the human gut microbiome. *Nature* **2014**, *505*, 559–563. [CrossRef]
48. Feise, R.J. Do multiple outcome measures require p-value adjustment? *BMC Med. Res. Methodol.* **2002**, *2*, 8. [CrossRef]
49. Friedewald, W.T.; Levy, R.I.; Fredrickson, D.S. Estimation of the concentration of low-density lipoprotein cholesterol in plasma, without use of the preparative ultracentrifuge. *Clin. Chem.* **1972**, *18*, 499–502. [CrossRef]

50. Mori, T.A.; Croft, K.D.; Puddey, I.B.; Beilin, L.J. An improved method for the measurement of urinary and plasma F_2-isoprostanes using gas chromatography-mass spectrometry. *Anal. Biochem.* **1999**, *268*, 117–125. [CrossRef]
51. Dobiášová, M.; Frohlich, J. The plasma parameter log (TG/HDL-C) as an atherogenic index: Correlation with lipoprotein particle size and esterification rate inapob-lipoprotein-depleted plasma (FERHDL). *Clin. Biochem.* **2001**, *34*, 583–588. [CrossRef]
52. Matthews, D.R.; Hosker, J.P.; Rudenski, A.S.; Naylor, B.A.; Treacher, D.F.; Turner, R.C. Homeostasis model assessment: Insulin resistance and beta-cell function from fasting plasma glucose and insulin concentration in man. *Diabetologia* **1985**, *28*, 412–419. [CrossRef] [PubMed]

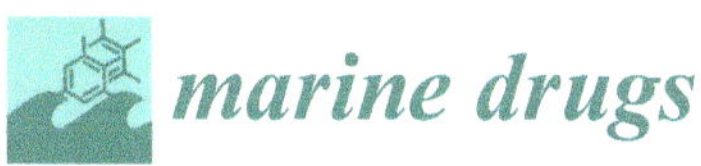

marine drugs

Article

Glucose Uptake and Oxidative Stress in Caco-2 Cells: Health Benefits from *Posidonia oceanica* (L.) Delile

Camilla Morresi [1,†], Marzia Vasarri [2,†], Luisa Bellachioma [3], Gianna Ferretti [1], Donatella Degl'Innocenti [2,4,*] and Tiziana Bacchetti [3]

[1] Department of Clinical Experimental Science and Odontostomatology-Biochemistry, Università Politecnica delle Marche, 60100 Ancona, Italy; m.morres@libero.it (C.M.); g.ferretti@univpm.it (G.F.)
[2] Department of Experimental and Clinical Biomedical Sciences, University of Florence, Viale Morgagni 50, 50134 Florence, Italy; marzia.vasarri@unifi.it
[3] Department of Life and Environmental Sciences-Biochemistry, Università Politecnica delle Marche, 60100 Ancona, Italy; luisabellachioma@gmail.com (L.B.); t.bacchetti@univpm.it (T.B.)
[4] Interuniversity Center of Marine Biology and Applied Ecology "G. Bacci" (CIBM), Viale N. Sauro 4, 57128 Livorno, Italy
* Correspondence: donatella.deglinnocenti@unifi.it
† These authors contributed equally to this work.

Abstract: *Posidonia oceanica* (L.) Delile is an endemic Mediterranean marine plant of extreme ecological importance. Previous in vitro and in vivo studies have demonstrated the potential antidiabetic properties of *P. oceanica* leaf extract. Intestinal glucose transporters play a key role in glucose homeostasis and represent novel targets for the management of diabetes. In this study, the ability of a hydroalcoholic *P. oceanica* leaf extract (POE) to modulate intestinal glucose transporters was investigated using Caco-2 cells as a model of an intestinal barrier. The incubation of cells with POE significantly decreased glucose uptake by decreasing the GLUT2 glucose transporter levels. Moreover, POE had a positive effect on the barrier integrity by increasing the Zonulin-1 levels. A protective effect exerted by POE against oxidative stress induced by chronic exposure to high glucose concentrations or tert-butyl hydroperoxide was also demonstrated. This study highlights for the first time the effect of POE on glucose transport, intestinal barrier integrity, and its protective antioxidant effect in Caco-2 cells. These findings suggest that the *P. oceanica* phytocomplex may have a positive impact by preventing the intestinal cell dysfunction involved in the development of inflammation-related disease associated with oxidative stress.

Keywords: *Posidonia oceanica*; AGEs; marine antioxidants; oxidative stress; intestinal glucose uptake; intestinal barrier integrity

Citation: Morresi, C.; Vasarri, M.; Bellachioma, L.; Ferretti, G.; Degl'Innocenti, D.; Bacchetti, T. Glucose Uptake and Oxidative Stress in Caco-2 Cells: Health Benefits from *Posidonia oceanica* (L.) Delile. *Mar. Drugs* **2022**, *20*, 457. https://doi.org/10.3390/md20070457

Academic Editor: Hideki Kishimura

Received: 20 June 2022
Accepted: 13 July 2022
Published: 14 July 2022

Publisher's Note: MDPI stays neutral with regard to jurisdictional claims in published maps and institutional affiliations.

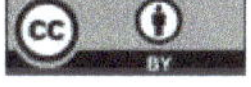

1. Introduction

Posidonia oceanica (L.) Delile is a seagrass of extreme ecological importance for the whole marine ecosystem, and it is the only species of the Posidoniaceae family endemic in the Mediterranean Sea [1,2]. Although *P. oceanica* leaves have been used in ancient times in traditional medical practices as a natural remedy for various health disorders, only more recent scientific studies have described its potential benefits for human health, including an anti-diabetic property [3]. For instance, Gokce et al. (2008) demonstrated that *P. oceanica* leaf extract has hypoglycemic properties in alloxan-induced diabetic rats [4]. Oral administration of its extract for 15 days dose-dependently decreased blood glucose in diabetic rats [4]. In addition, the hydroalcoholic extract of *P. oceanica* leaves (POE) was able to inhibit the in vitro glucose induced glycation of human serum albumin [5]. POE has also demonstrated antioxidant and anti-inflammatory properties in in vitro cellular models and in vivo animal models [6,7].

Overall, the POE biological effects have been related to the synergistic action of its individual constituents. A first UPLC characterization analysis showed that POE consists of 88% phenolic compounds, mostly represented by D-(+)-catechin, and less by gallic acid, ferulic acid, (−)-epicatechin, and chlorogenic acid [8] (Figure 1).

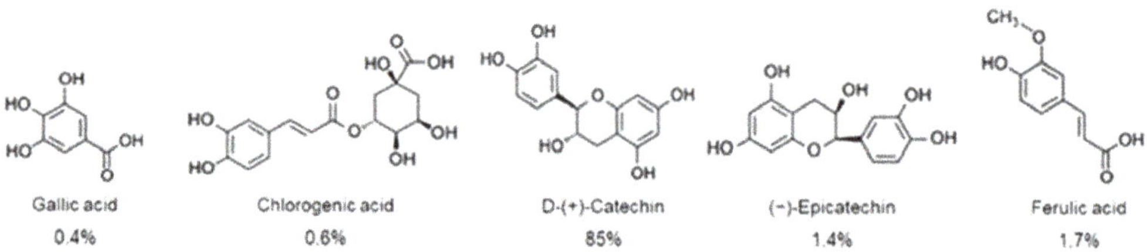

Figure 1. Phenolic compounds with relative percentages identified in *P. oceanica* leaf extract (POE) by UPLC analysis [8].

Among the biological properties of dietary polyphenols, growing attention has been devoted to their ability to modulate post-prandial increases in glucose levels and to modulate intestinal integrity and oxidative damage [9–14]. In fact, high post-prandial plasma glucose concentrations are associated with an increased risk of developing type 2 diabetes (T2D) and metabolic syndrome [15]. Intestinal glucose transporters such as sodium glucose co-transporter-1 (SGLT1) and glucose transporter 2 (GLUT2) play a role in glucose homeostasis and represent targets for the management of diabetes [16].

A Caco-2 cell monolayer is one of the most widely used in vitro model of the human intestinal barrier to study absorption [17,18]. This cellular model was used in this study to evaluate the effect of POE on the intestinal glucose uptake and its ability to modulate the levels of glucose transporters (SGLT1 and GLUT2). Furthermore, the intestinal barrier integrity is essential for the metabolic homeostasis. A dysfunction of the intestinal barrier is linked to inflammatory and dysmetabolic conditions, including diabetes [19].

In this study, the effect of POE on intestinal barrier integrity was verified by assessing transepithelial electrical resistance (TEER) across a monolayer of intestinal Caco-2 cells. The effect of POE on the level of Zonula occludens-1 (ZO-1), a protein involved in the regulation of intestinal barrier integrity, was also evaluated.

In addition, the potential protective effect of POE against oxidative stress has been studied in Caco-2 cells using tert-butyl hydroperoxide (TBHP) or chronic exposition to high glucose (HG) levels.

2. Results

2.1. Biochemical Characterization of P. oceanica Leaf Extract (POE)

POE was found to contain 3.4 ± 0.2 mg/mL of total polyphenols (TP) equivalent to gallic acid (mg GAE/mL). In addition, POE exhibited antioxidant and radical-scavenging activities of 0.9 ± 0.2 mg/mL and 8.9 ± 0.3 mg/mL ascorbic acid equivalents (mg AAE/mL), as evaluated by FRAP and DPPH assays, respectively (Table 1). The data obtained are consistent with those obtained in previous work [6,8], supporting the efficiency and reproducibility of the extraction method.

Table 1. Biochemical properties of POE in terms of total polyphenols (TP) antioxidant (FRAP assay) and radical scavenging activities (DPPH assay).

TP	3.4 ± 0.2 mg GAE/mL
FRAP	0.9 ± 0.2 mg AAE/mL
DPPH	8.9 ± 0.3 mg AAE/mL

2.2. Effect of POE on Cell Viability

No significant modifications of cell viability were observed in Caco-2 cells treated till to 24 h with increasing levels of POE (corresponding to polyphenol concentration ranging from 5 µg GAE/mL to 40 µg GAE/mL) (Supplementary Figure S1). These results confirm that POE did not exert a cytotoxic effect in our experimental conditions. Based on these results, all the following experiments were conducted using 15 µg GAE/mL POE.

2.3. Effect of POE on Glucose Transport under Sodium-Dependent or Sodium-Free Conditions

Caco-2 differentiated cells were used as a model of the intestinal barrier. The effect of POE on glucose uptake was investigated both in the presence or in the absence of sodium. In the presence of sodium, glucose transporters SGLT1 and GLUT2 are both active. In sodium-free conditions only GLUT2 is active.

As shown in Figure 2, POE treatment significantly ($p < 0.05$) decreased glucose transport, both in the presence (Figure 2A) and absence of sodium (Figure 2B).

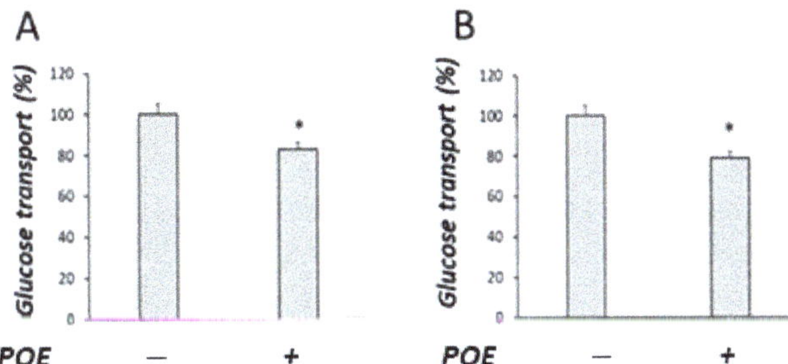

Figure 2. Effect of POE on glucose transport in Caco-2 differentiated cells. Glucose transport was evaluated under (**A**) sodium-dependent or (**B**) sodium-free conditions in differentiated Caco-2 cells treated with POE (15 µg GAE/mL) for 24 h. Values are presented as the mean ± SD of three determinations carried out in triplicate. Data are reported in terms of percentage with respect to control cells. *: $p < 0.05$.

To understand the decrease in glucose transport observed in POE-treated cells, the effect of POE on the expression of glucose transporters (SGLT1 and GLUT2) in Caco-2 differentiated cells was investigated by Western blot analysis (Figure 3A). POE treatment caused a significant ($p < 0.05$) decrease in the GLUT2 levels (68% ± 2.1%) with respect to control cells, as shown in Figure 3B. No modifications of the levels of transporter SGLT1 were observed in POE-treated cells compared with control cells (Figure 3C).

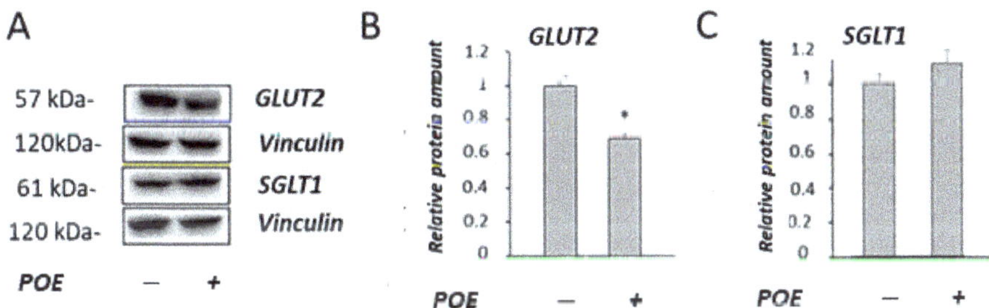

Figure 3. Effect of POE on the levels of glucose transporters. (**A**) Representative Western blot images of (**B**) GLUT2 and (**C**) SGLT1 glucose transporters in differentiated Caco-2 cells incubated in the absence or presence of POE (15 µg GAE/mL) for 24 h. Densitometric data are normalized to the Vinculin expression levels. Data are presented as the mean ± SD of three determinations. *: $p < 0.05$.

2.4. Effect of POE on Caco-2 Monolayer as a Model of Intestinal Barrier

The evaluation of transepithelial electrical resistance (TEER) across the monolayer of Caco-2 differentiated cells was used to assess the effect of POE on the integrity of the intestinal barrier.

As shown in Figure 4, POE treatment caused an increase in TEER across the Caco-2 cell monolayer. The effect was significant ($p < 0.05$) after 4 h and reached 118% of the initial value after 24 h of incubation compared with control cells.

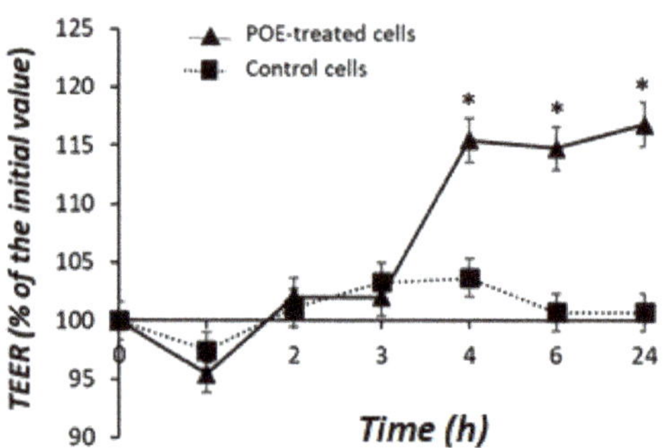

Figure 4. Effect of POE on Caco-2 monolayer cells. Transepithelial electrical resistance (TEER) in differentiated Caco-2 control cells or treated with POE (15 µg GAE/mL) for 24 h. Values are presented as the mean ± SD of three determinations carried out in triplicate. TEER values are reported in terms of percentage with respect the initial value. * Control vs. POE-treated cells. (*: $p < 0.05$).

Zonulin-1 (ZO-1) is a protein bound to the cytoskeleton and it has a pivotal role in tight junction (TJ) integrity. Therefore, to investigate the molecular mechanisms involved in the POE-induced increase in TEER, the levels of ZO-1 were determined by Western blot analysis (Figure 5A).

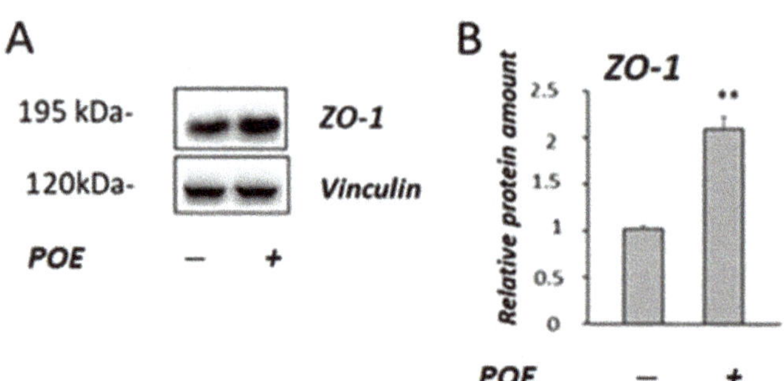

Figure 5. Effect of POE on the ZO-1 levels. (**A**) Representative Western blot images of ZO-1 in differentiated Caco-2 incubated in the absence or treated with POE (15 µg GAE/mL) for 24 h. (**B**) Densitometric data are normalized to Vinculin. Data are presented as the mean ± SD of five determinations. **: $p < 0.01$.

As shown in Figure 5B, a two-fold increase in the ZO-1 levels was observed in POE-treated Caco-2 cells compared with the untreated control cells ($p < 0.01$).

2.5. Effect of POE on High-Glucose-Induced Oxidative Stress

The chronic exposure to high glucose (HG) induces oxidative stress in Caco-2 cells, as previously described [20].

In this study, the potential protective role of POE (15 μg GAE/mL) on chronic HG-induced oxidative stress was investigated in Caco-2 cells. Cells not exposed to HG were used as control cells. A significant increase (1.95 ± 0.7 A.U.) in intracellular ROS production was confirmed in HG cells compared to control cells (1.02 ± 0.18 A.U.), in accordance with our previous study [20]. HG cells treated with POE showed a significant decrease in intracellular ROS production with respect to HG cells (Figure 6A). Figure 6B shows representative images of the fluorescence intensity indicative of ROS formation in POE-treated cells under HG conditions. The dose-dependent effect (0–40 μg GAE/mL) of POE on HG-induced intracellular ROS formation is reported in Supplementary Figure S2.

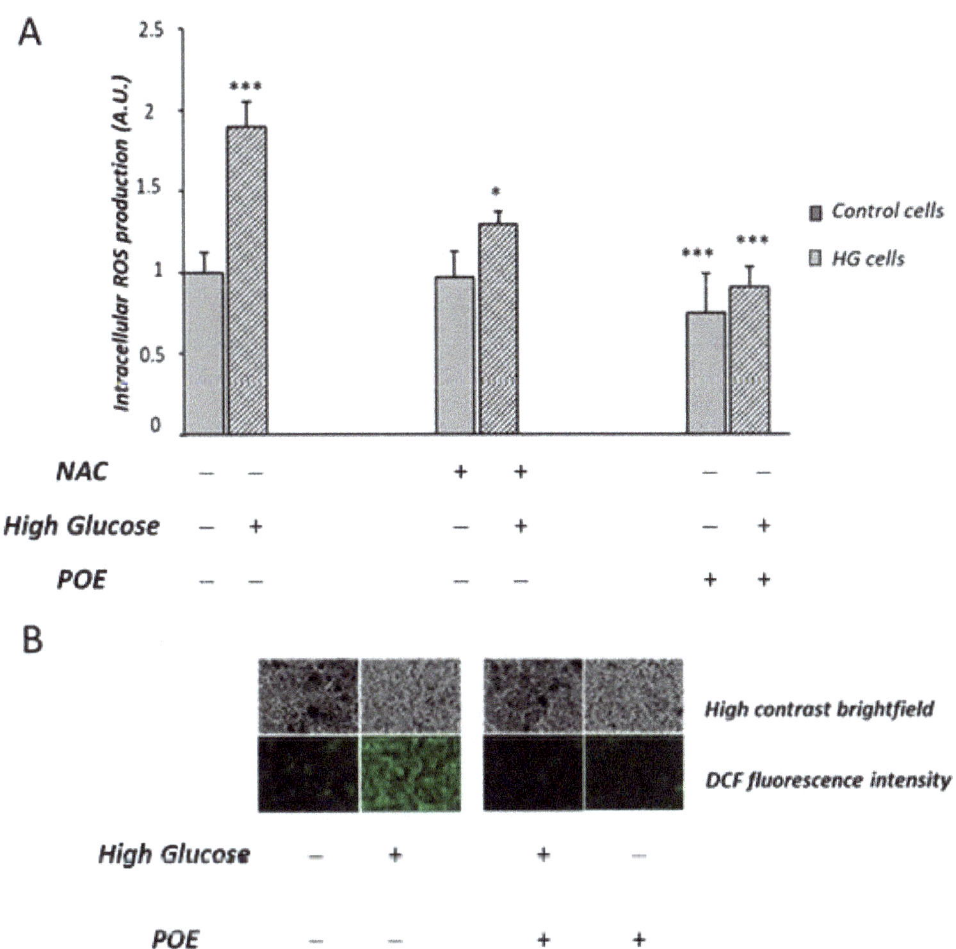

Figure 6. Effect of POE and *N*-acetylcysteine (NAC) on HG-induced intracellular ROS formation. (**A**) Intracellular ROS production was evaluated in Caco-2 cells incubated in the absence (control cells) or in the presence of high-glucose conditions (HG cells) for 1 week and co-incubated with POE (15 μg GAE/mL), and *N*-acetylcysteine (NAC) (50 μM) for the last 24 h. Values are represented as the mean ± SD of five determinations carried out in triplicate. *** Control vs. HG; * HG vs. HG + NAC; *** HG vs. POE; *** HG vs. HG + POE. (ANOVA: *: $p < 0.05$; ***: $p < 0.001$). (**B**) Fluorescent cells observed under a fluorescent microscope in the presence of POE (15 μg GAE/mL (Lionheart™ FX)).

HG cells treated with *N*-acetylcysteine (NAC) were used as the positive antioxidant control. The POE-induced mitigation of intracellular ROS production in HG cells was comparable to that induced by NAC (50 µM) (Figure 6A).

This finding suggests that POE exerts an antioxidant activity against HG-induced intracellular ROS production in Caco-2 cells.

The HG-induced intracellular ROS levels can cause an increase in advanced glycation end products (AGEs), due to the formation of highly reactive intermediates of the Maillard reaction, such as glycolaldehyde and glyoxal. These molecules are involved in cross-linking of proteins and are precursors of AGEs [21].

In this study, the glycolaldehyde (GA)-modified protein levels were also evaluated by Western blot analysis (Figure 7A) to investigate the effect of POE on AGEs formation in HG-treated cells. Higher levels of GA-modified proteins were observed in HG cells compared to control cells (Figure 7B), as previously described [20]. In the presence of POE, a significant ($p < 0.05$) decrease in GA-modified protein levels was observed in HG cells compared with untreated HG cells (Figure 7B). A slight decrease in the GA-modified protein levels was also observed in Caco-2 cells treated with POE compared with the untreated control cells (Figure 7B).

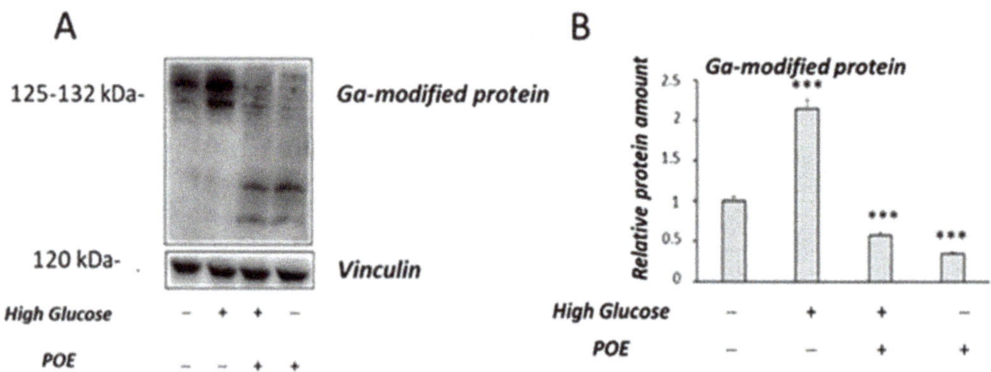

Figure 7. Effect of POE on GA-modified proteins levels in Caco-2 cells. (**A**) Representative Western blot images of GA-modified proteins. (**B**) Densitometric analysis of GA-modified proteins in Caco-2 control cells or HG cells in the absence or presence of POE (15 µg GAE/mL) for 24 h. Densitometric data are normalized to Vinculin. Results are presented as the mean ± SD of five determinations. *** Control vs. HG; *** Ctrl vs. POE; *** HG vs. POE; *** HG vs. HG + POE (ANOVA: ***: $p < 0.001$).

These results could explain the effect of POE on HG-induced cell toxicity. In fact, a significant decrease (about 40%) in cell viability was observed in HG cells compared with control cells. POE-treated cells exposed to chronic HG conditions had comparable viability to control cells (Supplementary Figure S3)

2.6. Effect of POE on Tert-Butyl Hydroperoxide-Induced Oxidative Stress

To further verify the potential antioxidant role of POE against intracellular ROS formation, the effect of POE was also investigated in Caco-2 cells acutely treated with the pro-oxidant agent tert-butyl hydroperoxide (TBHP).

As shown in Figure 8, TBHP induced a more than three-fold increase in intracellular ROS production with respect to control cells ($p < 0.001$). NAC was able to reduce intracellular ROS production in TBHP-treated cells ($p < 0.001$). POE showed a comparable effect to NAC in TBHP-treated cells (Figure 8).

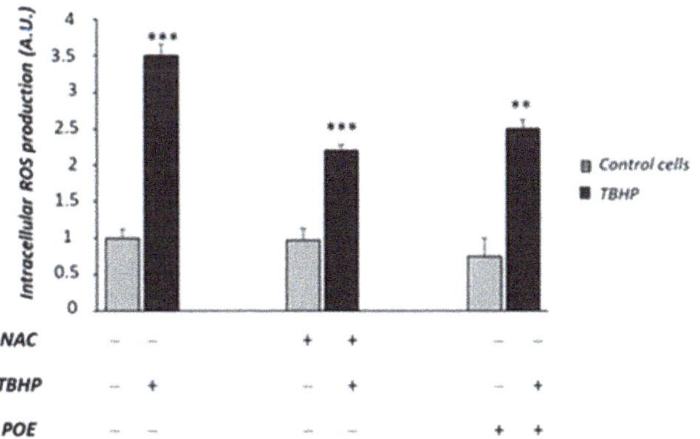

Figure 8. Effect of POE on TBHP-induced ROS formation in Caco-2 cells. Intracellular ROS production was evaluated in Caco-2 cells pre-incubated for 24 h with POE (15 µg GAE/mL) or NAC (50µM) and treated with TBHP (50 µM) for 90 min. Values are represented as the mean ± SD of five determinations carried out in triplicate. *** Control vs. TBHP; *** NAC + THBP vs. TBHP; ** POE + THBP vs. TBHP (ANOVA: **: $p < 0.01$; ***: $p < 0.001$).

3. Discussion

The Caco-2 cell line is extensively used as a model of the intestinal epithelial barrier. In particular, monolayers of differentiated Caco-2 cells are used for the investigation of the function and integrity of the intestinal barrier. Therefore, this cell model is often used to study the modulatory role that natural compounds (including polyphenols) may have on intestinal function [17,18]. Here, for the first time, POE, a polyphenol-rich phytocomplex, has been shown to inhibit glucose uptake, improve intestinal barrier integrity, and protect cells from oxidative stress in Caco-2 cells.

The inhibition of glucose uptake induced by POE was observed to the same extent in both the presence and absence of sodium. Moreover, a significant decrease in the GLUT2 levels in POE-treated cells was observed in our experimental conditions. On the contrary, no effect of POE on the SGLT1 protein levels was observed. These results suggest that the effect of POE on glucose could be mainly mediated by a modulation of the expression of glucose transporter GLUT2, in agreement with other studies that reported a reduction in the expression of intestinal glucose transporters by polyphenols [11]. In rat enterocytes, the apical membrane levels of both transporters can alter rapidly in response to cell signaling events [21,22]. GLUT2 has been detected at both the apical membrane and basolateral membrane of Caco-2 cells [23]. Further studies are required to address the effect of POE on cell signaling events and the cellular distribution of GLUT2 and SGLT1.

Elevated levels of intestinal glucose transporters have been reported in diabetic and obese animal models and this contributed directly to their hyperglycemic status [24,25]. Therefore, compounds that regulate glucose transporter expression may be useful as potential anti-hyperglycemic agents. Till today, this effect has been observed only in animal models. Gokce et al. (2008) have reported that the oral administration of a *P. oceanica* extract for 15 days (50, 150, and 250 mg/kg b.wt.) resulted in a dose-dependent decrease in blood glucose in alloxan-induced diabetic rats [4]. Further studies are needed to investigate the effects of POE intake on post-prandial glycaemia in normal and hyperglycemic subjects.

A dysfunctional intestinal barrier is associated also with dysmetabolic diseases, including diabetes and obesity [19,26,27]. Therefore, in this study, transepithelial electrical resistance (TEER) [28] and the levels of TJ proteins, such as Zonula occludens (ZO-1), have been evaluated to investigate the potential role of POE on the integrity of cell monolayer using differentiated Caco-2 cell, as a model of an intestinal barrier. A significant increase in TEER across the cellular monolayer in POE-treated cells was observed with respect to untreated control cells. Furthermore, POE demonstrated a positive effect on intestinal cells by increasing the levels of ZO-1. The protein ZO-1 is involved in the regulation of intestinal barrier integrity and plays a crucial role as a key molecule in cell-to-cell contact and in maintaining the structure of TJ and the epithelial barrier function [26]. TJ barrier integrity is essential for human health and metabolic homeostasis [26]. The effects of POE on ZO-1 are in agreement with previous studies, which demonstrated that polyphenols (such as catechins and phenolic acids) modulate intestinal barrier function and increase the expression of several TJ proteins, including ZO-1, in in vitro models [12,13]. Some in vivo studies have demonstrated that, in older subjects, a polyphenol-rich dietary pattern improves intestinal permeability, evaluated as the serum Zonulin levels [29]. However, further in vivo studies will be required to verify the protective effect of POE on the intestinal barrier integrity.

Intestinal cells are exposed to dietary pro-oxidants, AGEs, lipid peroxidation products, and are susceptible to oxidative damage [30–32]. In addition, previous studies have also shown that high-sugar diets cause increased oxidative stress and inflammation [31].

ROS-induced oxidative stress is widely considered as a possible upstream mechanism of high-glucose-induced cell damage [20]. These cellular alterations may cause a dysfunction of intestinal barrier and lead to the onset of the intestinal bowel diseases [30,31]. Previous studies have reported that POE has an antioxidant role against intracellular ROS formation in macrophages activated by LPS [6]. In our experimental conditions, POE shows a protective role against ROS-induced oxidative stress under chronic high-glucose conditions in Caco-2 cells. The antioxidant role of POE was also confirmed by an inhibitory action against the ROS formation induced, in the same cell model, by treatment with TBHP, a molecule commonly used to study cellular alterations resulting from oxidative stress [33].

Chronic exposure to high glucose evokes oxidative stress; the resulting high levels of intracellular ROS can promote AGEs formation. Indeed, previous studies have shown that highly reactive intermediates of the Maillard reaction, such as glycolaldehyde (GA) and glyoxal, are involved in cross-linking of proteins and are precursors of AGEs [34]. In this study, Caco-2 cells treated with POE showed a significant decrease in the GA protein levels in chronic high-glucose conditions. Since GA proteins are useful markers of oxidative stress [20], our findings further support the protective role of POE against oxidative stress induced by high glucose. Overall, these results are in agreement with our previous studies that described an in vitro role of POE against glucose-induced glycation of human serum albumin [5]. Moreover, other studies have demonstrated the ability of polyphenols to exert a protective effect against oxidative stress and formation of AGEs in Caco-2 cells [14]. In addition, previous studies have reported that some phenolic compounds exert a protective effect against oxidative stress, either by reducing ROS production during the glycation process or by trapping of dicarbonyl species [35].

In conclusion, the data reported in this study demonstrate that POE reduces glucose transport by lowering the GLUT2 levels and promotes intestinal barrier integrity by positively modulating the ZO-1 levels. Furthermore, POE has a protective antioxidant effect against high-glucose-induced damage, in terms of lower production of intracellular ROS and AGE-modified proteins.

Inhibition of glucose uptake in the small intestine may prevent post prandial hyperglycemia, which is one of the risk factors for diabetes and metabolic syndrome. Our findings suggest that POE may have a positive impact by preventing the intestinal cell dysfunction involved in the development of inflammation-related intestinal diseases associated with oxidative stress.

The in vitro effect of POE was observed at a concentration of polyphenols of 15 µg GAE/mL (88 µmol/L). It has been reported that the bioavailability of polyphenols is related to the structural properties of molecules. The total levels of polyphenols are present in plasma at <1 µmol/L concentrations, but they are present in the stomach and intestinal lumen at much higher concentrations after consumption of vegetables rich in polyphenols. Saura-Calixto et al. (2007) demonstrated that polyphenols could act as antioxidants in the intestine because they are present at millimolar concentrations after consumption of fruits and vegetables [36].

4. Materials and Methods

4.1. Reagents

Reagents for cell culture were obtained by Euroclone (Euroclone, Italy). All chemical reagents were purchased by Sigma Aldrich (Sigma, St. Louis, MO, USA). $2',7'$-Dichlorodihydrofluorescein diacetate (H_2DCFDA) was supplied by Invitrogen (Invitrogen, Carlsbad, CA, USA).

4.2. Preparation and Characterization of Posidonia oceanica (L.) Delile Extract

The hydroalcoholic extract of *P. oceanica* (POE) was obtained according to a previously described method [8]. Briefly, 1.84 mg of the dry extract from *P. oceanica* leaves were resuspended in 500 µL of 70% ethanol; POE was diluted and used in different experimental conditions.

4.3. Evaluation of Total Polyphenols in POE

Total polyphenol (TP) content in POE was evaluated using Folin–Ciocalteu's method, as previously described [8]. Briefly, for the determination of TP in POE, 100 µL of Folin–Ciocalteu (Folin–Ciocalteu phenol reagent diluted 1:10 in H_2O) was added to scalar volumes of POE. After a 5 min incubation at room temperature, 80 µL of 7.5% sodium carbonate solution was added for another 2 h. Absorbance at 595 nm was recorded with a microplate reader. Gallic acid (0.5 mg/mL) was used as a reference to determine the TP values. TP is expressed as mg of gallic acid equivalents (GAE) per mL.

4.4. Evaluation of Antioxidant and Radical Scavenging Activities of POE

The antioxidant and radical scavenging activities of POE were studied using ferric reducing/antioxidant potency (FRAP) and the 2,2-diphenyl-1-picrylhydrazyl (DPPH) radical [8]. Briefly, for determination of the antioxidant activity of POE by FRAP, 200 µL of Ferrozine™ reagent (10 mM Ferrozine™ in 40 mM HCl: 20 mM $FeCl_3$: 0.3 M acetate buffer pH 3.6 1:1:10 ratio) was added to scalar volumes of POE. After 4 min incubation at 37 °C, absorbance was measured at 595 nm at room temperature using a microplate reader.

For determination of the radical scavenging activities of POE, 100 µL of 95% methanol was added to scalar volumes of POE and mixed with 100 µL of freshly prepared DPPH solution (0.15 mg/mL in methanol). After a 30 min incubation in the dark at room temperature, absorbance was read at 490 nm with a microplate reader. Ascorbic acid (0.1 mg/mL) was used as a reference to determine the values of both the antioxidant and radical scavenging activity. These activities are expressed as mg of ascorbic acid equivalents (AAE) per mL.

4.5. Caco-2 Cells

Human colon epithelial cells, Caco-2 (ATCC®HTB-37™), were purchased from the American Type Culture Collection (Rockville, MD, USA). In our experiments, the Caco-2 cells were cultured in Dulbecco's Minimal Essential Medium (DMEM) supplemented with 10 mM nonessential amino acids, 10% (v/v) fetal bovine serum (FBS), 100 µg/mL streptomycin, 100 U/mL penicillin, and 2 mM glutamine (growth medium). Cells were incubated at 37 °C and 5% CO_2, and sub-cultured at 80–90% confluence every 3–4 days.

For differentiation, Caco-2 cells were seeded at a density of 1×10^5 cells/well in 12-well trans-well plate (12 mm, with 0.4 µm pore polycarbonate membrane Insert, Corning) and differentiated for 21 days in DMEM growth medium. The medium was replaced every 2–3 days for both the apical (AP) and basal (BL) sides of the trans-well filters. The integrity of cell monolayer was checked by measuring the trans-epithelial electrical resistance (TEER) before and after the experiments with an Epithelial Volt/Ohm Meter (EVOM).

4.6. Cell Viability Assay

Cell viability in Caco-2 cells treated in different experimental conditions was analyzed following the enzymatic reduction of 3-[4,5-dimethylthiazole-2-yl]-2,5-diphenyltetrazolium bromide (MTT) to MTT-formazan, catalyzed by mitochondrial succinate. Briefly, 100 μL of MTT solution (5 mg/mL) was added to each well. After 2 h, the incubation buffer was removed and the blue MTT–formazan product was extracted with DMSO (dimethyl sulfoxide). Supernatants were collected in a 96-well plate and the absorbance was measured at 540 nm (Microplate Rader) [37].

4.7. Evaluation of Glucose Transport in Caco-2 Cells

Glucose transport was evaluated in differentiated Caco-2 cells as described by Sharma et al. (2020) [12], applying some modifications. The transport was analyzed both in a sodium and non-sodium environment. Caco-2 cells were washed 2 times in HBBS (pH 7.5). Subsequently, POE (15 μg/mL) was co-incubated for 24 h in the apical compartment with 5 mM D-glucose prepared in DPBS. In the basolateral compartment was added DPBS. Similarly, sodium-free buffer was used for the sodium independent absorption experiment. Cells were incubated at 37 °C and 5% CO_2 for the duration of the experiment. To follow transport across the cell monolayer, 50 μL was collected in the basolateral compartment at time 0 and after 24 h. Glucose transport was measured using 65.8 mM of *p*-hydroxyacetophenonebenzoylhydrazone (PAHBH) added to the collected samples (30:1). The mixture was incubated for 10 min at 90 °C and then read in a 96-well plate reader at 410 nm. Glucose (0.01–5 mM) was used to create the standard curve. Data were expressed as % of glucose transport with respect to each specific control [38].

4.8. Evaluation of Caco-2 Monolayer Permeability

Monolayers of Caco-2 differentiated cells were incubated for 24 h in the presence or absence of POE (15 μg GAE/mL). Resistance measurement was performed by TEER. Cells were incubated at 37 °C and 5% CO_2 for the duration of the experiment. TEER was measured using an EVOM with a chopstick electrode (Millicell ERS-2, EMD Millipore, Billerica, MA, USA). The electrode was immersed at a 90° angle with one tip in the basolateral chamber and the other in the apical chamber. Care was taken to avoid electrode contact with the monolayer and triplicate measurements were recorded for each monolayer. An insert without cells was used as a blank and its mean resistance was subtracted from all samples. TEER measurements were registered hourly for 24 h. Results are reported as TEER % versus time [39].

4.9. Chronic High Glucose Caco-2 Cell Treatment

The chronic high glucose (HG) treatment of Caco-2 cells was carried out as previously described [20]. Briefly, cells were grown in 50 mM glucose for 1 week (high glucose, HG cells). Cells grown in growth medium without addition of glucose were used as control cells (Control cells). Medium was replaced two times a week. POE (15 μg GAE/mL) or *N*-acetyl-cysteine (NAC; 50 μM) was added to the media and co-incubated (in both HG and Control conditions) for the last 24 h.

4.10. Tert-Butyl Hydroperoxide (TBPH) Caco-2 Cell Treatment

Cells were pre-treated in the absence or in the presence of POE (15 μg GAE/mL) or NAC (50 μM) for 24 h. At the end of incubation cells were washed with cold PBS and incubated with TBHP (50 μM) for 90 min [40].

4.11. Intracellular ROS Detection

Intracellular ROS formation was evaluated in Caco-2 cells treated in the different experimental conditions using a 2′,7′-dichlorodihydrofluorescein diacetate (H_2DCFDA) fluorescent probe [20]. Cells were incubated for 45 min with pre-warmed PBS containing the fluorescent probe (25 μM). After incubation in the dark at 37 °C, cells were washed twice in PBS. Fluorescence of labeled cells was measured in a fluorescence plate reader at $\lambda_{ex}/\lambda_{em}$ (485/535 nm) (Multi-Mode Microplate Reader Synergy^{TM} HT, BioTek Instruments, Inc.). Data obtained in cells treated in different experimental condition were normalized to the results of the cell number. Data are expressed as arbitrary units of fluorescence (A.U.). An automated microscope (Lion hearth FX Automated live cell Imager, Biotek, BioTek Instruments, Inc., Santa Clara, CA, USA) was used for cellular imaging.

4.12. Western Blot Analysis

Total cell lysates (50 μg proteins) from the different experimental conditions were subjected to 12.5% sodium dodecyl sulfate polyacrylamide gel electrophoresis (SDS-PAGE) and transferred onto polyvinylidene fluoride (PVDF) membranes.

After regular blocking and washing, the membranes were incubated with specific primary antibodies over night at 4 °C.

For the determination of glucose receptors and tight junction levels: rabbit polyclonal anti-GLUT2 antibody (JJ20-21 Invitrogen, USA, diluted 1:500), rabbit polyclonal anti-SGLT1 antibody (Pa5-84085 Invitrogen, USA, diluted 1:200), and rabbit polyclonal anti ZO-1 antibody (GTX108587 GENETEX, Irvine, California, USA, diluted 1:200).

For the determination of glycolaldehyde-modified proteins (GA-modified proteins) levels: goat polyclonal anti-AGE antibody (Ab9890 Merck KGaA, Darmstadt, Germany, diluted 1:2000). Vinculin was used as the loading control (sc-25336 Santa Cruz Biotechnology, Dallas, TX, USA, diluted 1:200)

Donkey anti-goat (AP186P Sigma-Aldrich, Merck KGaA, Darmstadt, Germany, diluted 1:100,000), goat anti-mouse (sc-2005 Santa Cruz Biotechnology, Dallas, TX, USA, diluted 1:100,000), and goat anti-rabbit (12-348Sigma-Aldrich, Darmstadt, Germany, diluted 1:150,000) secondary antibodies HRP (Horseradish Peroxidase) were used in accordance with the manufacturer's instructions.

Protein bands were developed by the enhanced SuperSignal West Femto Maximum Sensitivity Substrate (Thermo Fisher Scientific, Waltham, MA, USA). The chemiluminescent signal was acquired using ChemiDoc XRS+ System (Bio-Rad Laboratories, Hercules, CA, USA) and analyzed by using Image J software (Version 1.50i, National Institute of Health, Bethesda, MD, USA).

4.13. Statistical Analysis

The experiments were performed on a minimum of three independent determinations, carried out in triplicate, and the results are reported as the means $\pm$ SD.

For comparison between the two groups, a *t*-test was used, and differences were considered to be significantly different if $p < 0.05$ (GraphPad PRISM 8.2). One-way analysis of variance (ANOVA) was carried out in GraphPad PRISM 8.2 software to evaluate any statistical difference among more than two different samples. Differences were considered to be significantly different if $p < 0.05$ (Tukey's post-hoc multiple-comparison test).

5. Conclusions

The effect of natural compounds on glucose transporters and their protective effects against oxidative stress have been previously demonstrated in several experimental models. For the first time, this study highlights the ability of POE to reduce glucose transport by lowering the GLUT2 levels, to promote intestinal barrier integrity by modulating ZO-1 levels, and to have a protective antioxidant effect against glucose-induced damage in Caco-2 cells. This is the first study to investigate the behavior of a complex pool of POE phenolic compounds, rather than a single molecule, on differentiated human intestinal Caco-2 cells. We suggest that the biological properties exerted by POE could be related to synergistic effects of its constituents.

In the face of the incessant demand for new alternative natural antioxidants, as well as anti-inflammatory and antidiabetic agents, the cell-safe POE profile makes this phyto-complex an excellent candidate for continuing to investigate the potential use of POE in the management of chronic diseases, including diabetes, in support of practices described in traditional medicine. Therefore, our results lay the foundation for further in vitro and in vivo studies to verify the antioxidant and antidiabetic role of *P. oceanica*.

Supplementary Materials: The following supporting information can be downloaded at: https://www.mdpi.com/article/10.3390/md20070457/s1, Figure S1: Effect of POE on Caco-2 cells viability; Figure S2: Effect of POE on HG-induced intracellular ROS formation; Figure S3: Effect of POE on HG-induced cell toxicity.

Author Contributions: Conceptualization, D.D., T.B. and G.F.; methodology, C.M., M.V. and L.B.; writing—original draft preparation, D.D., M.V., T.B. and C.M.; writing—review and editing, D.D., T.B. and G.F.; funding acquisition, D.D., T.B. and G.F. All authors have read and agreed to the published version of the manuscript.

Funding: Fondi di Ateneo 2021 D.D., T.B and G.F.

Institutional Review Board Statement: Not applicable.

Data Availability Statement: Not applicable.

Acknowledgments: The authors thank the authorized staff of the Interuniversity Center for Marine Biology and Applied Ecology "G. Bacci" (CIBM) (Leghorn, Italy) for kindly providing leaves of *P. oceanica*.

Conflicts of Interest: The authors declare no conflict of interest.

References

1. Personnic, S.; Boudouresque, C.F.; Astruch, P.; Ballesteros, E.; Blouet, S.; Bellan-Santini, D.; Bonhomme, P.; Thibault-Botha, D.; Feunteun, E.; Harmelin-Vivien, M.; et al. An ecosystem-based approach to assess the status of a Mediterranean ecosystem, the *Posidoniaoceanica* seagrass meadow. *PLoS ONE* **2014**, *9*, e98994. [CrossRef] [PubMed]
2. Pergent-Martini, C.; Pergent, G.; Monnier, B.; Boudouresque, C.F.; Mori, C.; Valette-Sansevin, A. Contribution of *Posidoniaoceanica* meadows in the context of climate change mitigation in the Mediterranean Sea. *Mar. Environ. Res.* **2021**, *165*, 105236. [CrossRef] [PubMed]
3. Vasarri, M.; De Biasi, A.M.; Barletta, E.; Pretti, C.; Degl'Innocenti, D. An Overview of New Insights into the Benefits of the Seagrass *Posidoniaoceanica* for Human Health. *Mar. Drugs* **2021**, *19*, 476. [CrossRef] [PubMed]
4. Gokce, G.; Haznedaroglu, M.Z. Evaluation of antidiabetic, antioxidant and vasoprotective effects of Posidonia oceanica extract. *J. Ethnopharmacol.* **2008**, *115*, 122–130. [CrossRef]
5. Vasarri, M.; Barletta, E.; Ramazzotti, M.; Degl'Innocenti, D. In vitro anti-glycation activity of the marine plant *Posidonia oceanica* (L.) Delile. *J. Ethnopharmacol.* **2020**, *259*, 112960. [CrossRef]
6. Vasarri, M.; Leri, M.; Barletta, E.; Ramazzotti, M.; Marzocchini, R.; Degl'Innocenti, D. Anti-inflammatory properties of the marine plant *Posidonia oceanica* (L.) Delile. *J. Ethnopharmacol.* **2020**, *247*, 112252. [CrossRef]
7. Micheli, L.; Vasarri, M.; Barletta, E.; Lucarini, E.; Ghelardini, C.; Degl'Innocenti, D.; Di Cesare Mannelli, L. Efficacy of *Posidonia oceanica* Extract against Inflammatory Pain: In Vivo Studies in Mice. *Mar. Drugs.* **2021**, *19*, 48. [CrossRef]
8. Barletta, E.; Ramazzotti, M.; Fratianni, F.; Pessani, D.; Degl'Innocenti, D. Hydrophilic extract from *Posidonia oceanica* inhibits activity and expression of gelatinases and prevents HT1080 human fibrosarcoma cell line invasion. *Cell. Adh. Migr.* **2015**, *9*, 422–431. [CrossRef]
9. Johnston, K.; Sharp, P.; Clifford, M.; Morgan, L. Dietary polyphenols decrease glucose uptake by human intestinal Caco-2 cells. *FEBS Lett.* **2005**, *579*, 1653–1657. [CrossRef]
10. Ni, D.; Ai, Z.; Munoz-Sandoval, D.; Suresh, R.; Ellis, P.R.; Yuqiong, C.; Sharp, P.A.; Butterworth, P.J.; Yu, Z.; Corpe, C.P. Inhibition of the facilitative sugar transporters (GLUTs) by tea extracts and catechins. *FASEB J.* **2020**, *34*, 9995–10010. [CrossRef]
11. Kwon, O.; Eck, P.; Chen, S.; Corpe, C.P.; Lee, J.; Kruhlak, M.; Levine, M. Inhibition of the intestinal glucose transporter GLUT2 by flavonoids. *FASEB J.* **2007**, *21*, 366–377. [CrossRef] [PubMed]
12. Sharma, S.; Tripathi, P.; Sharma, J.; Dixit, A. Flavonoids modulate tight junction barrier functions in hyperglycemic human intestinal Caco-2 cells. *Nutrition* **2020**, *78*, 110792. [CrossRef] [PubMed]
13. Bernardi, S.; Del Bo', C.; Marino, M.; Gargari, G.; Cherubini, A.; Andrés-Lacueva, C.; Hidalgo-Liberona, N.; Peron, G.; González-Dominguez, R.; Kroon, P.; et al. Polyphenols and Intestinal Permeability: Rationale and Future Perspectives. *J. Agric. Food. Chem.* **2020**, *68*, 1816–1829. [CrossRef] [PubMed]
14. Cianfruglia, L.; Morresi, C.; Bacchetti, T.; Armeni, T.; Ferretti, G. Protection of Polyphenols against Glyco-Oxidative Stress: Involvement of Glyoxalase Pathway. *Antioxidants* **2020**, *9*, 1006. [CrossRef]
15. Ludwig, S. The Glycemic Index: Physiological mechanisms relating to obesity. Diabetes and cardiovascular disease. *J. Am. Med. Assoc.* **2002**, *287*, 2414–2423. [CrossRef]

16. Koepsell, H. Glucose transporters in the small intestine in health and disease. *Pflugers Arch.* **2020**, *472*, 1207–1248. [CrossRef]
17. De Angelis, I.; Turco, L. Caco-2 cells as a model for intestinal absorption. *Curr. Protoc. Toxicol.* **2011**, *20*, 20.6. [CrossRef]
18. Ding, X.; Hu, X.; Chen, Y.; Xie, J.; Ying, M.; Wang, Y.; Yu, Q. Differentiated Caco-2 cell models in food-intestine interaction study: Current applications and future trends. *Trends Food Sci. Technol.* **2021**, *107*, 455–465. [CrossRef]
19. Vancamelbeke, M.; Vermeire, S. The intestinal barrier: A fundamental role in health and disease. *Expert. Rev. Gastroenterol. Hepatol.* **2017**, *11*, 821–834. [CrossRef]
20. Morresi, C.; Cianfruglia, L.; Sartini, D.; Cecati, M.; Fumarola, S.; Emanuelli, M.; Armeni, T.; Ferretti, G.; Bacchetti, T. Effect of High Glucose-Induced Oxidative Stress on Paraoxonase 2 Expression and Activity in Caco-2 Cells. *Cells* **2019**, *8*, 1616. [CrossRef]
21. Kellett, G.L.; Helliwell, P.A. The diffusive component of intestinal glucose absorption is mediated by the glucose-induced recruitment of GLUT2 to the brush-border membrane. *Biochem. J.* **2000**, *350*, 155–162. [CrossRef] [PubMed]
22. Roder, P.V.; Geillinger, K.E.; Zietek, T.S.; Thorens, B.; Koepsell, H.; Daniel, H. The role of SGLT1 and GLUT2 in intestinal glucose transport and sensing. *PLoS ONE* **2014**, *9*, e89977. [CrossRef] [PubMed]
23. Tobin, V.; Le Gall, M.; Fioramonti, X.; Stolarczyk, E.; Blazquez, A.G.; Klein, C.; Prigent, M.; Serradas, P.; Cuif, M.H.; Magnan, C.; et al. Insulin internalizes GLUT2 in the enterocytes of healthy but not insulin-resistant mice. *Diabetes* **2008**, *57*, 555–562. [CrossRef] [PubMed]
24. Corpe, C.P.; Basaleh, M.M.; Affleck, J.; Gould, G.; Jess, T.J.; Kellet, G.L. The regulation of GLUT5 and GLUT2 activity in the adaptation of intestinal brush-border fructose transport in diabetes. *Pflugers Arch.* **1996**, *432*, 192–201. [CrossRef] [PubMed]
25. Ait-Omar, A.; Monteiro-Sepulveda, M.; Poitou, C.; Le Gall, M.; Cotillard, A. GLUT2 accumulation in enterocyte apical and intracellular membranes: A study in morbidly obese human subjects and ob/ob and high fat-fed mice. *Diabetes* **2011**, *60*, 2598–2607. [CrossRef] [PubMed]
26. Fasano, A. Zonulin and Its Regulation of Intestinal Barrier Function: The Biological Door to Inflammation, Autoimmunity, and Cancer. *Physiol. Rev.* **2011**, *91*, 151–175. [CrossRef]
27. Thaiss, C.A.; Levy, M.; Grosheva, I.; Zheng, D.; Soffer, E.; Blacher, E.; Braverman, S.; Tengeler, A.C.; Barak, O.; Elazar, O.; et al. Hyperglycemia drives intestinal barrier dysfunction and risk for enteric infection. *Science* **2018**, *359*, 1376–1383. [CrossRef]
28. Srinivasan, B.; Kolli, A.R.; Esch, M.B.; Abaci, H.E.; Shuler, M.L.; Hickman, J.J. TEER Measurement techniques for In Vitro barrier model systems. *J. Lab. Autom.* **2015**, *20*, 107–126. [CrossRef]
29. Del Bo, C.; Bernardi, S.; Cherubini, A.; Porrini, M.; Gargari, G.; Hidalgo-Liberona, N.; Gonzalez-Dominguez, R.; Zamora-Ros, R.; Peron, G.; Marino, M.; et al. A polyphenol-rich dietary pattern improves intestinal permeability, evaluated as serum zonulin levels, in older subjects: The MaPLE randomised controlled trial. *Clin. Nutr.* **2021**, *40*, 3006–3018. [CrossRef]
30. Bhattacharyya, A.; Chattopadhyay, R.; Mitra, S.; Crowe, S.E. Oxidative stress: An essential factor in the pathogenesis of gastrointestinal mucosal diseases. *Physiol. Rev.* **2014**, *94*, 329–354. [CrossRef]
31. Sottero, B.; Rossin, D.; Poli, G.; Biasi, F. Lipid Oxidation Products in the Pathogenesis of Inflammation-related Gut Diseases. *Curr. Med. Chem.* **2018**, *25*, 1311–1326. [CrossRef] [PubMed]
32. Jiang, S.; Liu, H.; Li, C. Dietary Regulation of Oxidative Stress in Chronic Metabolic Diseases. *Foods* **2021**, *10*, 1854. [CrossRef] [PubMed]
33. Kučera, O.; Endlicher, R.; Roušar, T.; Lotková, H.; Garnol, T.; Drahota, Z.; Červinková, Z. The Effect of tert-butyl hydroperoxide-induced oxidative stress on lean and steatotic rat hepatocytes in vitro. *Oxid. Med. Cell Longev.* **2014**, *2014*, 752506. [CrossRef] [PubMed]
34. Brings, S.; Fleming, T.; Freichel, M.; Muckenthaler, M.U.; Herzig, S.; Nawroth, P.P. Dicarbonyls and Advanced Glycation End-Products in the Development of Diabetic Complications and Targets for Intervention. *Int. J. Mol. Sci.* **2017**, *18*, 984. [CrossRef] [PubMed]
35. Yeh, W.J.; Hsia, S.M.; Lee, W.H.; Wu, C.H. Polyphenols with antiglycation activity and mechanisms of action: A review of recent findings. *J. Food Drug Anal.* **2017**, *25*, 84–92. [CrossRef]
36. Saura-Calixto, F.; Serrano, J.; Goñibc, I. Intake and bioaccessibility of total polyphenols in a whole diet. *Food Chem.* **2007**, *101*, 492–501. [CrossRef]
37. Riss, T.L.; Moravec, R.A.; Niles, A.L.; Duellman, S.; Benink, H.A.; Worzella, T.J.; Minor, L. Cell Viability Assays. In *Assay Guidance Manual*; Markossian, S., Grossman, A., Brimacombe, K., Arkin, M., Auld, D., Austin, C.P., Baell, J., Chung, T.D.Y., Coussens, N.P., Dahlin, J.L., et al., Eds.; Eli Lilly & Company and the National Center for Advancing Translational Sciences: Bethesda, MD, USA, 2004.
38. Moretti, R.; Thorson, J.S. A comparison of sugar indicators enables a universal high-throughput sugar-1-phosphate nucleotidyl-transferase assay. *Anal. Biochem.* **2008**, *377*, 251–258. [CrossRef]
39. Putt, K.; Pei, R.; White, H.; Bolling, B. Yogurt inhibits intestinal barrier dysfunction in Caco-2 cells by increasing tight junctions. *Food Funct.* **2017**, *8*, 406–414. [CrossRef]
40. Bacchetti, T.; Morresi, C.; Bellachioma, L.; Ferretti, G. Antioxidant and Pro-Oxidant Properties of Carthamus Tinctorius, Hydroxy Safflor Yellow A, and Safflor Yellow A. *Antioxidants* **2020**, *9*, 119. [CrossRef]

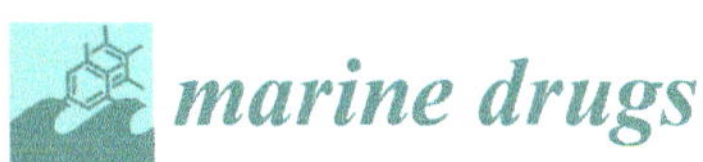 *marine drugs*

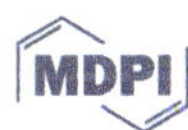

Article

Chlorella vulgaris Extracts as Modulators of the Health Status and the Inflammatory Response of Gilthead Seabream Juveniles (*Sparus aurata*)

Bruno Reis [1,2,3,4,*], Lourenço Ramos-Pinto [1], Sara A. Cunha [5], Manuela Pintado [5], Joana Laranjeira da Silva [6], Jorge Dias [2], Luís Conceição [2], Elisabete Matos [3,7] and Benjamín Costas [1,*]

[1] Centro Interdisciplinar de Investigação Marinha e Ambiental (CIIMAR), Universidade do Porto, Avenida General Norton de Matos, Terminal de Cruzeiros do Porto de Leixões, 4450-208 Matosinhos, Portugal; lourenco.pinto@ciimar.up.pt
[2] SPAROS Lda., Área Empresarial de Marim, Lote C, 8700-221 Olhão, Portugal; jorgedias@sparos.pt (J.D.); luisconceicao@sparos.pt (L.C.)
[3] Sorgal S.A., EN 109-Lugar da Pardala, 3880-728 São João de Ovar, Portugal
[4] Instituto de Ciências Biomédicas Abel Salazar (ICBAS-UP), Universidade do Porto, Rua de Jorge Viterbo Ferreira 228, 4050-313 Porto, Portugal
[5] CBQF—Centro de Biotecnologia e Química Fina—Laboratório Associado, Escola Superior de Biotecnologia, Universidade Católica Portuguesa Rua Diogo Botelho 1327, 4169-005 Porto, Portugal; scunha@ucp.pt (S.A.C.); mpintado@ucp.pt (M.P.)
[6] Allmicroalgae, Natural Products SA, Industrial Microalgae Production, Apartado 9, 2449-909 Pataias, Portugal; joana.g.silva@allmicroalgae.com
[7] B2E Associação para a Bioeconomia Azul—Laboratório Colaborativo, Av. Liberdade, UPTEC Mar, 4450-718 Leça da Palmeira, Portugal; ematos@b2e.pt
[*] Correspondence: breis@ciimar.up.pt (B.R.), bcostas@ciimar.up.pt (B.C.), Tel.. +351-223-401-840 (B.R.); +351-223-401-838 (B.C.)

Citation: Reis, B.; Ramos-Pinto, L.; Cunha, S.A.; Pintado, M.; da Silva, J.L.; Dias, J.; Conceição, L.; Matos, E.; Costas, B. *Chlorella vulgaris* Extracts as Modulators of the Health Status and the Inflammatory Response of Gilthead Seabream Juveniles (*Sparus aurata*). *Mar. Drugs* 2022, 20, 407. https://doi.org/10.3390/md20070407

Academic Editors: Donatella DeglInnocenti and Marzia Vasarri

Received: 28 April 2022
Accepted: 16 June 2022
Published: 21 June 2022

Publisher's Note: MDPI stays neutral with regard to jurisdictional claims in published maps and institutional affiliations.

Abstract: This study aimed to evaluate the effects of short-term supplementation, with 2% *Chlorella vulgaris* (*C. vulgaris*) biomass and two 0.1% *C. vulgaris* extracts, on the health status (experiment one) and on the inflammatory response (experiment two) of gilthead seabream (*Sparus aurata*). The trial comprised four isoproteic (50% crude protein) and isolipidic (17% crude fat) diets. A fishmeal-based (FM), practical diet was used as a control (CTR), whereas three experimental diets based on CTR were further supplemented with a 2% inclusion of C. vulgaris biomass (Diet D1); 0.1% inclusion of C. vulgaris peptide-enriched extract (Diet D2) and finally a 0.1% inclusion of C. vulgaris insoluble fraction (Diet D3). Diets were randomly assigned to quadruplicate groups of 97 fish/tank (IBW: 33.4 ± 4.1 g), fed to satiation three times a day in a recirculation seawater system. In experiment one, seabream juveniles were fed for 2 weeks and sampled for tissues at 1 week and at the end of the feeding period. Afterwards, randomly selected fish from each group were subjected to an inflammatory insult (experiment two) by intraperitoneal injection of inactivated gram-negative bacteria, following 24 and 48 h fish were sampled for tissues. Blood was withdrawn for haematological procedures, whereas plasma and gut tissue were sampled for immune and oxidative stress parameters. The anterior gut was also collected for gene expression measurements. After 1 and 2 weeks of feeding, fish fed D2 showed higher circulating neutrophils than seabream fed CTR. In contrast, dietary treatments induced mild effects on the innate immune and antioxidant functions of gilthead seabream juveniles fed for 2 weeks. In the inflammatory response following the inflammatory insult, mild effects could be attributed to *C. vulgaris* supplementation either in biomass form or extract. However, the *C. vulgaris* soluble peptide-enriched extract seems to confer a protective, anti-stress effect in the gut at the molecular level, which should be further explored in future studies.

Keywords: functional feeds; protein hydrolysate; innate immunity; fish robustness

---

1. Introduction

In intensive farming facilities, fish are reared at high densities, which may increase stress and susceptibility to diseases, resulting in lower production yields. Consequently, there is an increasing pressure for disease management strategies, beyond the use of antibiotics or vaccination. In this sense, health promoting feeds designed not only to fulfil the nutrient requirements but also to strengthen the immune system are viewed as a way to reduce aquaculture dependency on chemotherapeutics and to mitigate its negative environmental effects [1,2]. Novel applications based on algal products are a fast emerging and a developing area, expected to reach 56.5 billion US$ by 2027 with a compound annual growth rate of 6% in the period from 2019 to 2027 [3]. The ability to grow in different environments and conditions as well as to produce large numbers of secondary metabolites makes microalgae a suitable raw material for different applications. These organisms are regarded as sustainable alternative sources of bioactive compounds, mostly sought out for the development of functional feeds, foods and health products [4–6].

Chlorella vulgaris is a green microalga with a wide distribution in freshwater, marine and terrestrial environments that is capable of rapid growth under autotrophic, mixotrophic and heterotrophic conditions [7]. These characteristics made *C. vulgaris* a successful candidate for large-scale cultivation and commercial production [8]. As with other microalgae species, *C. vulgaris* produces a different array of health-promoting biomolecules [9,10]. Notably, natural pigments such as lutein and astaxanthin extracted from *Chlorella* sp. show immunostimulatory and antioxidant protective effects [4,11,12]. Furthermore, these microalgae are characterised by a very high crude protein content (>50%) and a balanced amino acid (AA) profile, synthesising all essential AA in a considerable amount [4]. Already, *C. vulgaris* biomass has been successfully used in aquafeeds as a source of protein, improving growth performance, oxidative status and immune response in several fish species [13–17]. For instance, dietary supplementation of *Chlorella sp.* at 0.4 to 1.2%, stimulated the innate immunity of gibel carp (*Carassius auratus gibelio*), namely by increasing IgM, IgD, Interleukin-22 and chemokine levels [18]. Also, Zahran and Risha [16] reported that feed supplementation with powdered *C. vulgaris* protected Nile tilapia against arsenic-induced immunosuppression and oxidative stress.

Nonetheless, as with other algal biomasses, at high fishmeal replacement levels, studies start to report impaired growth performances [19,20]. Microalgae generally show thick cell walls that hinder the access of fish gut enzymes to intracellular nutrients. Hence, algae nutritional value increases if access is provided to macro and micronutrients [21–23]. Hydrolyses improve digestibility through the application of chemical or enzymatic methods to disrupt the cell wall and hydrolyse intact proteins [24]. The enzymatic method is sometimes advantageous because of milder processing conditions and peptide bond specificity, giving rise to digestible peptides believed to be more effective than the whole protein or the free AA [24,25]. Peptide bioactivity is influenced by molecular weight and peptide chain size [26]. In fact, low molecular weight peptides (<3 kDa) are described as having immune-stimulating or anti-inflammatory properties [26–28].

Several studies, have evaluated marine protein hydrolysates (MPH) as a dietary ingredient and their effects on growth performance, immune response and disease resistance in fish [26]. Results are promising, as the dietary inclusion of MPH has been shown to induce growth, antioxidant activity and fish immunity [28–32] as well as improve fish immune response and disease resistance to specific bacterial infections [27,33–35]. Moreover, regarding microalgae, different *C. vulgaris* protein hydrolysates and extracts have already been studied concerning its different bioactivities, namely, anticancer and antibacterial effects [36], as well as antioxidant and immune modulatory properties [37]. Results mentioned above suggest that *C. vulgaris* has the potential to act as a dietary supplement with nutraceutical properties and to stimulate the immune system. Therefore, the present study aimed to evaluate the effects of short-term dietary supplementation, with a 2% *C. vulgaris* biomass and a 0.1% supplementation with *C. vulgaris* soluble peptide-enriched extract, on the immune and the oxidative stress defences (health status; experiment one) and on the inflammatory response after an inflammatory insult (experiment two) of gilthead seabream (*Sparus aurata*).

2. Results

2.1. Haematology/Peripheral Leucocyte Responses

In experiment one, total WBC and RBC as well as MCH did not change significantly among different dietary treatments at both 1 and 2 weeks of feeding (Table 1). However, fish fed D2 presented a higher haemoglobin (Hb) concentration than D1 and D3 fed fish (Table 1). Differential leucocyte counts showed different modulation patterns between dietary treatments regardless of the sampling point (Table 2). For instance, the D1 fed group showed lower lymphocyte numbers at both 1 and 2 weeks, when compared to the other dietary treatments (Table 2). Whereas peripheral neutrophils increased in D2 fed fish compared to those fed CTR (Table 2). Circulating monocytes were not significantly modulated by dietary treatments at either 1 or 2 weeks of feeding.

Table 1. Haemoglobin, mean corpuscular haemoglobin (MCH), red blood cells (RBC) and white blood cells (WBC) in gilthead seabream juveniles after 1 and 2 weeks of feeding (experiment one). Data are the mean $\pm$ SEM ($n = 12$).

Haematology	1 Week				2 Weeks			
Diets	CTR	D1	D2	D3	CTR	D1	D2	D3
Haemoglobin (g·dL^{-1})	0.69 ± 0.05	0.65 ± 0.04	0.81 ± 0.04	0.61 ± 0.03	0.68 ± 0.06	0.65 ± 0.02	0.74 ± 0.05	0.67 ± 0.05
MCH (pg·cell^{-1})	2.24 ± 0.31	1.89 ± 0.16	2.29 ± 0.23	1.87 ± 0.16	3.31 ± 0.39	3.12 ± 0.19	3.61 ± 0.19	3.24 ± 0.18
WBC (10^4·µL^{-1})	1.85 ± 0.05	1.84 ± 0.12	1.96 ± 0.06	1.86 ± 0.05	3.96 ± 0.18	4.19 ± 0.21	3.73 ± 0.23	3.89 ± 0.19
RBC (10^6·µL^{-1})	3.25 ± 0.26	3.46 ± 0.21	3.79 ± 0.39	3.64 ± 0.20	1.93 ± 0.09	2.13 ± 0.16	2.06 ± 0.12	1.91 ± 0.11

2-Way ANOVA							
	Time		Diet				Diet × Time
	1 week	2 weeks	CTR	D1	D2	D3	
Haemoglobin (g·dL^{-1})	-	-	AB	B	A	B	ns
MCH (pg·cell^{-1})	A	B	-	-	-	-	ns
WBC (10^4·µL^{-1})	B	A	-	-	-	-	ns
RBC (10^6·µL^{-1})	A	B	-	-	-	-	ns

Different capital letters represent significant differences in time regardless of diet and between diets regardless of time ($p < 0.05$), ns (not significant).

Table 2. Absolute values of peripheral blood leucocytes (thrombocytes, Lymphocytes, monocytes and neutrophils) in gilthead seabream juveniles after 1 and 2 weeks of feeding (experiment one). Data are the mean $\pm$ SEM ($n = 12$).

Peripheral Leucocytes	1 Week				2 Weeks			
Diets	CTR	D1	D2	D3	CTR	D1	D2	D3
Thrombocytes (10^4·µL^{-1})	1.17 ± 0.08	1.30 ± 0.07	1.29 ± 0.12	1.26 ± 0.05	2.78 ± 0.18	3.24 ± 0.17	2.58 ± 0.17	2.66 ± 0.16
Lymphocytes (10^4·µL^{-1})	0.57 ± 0.07	0.37 ± 0.04	0.62 ± 0.05	0.56 ± 0.03	1.15 ± 0.12	0.84 ± 0.07	1.05 ± 0.15	1.17 ± 0.08
Monocytes (10^4·µL^{-1})	0.01 ± 0.00	0.02 ± 0.00	0.02 ± 0.01	0.02 ± 0.01	0.02 ± 0.01	0.03 ± 0.01	0.02 ± 0.00	0.02 ± 0.01
Neutrophils (10^4·µL^{-1})	0.01 ± 0.00	0.01 ± 0.01	0.04 ± 0.01	0.02 ± 0.01	0.02 ± 0.01	0.06 ± 0.02	0.06 ± 0.01	0.06 ± 0.01

2-Way ANOVA							
	Time		Diet				Diet × Time
	1 week	2 weeks	CTR	D1	D2	D3	
Thrombocytes (10^4·µL^{-1})	B	A	-	-	-	-	ns
Lymphocytes (10^4·µL^{-1})	B	A	A	B	A	A	ns
Monocytes (10^4·µL^{-1})	-	-	-	-	-	-	ns
Neutrophils (10^4·µL^{-1})	B	A	B	AB	A	AB	ns

Different capital letters represent significant differences in time regardless of diet and between diets regardless of time ($p < 0.05$), ns (not significant).

After the inflammatory insult (experiment two), Hb increased at 24 h following inoculation with the inactivated bacteria, while MCH, total WBC and RBC remained unchanged

(Table 3). Peripheral lymphocyte numbers decreased at 24 h compared to 0 h, returning to resting values at 48 h (Table 4). Circulating neutrophil levels increased at 24 h and 48 h following pathogen inoculation compared to time 0 h (Table 4). Total thrombocyte and monocyte concentrations were unaffected (Table 4).

2.2. Plasma Humoral Parameters

In experiment one, plasma humoral parameters (NO production, antiprotease and peroxidase activities) remained unaffected by the different dietary treatments at both sampling points (Figure 1A–C). However, antiprotease activity increased from 1 to 2 weeks of feeding, while peroxidase followed an opposite trend.

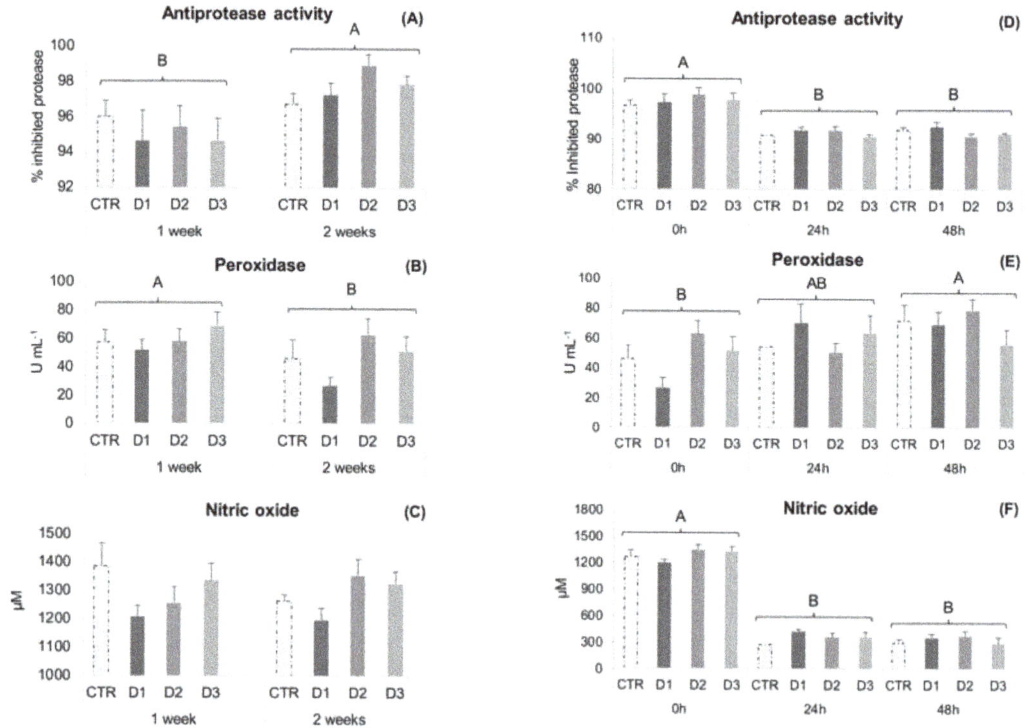

Figure 1. Plasma immune parameters of gilthead seabream juveniles. Experiment one: (**A**) Antiprotease activity; (**B**) Peroxidase activity; (**C**) Nitric oxide. Data are the mean ± SEM ($n = 12$). Experiment two: (**D**) Antiprotease activity; (**E**) Peroxidase activity; (**F**) Nitric oxide. Data are the mean ± SEM ($n = 9$). Different capital letters represent significant differences in time regardless diet ($p < 0.05$).

Following heat-inactivated bacteria inoculation, peroxidase activity increased after 48 h (Figure 1E), while both NO concentration and antiprotease activity decreased at 24 and 48 h (Figure 1D,F).

Table 3. Haemoglobin, mean corpuscular haemoglobin (MCH), red blood cells (RBC) and white blood cells (WBC) in gilthead seabream juveniles following an inflammatory insult after 2 weeks of feeding (experiment two). Data are the mean $\pm$ SEM ($n = 9$).

Haematology	0 h				24 h				48 h			
Diets	CTR	D1	D2	D3	CTR	D1	D2	D3	CTR	D1	D2	D3
Haemoglobin ($g \cdot dL^{-1}$)	0.68 ± 0.06	0.65 ± 0.02	0.74 ± 0.05	0.67 ± 0.05	0.87 ± 0.10	0.79 ± 0.10	0.96 ± 0.08	0.78 ± 0.09	0.57 ± 0.05	0.83 ± 0.08	0.73 ± 0.05	0.69 ± 0.03
MCH ($pg \cdot cell^{-1}$)	3.31 ± 0.39	3.12 ± 0.19	3.61 ± 0.19	3.24 ± 0.18	3.60 ± 0.28	3.82 ± 0.33	3.98 ± 0.33	3.79 ± 0.34	3.09 ± 0.28	3.93 ± 0.33	3.43 ± 0.16	3.54 ± 0.13
WBC ($10^4 \cdot \mu L^{-1}$)	3.96 ± 0.18	4.19 ± 0.21	3.73 ± 0.23	3.89 ± 0.19	4.04 ± 0.28	4.23 ± 0.28	4.09 ± 0.42	4.11 ± 0.32	4.56 ± 0.29	4.69 ± 0.26	4.19 ± 0.35	4.42 ± 0.35
RBC ($10^6 \cdot \mu L^{-1}$)	1.93 ± 0.09	2.13 ± 0.16	2.06 ± 0.12	1.91 ± 0.11	2.20 ± 0.14	2.11 ± 0.12	2.34 ± 0.13	2.05 ± 0.09	1.86 ± 0.11	2.23 = 0.10	2.13 ± 0.10	1.97 ± 0.09

	2-Way ANOVA							
	Time			Diet				Diet × Time
	0 h	24 h	48 h	CTR	D1	D2	D3	
Haemoglobin	B	A	B	-	-	-	-	ns
MCH	-	-	-	-	-	-	-	ns
WBC	-	-	-	-	-	-	-	ns
RBC	-	-	-	-	-	-	-	ns

Different capital letters represent significant differences in time regardless of diet ($p < 0.05$), ns (not significant).

Table 4. Absolute values of peripheral blood leucocytes (thrombocytes, Lymphocytes, monocytes and neutrophils) in gilthead seabream juveniles following an inflammatory insult after 2 weeks of feeding (experiment two). Data are the mean $\pm$ SEM ($n = 9$).

Peripheral Leucocytes	0 h				24 h				48 h			
Diets	CTR	D1	D2	D3	CTR	D1	D2	D3	CTR	D1	D2	D3
Thrombocytes ($10^4 \cdot \mu L^{-1}$)	2.78 ± 0.18	3.24 ± 0.17	2.58 ± 0.17	2.66 ± 0.16	3.06 ± 0.16	3.05 ± 0.24	3.33 ± 0.29	3.26 ± 0.28	3.14 ± 0.33	3.10 ± 0.16	2.88 ± 0.19	2.93 ± 0.20
Lymphocytes ($10^4 \cdot \mu L^{-1}$)	1.15 ± 0.12	0.84 ± 0.07	1.05 ± 0.15	1.17 ± 0.08	0.75 ± 0.13	0.88 ± 0.13	0.76 ± 0.14	0.60 ± 0.10	1.09 ± 0.12	1.00 ± 0.12	0.93 ± 0.15	0.87 ± 0.07
Monocytes ($10^4 \cdot \mu L^{-1}$)	0.02 ± 0.01	0.03 ± 0.01	0.02 ± 0.00	0.02 ± 0.01	0.03 ± 0.01	0.05 ± 0.02	0.02 ± 0.01	0.03 ± 0.01	0.01 ± 0.01	0.02 ± 0.01	0.02 ± 0.01	0.04 ± 0.01
Neutrophils ($104 \cdot \mu L^{-1}$)	0.02 ± 0.01	0.06 ± 0.02	0.06 ± 0.01	0.06 ± 0.01	0.16 ± 0.05	0.18 ± 0.04	0.14 ± 0.04	0.18 ± 0.06	0.09 ± 0.02	0.21 ± 0.07	0.20 ± 0.06	0.25 ± 0.05

	2-Way ANOVA							
	Time			Diet				Diet $\times$ Time
	0 h	24 h	48 h	CTR	D1	D2	D3	
Thrombocytes	-	-	-	-	-	-	-	ns
Lymphocytes	A	B	A	-	-	-	-	ns
Monocytes	-	-	-	-	-	-	-	ns
Neutrophils	B	A	A	-	-	-	-	ns

Different capital letters represent significant differences in time regardless of diet ($p < 0.05$), ns (not significant).

2.3. Gut Innate Immune and Oxidative Stress Biomarkers

Peroxidase, NO production and SOD activity remained unchanged during the health status experiment in gut samples (Figure 2A–C). Nonetheless, D2 fed fish showed increased gut lipid peroxidation compared to D3 and CTR (Figure 3A), and catalase activity increased from 1 to 2 weeks of feeding.

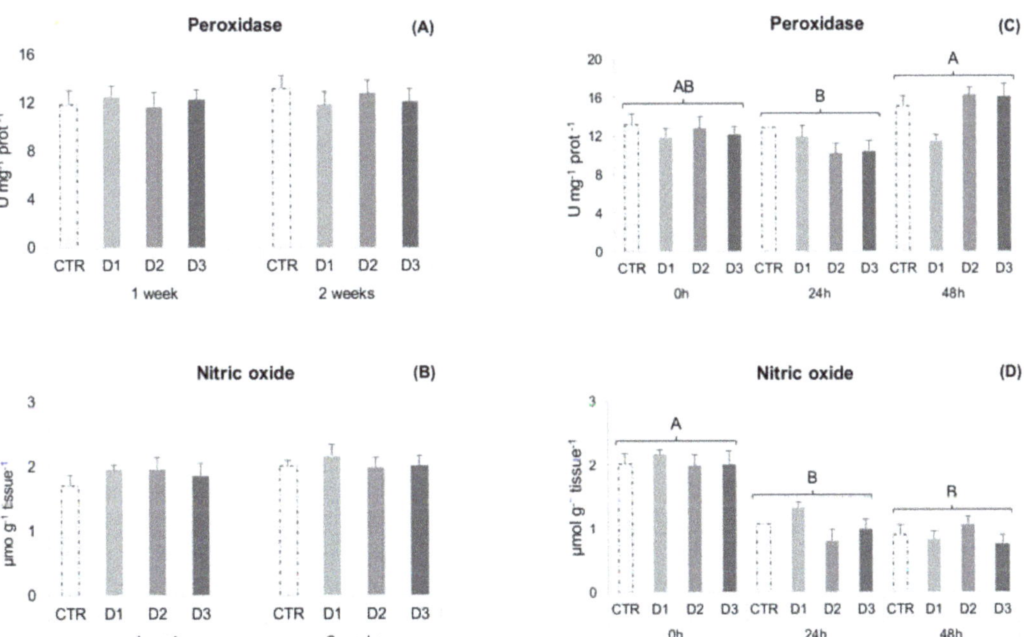

Figure 2. Gut immune parameters of gilthead seabream juveniles. Experiment one: (**A**) Peroxidase activity; (**B**) Nitric oxide (NO). Data are the mean ± SEM (*n* = 12). Experiment two: (**C**) Peroxidase activity; (**D**) Nitric oxide (NO). Data are the mean ± SEM (*n* = 9) Different capital letters represent significant differences in time regardless of diet ($p < 0.05$).

In experiment two, all measured parameters changed over time. Peroxidase activity increased from 24 to 48 h and NO production decreased after 24 and 48 h (Figure 2C,D). Antioxidant defences, such as catalase activity decreased 48 h after inoculation (Figure 3E), while lipid peroxidation increased at 24 and 48 h (Figure 3D). Superoxide dismutase activity increased at 24 h post-stimulus and D1 fed fish had higher activity than D3, irrespective of the sampling point (Figure 3F).

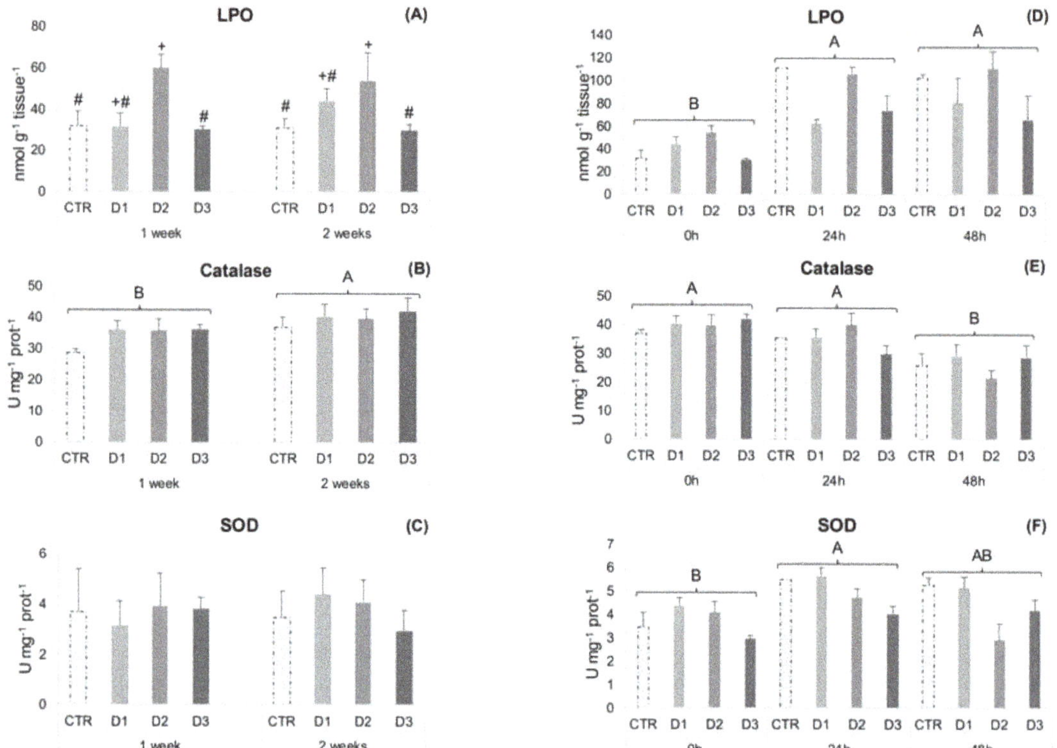

Figure 3. Gut oxidative stress parameters of gilthead seabream juveniles. Experiment one: (**A**) Lipid peroxidation (LPO); (**B**) Catalase activity; (**C**) Superoxide dismutase activity (SOD). Data are the mean $\pm$ SEM (n = 12). Experiment two: (**D**) Lipid peroxidation (LPO); (**E**) Catalase activity; (**F**) Superoxide dismutase activity (SOD). Data are the mean $\pm$ SEM (n = 9). Different symbols represent significant differences between diets regardless of time ($p < 0.05$). Different capital letters represent significant differences in time regardless of diet ($p < 0.05$).

2.4. Gut Gene Expression Analysis

To evaluate the expression of gut health, immunity and oxidative stress related genes (Tables 5 and 6), total RNA was isolated from fish anterior intestine. In experiment one, target genes transcriptomic analysis was not able to ascertain differences attributable to the dietary treatments, which could be related to the high intraspecific variability for some target genes (Table 5). However, cd8α, hsp70 and muc2 genes expression increased from 1 to 2 weeks.

Following the inflammatory insult, changes attributed to dietary treatments were also not found in the majority of analysed genes, except for hsp70, which was down-regulated at 24 h in D2 fed fish (Table 6). Furthermore, tlr1 gene expression was up-regulated and gpx was down-regulated at 24 h in all dietary treatments.

Table 5. Relative gene expression profiling of anterior intestine in gilthead seabream juveniles after 1 and 2 weeks of feeding (experiment one). Data are the mean ± SEM ($n = 12$). All data values for each gene were in reference to the expression level of CTR.

		Relative mRNA Expression										
Trial 1	**Diets**	*il1-β*	*il-34*	*tlr1*	*cd8α*	*igm*	*hepc*	*hsp70*	*gpx*	*sod(mn)*	*muc2*	*muc13*
1 week	CTR	1.09 ± 0.15	1.20 ± 0.16	1.05 ± 0.10	1.52 ± 0.43	1.09 ± 0.13	1.58 ± 0.45	1.04 ± 0.09	1.11 ± 0.13	1.06 ± 0.12	1.34 ± 0.29	1.11 ± 0.17
	D1	1.06 ± 0.22	1.18 ± 0.16	1.27 ± 0.12	0.94 ± 0.27	1.17 ± 0.43	1.58 ± 0.52	1.38 ± 0.25	1.49 ± 0.29	1.28 ± 0.14	1.04 ± 0.27	1.27 ± 0.15
	D2	1.41 ± 0.18	1.37 ± 0.12	1.12 ± 0.16	1.22 ± 0.34	2.01 ± 0.63	1.13 ± 0.32	1.67 ± 0.28	1.79 ± 0.26	1.12 ± 0.14	1.35 ± 0.22	1.17 ± 0.14
	D3	1.15 ± 0.09	1.18 ± 0.12	1.28 ± 0.16	1.67 ± 0.58	1.31 ± 0.57	0.99 ± 0.19	1.77 ± 0.38	1.50 ± 0.23	1.46 ± 0.20	1.28 ± 0.18	1.34 ± 0.20
2 weeks	CTR	1.54 ± 0.47	1.08 ± 0.15	1.31 ± 0.34	1.23 ± 0.29	1.67 ± 0.50	3.17 ± 1.50	1.04 ± 0.16	1.67 ± 0.41	1.18 ± 0.20	1.93 ± 0.99	1.58 ± 0.58
	D1	1.61 ± 0.62	1.93 ± 0.37	1.94 ± 0.37	1.84 ± 0.42	7.39 ± 3.31	3.45 ± 1.04	1.40 ± 0.25	2.26 ± 0.33	2.25 ± 0.51	3.11 ± 0.68	1.89 ± 0.24
	D2	1.59 ± 0.47	1.43 ± 0.37	2.44 ± 0.65	2.02 ± 0.65	4.16 ± 1.53	3.43 ± 2.61	0.77 ± 0.27	1.78 ± 0.70	1.02 ± 0.29	1.86 ± 0.60	1.59 ± 0.57
	D3	1.31 ± 0.42	1.77 ± 0.54	2.09 ± 0.44	1.70 ± 0.55	3.70 ± 1.58	1.49 ± 0.52	1.56 ± 0.77	1.92 ± 0.50	1.66 ± 0.65	2.19 ± 0.63	1.92 ± 0.69
2 way-ANOVA		*il1-β*	*il-34*	*tlr1*	*cd8α*	*igm*	*hepc*	*hsp70*	*gpx*	*sod(mn)*	*muc2*	*muc13*
Sig.	Time	ns	ns	ns	0.024	ns	ns	0.009	ns	ns	0.046	ns
	Diet	ns	ns	ns	0.747	ns	ns	0.541	ns	ns	0.569	ns
	Time × Diet	ns	ns	ns	0.405	ns	ns	0.106	ns	ns	0.156	ns
Diet	CTR	-	-	-	-	-	-	-	-	-	-	-
	D1	-	-	-	-	-	-	-	-	-	-	-
	D2	-	-	-	-	-	-	-	-	-	-	-
	D3	-	-	-	-	-	-	-	-	-	-	-
Time	1 week	-	-	-	B	-	-	B	-	-	B	-
	2 weeks	-	-	-	A	-	-	A	-	-	A	-

Different capital letters represent significant differences in time regardless of diet ($p < 0.05$).

Table 6. Relative gene expression profiling of anterior intestine in gilthead seabream juveniles following an inflammatory insult after 2 weeks of feeding (experiment two). Data are the mean $\pm$ SEM ($n = 9$). All data values for each gene were in reference to the expression level of 0 h CTR fish.

		Relative mRNA Expression										
Trial 2	Diets	*il1-β*	*il-34*	*tlr1*	*cd8α*	*igm*	*hepc*	*hsp70*	*gpx*	*sod(mn)*	*muc2*	*muc13*
0 h	CTR	1.54 ± 0.47	1.08 ± 0.15	1.23 ± 0.34	1.31 ± 0.29	1.67 ± 0.50	3.17 ± 1.50	1.04 ± 0.16	1.67 ± 0.41	1.18 ± 0.20	1.93 ± 0.99	1.58 ± 0.58
	D1	1.61 ± 0.62	1.93 ± 0.37	1.84 ± 0.37	1.94 ± 0.42	7.39 ± 3.31	3.45 ± 1.04	1.40 ± 0.25	2.26 ± 0.33	2.25 ± 0.51	3.11 ± 0.68	1.89 ± 0.24
	D2	1.59 ± 0.47	1.43 ± 0.37	2.02 ± 0.65	2.44 ± 0.65	4.16 ± 1.53	3.43 ± 2.61	0.77 ± 0.27 *#	1.78 ± 0.70	1.02 ± 0.29	1.86 ± 0.60	1.59 ± 0.57
	D3	1.31 ± 0.42	1.77 ± 0.54	1.70 ± 0.44	2.09 ± 0.55	3.70 ± 1.58	1.49 ± 0.52	1.56 ± 0.77	1.92 ± 0.50	1.66 ± 0.65	2.19 ± 0.63	1.92 ± 0.69
24 h	CTR	0.98 ± 0.17	2.20 ± 0.36	2.19 ± 0.38	1.95 ± 0.50	6.18 ± 2.70	2.31 ± 0.83	1.41 ± 0.19 [a]	1.59 ± 0.61	1.22 ± 0.30	2.98 ± 0.52	1.71 ± 0.31
	D1	0.58 ± 0.22	0.85 ± 0.36	3.47 ± 1.06	0.80 ± 0.37	1.53 ± 0.87	1.77 ± 0.57	0.68 ± 0.22 [ab]	1.14 ± 0.36	1.27 ± 0.51	3.31 ± 1.19	1.13 ± 0.38
	D2	0.80 ± 0.26	1.75 ± 1.11	2.38 ± 0.59	1.31 ± 0.80	0.77 ± 0.24	1.25 ± 0.41	0.34 ± 0.14 [b*]	0.89 ± 0.32	0.62 ± 0.25	3.70 ± 2.22	0.94 ± 0.25
	D3	0.96 ± 0.41	1.80 ± 0.57	2.13 ± 0.29	1.95 ± 0.53	4.90 ± 4.01	1.77 ± 0.42	1.25 ± 0.22 [ab]	0.69 ± 0.20	0.98 ± 0.24	3.06 ± 0.77	2.83 ± 1.22
48 h	CTR	0.60 ± 0.07	1.49 ± 0.26	0.90 ± 0.14	2.11 ± 0.55	5.64 ± 1.59	3.70 ± 1.84	3.28 ± 1.47	1.86 ± 0.42	2.40 ± 0.51	2.27 ± 0.52	2.56 ± 0.87
	D1	0.51 ± 0.11	1.08 ± 0.28	1.42 ± 0.33	1.37 ± 0.29	1.11 ± 0.47	1.13 ± 0.34	0.83 ± 0.16	0.84 ± 0.20	0.81 ± 0.22	1.42 ± 0.42	1.02 ± 0.24
	D2	0.84 ± 0.21	1.35 ± 0.20	0.78 ± 0.10	2.51 ± 0.27	1.54 ± 0.34	3.20 ± 0.82	1.12 ± 0.2 [#]	1.07 ± 0.19	1.27 ± 0.18	2.60 ± 0.47	2.34 ± 0.48
	D3	1.94 ± 1.49	1.44 ± 0.38	1.00 ± 0.27	2.39 ± 1.14	2.59 ± 1.08	4.63 ± 2.31	1.50 ± 0.50	1.64 ± 0.20	1.46 ± 0.60	2.78 ± 0.78	1.75 ± 0.52
Two way-ANOVA		*il1-β*	*il-34*	*tlr1*	*cd8α*	*igm*	*hepc*	*hsp70*	*gpx*	*sod(mn)*	*muc2*	*muc13*
Sig.	Time	ns	ns	<0.001	ns	ns	ns	0.030	0.006	ns	ns	ns
	Diet	ns	ns	ns	ns	ns	ns	<0.001	ns	ns	ns	ns
	Time × Diet	ns	ns	ns	ns	ns	ns	0.028	ns	ns	ns	ns
Diet	CTR	-	-	-	-	-	-	-	-	-	-	-
	D1	-	-	-	-	-	-	-	-	-	-	-
	D2	-	-	-	-	-	-	-	-	-	-	-
	D3	-	-	-	-	-	-	-	-	-	-	-
Time	*0 h*	-	-	B	-	-	-	-	A	-	-	-
	24 h	-	-	A	-	-	-	-	B	-	-	-
	48 h	-	-	B	-	-	-	-	AB	-	-	-

Different superscript letters represent significant differences between diets within the same time ($p < 0.05$). Different superscript symbols represent significant differences in time within the same diet ($p < 0.05$). Different capital letters represent significant differences in time regardless of diet ($p < 0.05$).

3. Discussion

A main feature of *C. vulgaris* is its protein content and its balanced AA profile, making it a potential source of bioactive peptides. However, the presence of rigid cell walls limits the fish's ability to access and to utilise the different nutrients inside microalgae cells. In the present study, cell wall disruption was obtained through a combination of chemical and enzymatic processes and the protein fraction was hydrolysed using a serine protease. Protein hydrolysates seem more effective than either intact protein or free AA in different applications for nutrition [25,38]. The current study was devised using two different approaches. First, there was a 2-week feeding trial to evaluate the health status of the fish, aiming to develop future prophylactic strategies (experiment one). After 2 weeks of feeding, fish were subjected to an inflammatory insult to evaluate the inflammatory response (experiment two) and to better discriminate any immunomodulatory effect from the different dietary treatments.

The overall haematological profile from the health status experiment showed some changes, mainly exerted by *C. vulgaris* biomass and peptide-enriched extract supplemented diets (D1 and D2 diets). Fish fed diet D1 showed lower lymphocyte numbers (Table 2). Accordingly, in a previous experiment with poultry, where different preparations of *C. vulgaris* were used, animals fed a supplemented diet with 1% chlorella powder showed decreased lymphocyte numbers [39]. Nonetheless, fish fed D2 diet not only had comparable lymphocyte numbers to CTR, but also showed a higher neutrophil concentration (Table 2). These higher circulating myeloid cell numbers in the D2 group might be of relevance during early responses to infection. Bøgwald et al. [40] have shown that medium-size peptides (500–3000 Da) from cod muscle protein hydrolysate, stimulated in vivo respiratory burst activity in Atlantic salmon (*Salmo salar*) head-kidney leucocytes. In the present study, the peptide-enriched extract protein/peptide profile (Figure S1) is mainly composed of small to medium size particles (<1200 Da) [41]. Size and molecular weight (MW) seem to be particularly important for peptide immunomodulatory activities, with small- to medium-sized particles showing the highest activity [26,28,40,42]. However, an increased leucocyte response in fish fed the D2 diet did not translate into an improved plasma humoral parameters response (NO concentration, antiprotease and peroxidase activities) at 1 or 2 weeks (Figure 1A–C), although those values tended to increase in seabream fed D2 and D3. Accordingly, former studies conducted on Coho salmon (*Oncorhynchus kisutch*) and turbot (*Scophthalmus maximus*) did not show any significant impacts on several innate immune defence mechanisms, when fish were fed MPH supplemented diets [43,44]. Nonetheless, beneficial effects have been reported in different fish species [26]. Khosravi et al. [33] supplemented red seabream (*Pagrus major*) and olive flounder (*Paralichthys olivaceus*) feeds with 2% krill and tilapia protein hydrolysates and supplementation improved lysozyme activity and respiratory burst in both species. Protein hydrolysates were mainly composed of small- (<500 Da) to medium-sized peptides (500–5000 Da). Furthermore, diet D2 shows a higher Hb concentration than D1 and D3 fed fish. The extraction method employed in a *C. vulgaris* biomass to obtain the soluble extract (diet D2) might increase iron availability, since most of the intracellular iron is associated with soluble proteins and iron is an essential element for Hb production [45].

In the present study, when fish were subjected to an inflammatory insult (experiment two), an immune response after the stimulus was observed through the time-dependent response pattern of peripheral leucocytes, plasma and gut immune parameters. Peripheral cell dynamics were significantly changed at 24 h post-stimulus, translating into a sharp increase in circulating neutrophils and a significant decrease in lymphocytes (Table 4), indicating that cells were differentiating and being recruited to the site of inflammation. Also, Hb concentration increased (Table 3) in line with a higher metabolic expenditure due to the inflammatory response, and peroxidase activity showed a clear augmentation following inflammation (Figure 1E). Even though circulating neutrophil numbers tended to increase in D1, 2 and 3 dietary treatments at 48 h following inflammation (Table 4), it was not possible to ascertain a clear Chlorella whole-biomass or extracts effect, a fact that could be related to high intraspecific variability in response to the stimulus and that reinforces the need for further studies to unravel the potential of these extracts.

Hydrogen peroxide and oxygen radicals are physiologically generated within cellular compartments and their build-up leads to tissue oxidative stress and damage [46]. Free radical effects are controlled endogenously by antioxidant enzymes and non-enzymatic antioxidants and also by exogenous dietary antioxidants that prevent oxidative damage. Chlorella sp. contain several phytochemicals, namely carotenoids, chlorophyll, flavonoids and polyphenols, which exhibit antioxidant activities [47,48]. Earlier studies showed a significant increase in serum SOD activity in gibel carp fed diets containing 0.8–2.0% dry Chlorella powder [20]. Rahimnejad et al. [14] reported increased plasma CAT activity and total antioxidant capacity (TAC) in olive flounder fed diets with 5% and 10% defatted *C. vulgaris* meal. As with other microalgae species, the antioxidant potential of *C. vulgaris* has been mainly assessed on serum and liver, though information is still scarce at the intestinal level. The intestinal epithelium, a highly selective barrier between the animal and the external environment, is constantly exposed to dietary and environmental oxidants. Consequently, it is more prone to oxidative stress and damage, which can impact gut functionality and health [49,50]. The dietary effects of microalgae biomass inclusion have been previously assessed on the intestine of gilthead seabream. Fish were fed diets supplemented with 0.5, 0.75 and 1.5% *Nannochloropsis gaditana* biomass and no signs of nutritional modulation were found for intestinal SOD and CAT transcription [51]. In the present study, D2 fed fish showed higher gut LPO than CTR and D3 at the end of experiment one (Figure 3A), which could be related to the extraction method employed, since most of the pigments present in the *C. vulgaris* biomass are not present in the peptide-enriched extract, diminishing the availability of exogenous dietary antioxidants. As pigments are mostly hydrophobic, they are extracted alongside the lipid fraction present in the insoluble extract (Diet D3). Regarding the activities of key enzymes involved in intestinal redox homeostasis (CAT and SOD), these remained unchanged among experimental groups. Castro et al. [17] replaced 100% FM by *C. vulgaris* biomass in plant protein rich diets for seabass (*Dicentrarchus labrax*) and found no differences in intestinal LPO, tGSH and GSH levels between dietary treatments. However, they reported lower SOD activity and higher GSSG levels in microalgae-enriched diets, suggesting an increased risk for oxidative stress when fish are subjected to pro-oxidative conditions. Such conditions might arise during an inflammatory insult. However, in experiment two of the present study, lipid peroxidation increased at 24 and 48 h (Figure 3D) post-stimulus but to the same extent for all the dietary treatments. It could be hypothesised that fish fed the D2 diet were able to cope with acute inflammation in a similar manner as the other experimental groups, despite their higher intestinal oxidative state. In other studies, *C. vulgaris* powdered biomass has been found to counteract the pro-oxidative effects of arsenic induced toxicity in both the gills and the liver of tilapia [16]. Furthermore, Grammes et al. [51] reported that substituting FM by *C. vulgaris* in aquafeeds containing 20% soybean meal (SBM) is an effective strategy to counteract soybean meal-induced enteropathy (SBMIE) in Atlantic salmon. Likely, this was by maintaining the integrity of the intestinal epithelial barrier and therefore preventing innate immune response activation and ROS generation [52,53].

In the present study, anterior gut transcriptional changes were also evaluated to determine the effect of dietary treatments on the expression patterns of different structural (muc2 and muc13), antioxidant (hsp70; gpx and sod(mn)) and immune related genes (il1β; il34; tlr1; cd8α; igm and hepc). The transcriptomic approach employed was not able to ascertain a clear dietary modulation, at least for the great majority of genes under evaluation in both experiments one and two. However, after the inflammatory insult, the hsp70 gene was down regulated in the D2 fed group after 24 h compared to those fed CTRL (Table 6). Heat shock protein 70 (HSP70) maintains cell integrity and function, and it promotes cell survival under stressful conditions [54]. Leduc et al. [28] reported that genes involved in cellular damage response and repair were also under-expressed in seabass fed a mix of tilapia (TH) and shrimp (SH) protein hydrolysates (5% dry matter diet), mainly composed of low molecular weight peptides. In the same study, fish that were fed the SH alone showed up-regulation of intestinal immune-related genes. Although composed of small-sized peptides, TH did not show the same pattern of stimulation, following what was observed in the current work. According to the authors, the immune-stimulatory effect of the SH was due to low molecular weight peptides, but also to its origin and its degree of hydrolysis [28]. Bioactive peptides are inactive when they are part of the native protein sequence; and, after hydrolysis, bioactivity can be gained depending on specific AA sequences and the size of the newly formed peptides [25]. Nevertheless, in the present study, the observed down-regulation of hsp70 gene expression in the gut of seabream fed D2 suggests a certain degree of anti-stress and/or antioxidant properties from the *C. vulgaris* peptide-enriched extract, in line with that hypothesized above.

In summary, the *C. vulgaris* peptide-enriched extract tested in the present study seems to confer a dual modulatory effect at both peripheral (blood) and local (gut) levels. In particular, it drives the proliferation of circulating neutrophils in resting seabream, which could be of assistance to fight against opportunistic pathogens. Following an inflammatory insult, this peptide-enriched extract may protect the gut against stress, and it should be considered for further studies.

4. Materials and Methods

4.1. C. vulgaris Hydrolysates Production

C. vulgaris was supplied, as powder, by AllMicroalgae—Natural Products, SA (Pataias, Portugal). The *C. vulgaris* hydrolysates were produced by an acid pre-treatment followed by an enzymatic hydrolysis, using a previously optimised method [41]. Briefly, C. vulgaris (Table 7) was mixed with an acetic acid solution (2% in deionised water) in a ratio of microalgae:water of 1:3 (*w/v*). The mixture was incubated for 1 h at 50 °C and 125 rpm in an orbital shaker (ThermoFisher Scientific, Waltham, MA, USA, MaxQ™ 6000). Then, deionised water was added until microalgae:water ratio reached 1:10 and the pH was adjusted to 7.5. For the enzymatic hydrolysis, first, 5% cellulase was added and the mixture was incubated for 2 h at 50 °C and 125 rpm. Secondly, 3.9% subtilisin was added and the mixture was incubated for 2 h at 40 °C at 125 rpm. During the enzymatic hydrolysis, pH was constantly verified and adjusted to 7.5, mainly in the subtilisin hydrolysis step. To stop the hydrolysis reaction, the mixture was incubated at 90 °C for 10 min to inactivate the enzymes. The resulting solution was centrifuged at $5000 \times g$ for 20 min, and both the water-soluble peptide-enriched supernatant (Table 8) and the pellet were collected and freeze-dried for further analysis.

Table 7. Microalgae *Chlorella vulgaris* biomass composition (prior to extraction).

Nutrients	Quantity (g/100 g)
Crude Protein	52.2
Crude Fat	7.9
Carbohydrates	10.9
Fibers	15.5
Mineral matter	11.1
Moisture	2.4

Table 8. *Chlorella vulgaris* soluble extract protein concentration and in vitro bioactivities.

	Chlorella vulgaris **Soluble Extract**
% Protein	11.71 ± 1.75
Antioxidant activity (ORAC) (μmol TE/g of extract)	462.83 ± 39.97
Anti-hypertensive activity (iACE) (IC$_{50}$ μg protein mL^{-1})	$286.0 + 55.00$
Anti-diabetic activity (% of inhibition of α-Glucosidase enzyme in a solution with 30 mg mL^{-1} of soluble extract)	31.36 ± 3.90

4.2. Diet Composition

The trial comprised 4 isoproteic (50% protein in dry matter (DM)), isolipidic (17% fat in DM) and isoenergetic (23 kJ/g) dietary treatments. A fishmeal-based (FM), practical diet was used as a control (CTR), whereas three experimental diets based on CTR were further supplemented with a 2% inclusion of *C. vulgaris* powdered biomass (Diet D1); 0.1% inclusion of *C. vulgaris* peptide-enriched extract (Diet D2) and finally 0.1% inclusion of *C. vulgaris* insoluble residue (Diet D3) (Table 9). Diets were manufactured by SPAROS (Olhão, Portugal). All powder ingredients were initially mixed and ground (<200 micron) in a micropulverizer hammer mill (SH1, Hosokawa-Alpine, Germany). Subsequently, the oils were added to the powder mixtures, which were humidified with 25% water and agglomerated by a low-shear and a low-temperature extrusion process (ITALPLAST, Parma, Italy). The resulting pellets of 2.0 mm were dried in a convection oven for 4 h at 55 °C (OP 750-UF, LTE Scientifics, Oldham, UK). Diets were packed in sealed plastic buckets and shipped to the research site (CIIMAR, Matosinhos, Portugal), where they were stored in a temperature-controlled room.

Table 9. Ingredients and proximate composition of experimental diets.

Ingredients (%)	CTR	D1	D2	D3
Fishmeal Super Prime [1]	10.00	10.00	10.00	10.00
Fish gelatin [2]	2.00	2.00	2.00	2.00
Soy protein concentrate [3]	10.00	10.00	10.00	10.00
Wheat gluten [4]	7.00	7.00	7.00	7.00
Corn gluten [5]	15.00	15.00	15.00	15.00
Soybean meal [6]	20.00	20.00	20.00	20.00
Rapeseed meal [7]	5.25	5.25	5.25	5.25
Sunflower meal [8]	5.00	5.00	5.00	5.00
Wheat meal [9]	7.00	5.00	7.00	7.00
Fish oil [10]	4.90	4.90	4.90	4.90
Soybean oil [11]	9.10	9.10	9.10	9.10
Premix 1% [12]	1.00	1.00	1.00	1.00
Binder (Celatom—Diatomite) [13]	1.00	1.00	1.00	1.00
MAP (Monoammonium phosphate) [14]	1.50	1.50	1.50	1.50
L-Lysine [15]	1.00	1.00	1.00	1.00
L-Threonine [16]	0.10	0.10	0.10	0.10
DL-Methionine [17]	0.15	0.15	0.15	0.15
Chlorella whole biomass—Algafarm [18]	0.00	2.00	0.00	0.00
Chlorella—soluble fraction [19]	0.00	0.00	0.10	0.00
Chlorella—Insoluble residue [20]	0.00	0.00	0.00	0.10

[1] 66.3% CP, 11.5% CF, Pesquera Diamante, Peru; [2] 94% WEISHARDT, Slovakia; [3] 62.2% CP, 0.7% CF, Soycomil P, ADM, Netherlands; [4] 80.4% CP, 5.8% CF, VITAL, Roquette, France; [5] 61.2% CP, 5.2% CF, COPAM, Portugal; [6] Dehulled solvent extracted: 47.4% CP, 2.6% CF, Cargill, Spain; [7] Solvent extracted: 34.3% CP, 2.1% CF, Ribeiro e Sousa Lda, Portugal; [8] Solvent extracted: 29.1% CP, 1.8% CF, Ribeiro e Sousa Lda, Portugal; [9] 11.7% CP, 1.6% CF, Molisur, Spain; [10] 98.1% CF (16% EPA; 12% DHA), Sopropêche, France; [11] 98.6%, JC Coimbra, Portugal; [12] Vitamins (IU or mg/Kg diet): DL-alphatocopherol acetate, 100 mg; sodium menadione bisulphate, 25 mg; retinyl acetate, 20,000 IU; DL-cholecalciferol, 2000 IU; thiamine, 30 mg; riboflavin, 30 mg; pyridoxine, 20 mg; cyanocobalamin, 0.1 mg; nicotidin acid, 200 mg; folic acid, 15 mg; ascorbic acid, 1000 mg; inositol, 500 mg; biotin, 3 mg; calcium panthotenate, 100 mg; choline chloride, 1000 mg, betaine, 500 mg. Minerals (g or mg/kg diet): cobalt carbonate, 0.65 mg; copper sulphate, 9 mg; ferric sulphate, 6 mg; potassium iodide, 0.5 mg; manganese oxide, 9.6 mg; sodium selenite, 0.01 mg; zinc sulphate. 7.5 mg; sodium chloride, 400 mg; calcium carbonate, 1.86 g; excipient wheat middling's, Premix Lda, Portugal; [13] CELATOM FP1SL (diatomite), Angelo Coimbra S.A., Portugal; [14] Windmill AQUAPHOS (26% P), ALIPHOS, Netherlands; [15] 99% Lys, Ajinomoto EUROLYSINE S.A.S, France; [16] 98.5% Thr, Ajinomoto EUROLYSINE S.A.S, France; [17] 99% Met, Rodhimet NP99, ADISSEO, France; [18] *Chlorella vulgaris* lyophilized biomass, Allmicroalgae, Portugal; [19,20] *Chlorella vulgaris* aqueous and insoluble extracts, CBQF—Escola Superior de Biotecnologia, Universidade Católica Portuguesa, Portugal.

4.3. Bacterial Growth and Inoculum Preparation

Photobacterium damselae subsp. piscicida (Phdp), strain PP3, was used for the inflammatory insult. Bacteria were routinely cultured at 22 °C in tryptic soy broth (TSB) or tryptic soy agar (TSA) (both from BD Difco™, Franklin Lakes, NJ, USA) supplemented with NaCl to a final concentration of 1% (w/v) (TSB-1 and TSA-1, respectively) and stored at $-80\ ^\circ$C in TSB-1 supplemented with 15% (v/v) glycerol. To prepare the inoculum for injection into the fish peritoneal cavities, stocked bacteria were cultured for 48 h at 22 $^\circ$C on TSA-1. Afterwards, exponentially growing bacteria were collected and resuspended in sterile HBSS and adjusted against its growth curve to 1×10^7 colony forming units (cfu) mL^{-1}. Plating serial dilutions of the suspensions onto TSA-1 plates and counting the number of cfu following incubation at 22 $^\circ$C confirmed bacterial concentration of the inocula. Bacteria were then killed by heat at 70 $^\circ$C for 10 min. Loss of bacterial viability following heat exposure was confirmed by plating resulting cultures on TSA-1 plates and failing to see any bacterial growth.

4.4. Fish Rearing Conditions and Feeding Scheme

The experiment was carried out in compliance with the Guidelines of the European Union Council (Directive 2010/63/EU) and Portuguese legislation for the use of laboratory animals at CIIMAR aquaculture and animal experimentation facilities in Matosinhos, Portugal. The protocol was approved by the CIIMAR Animal Welfare Committee in 29/04/2020 with the reference 0421/000/000/2020 from Direção Geral de Alimentação e Veterinária (DGAV). Seawater flow was kept at 4 L min^{-1} (mean temperature 22.4 $\pm$ 1 $^\circ$C; mean salinity 35.2 $\pm$ 0.7 ‰) in a recirculation system with aeration (mean dissolved oxygen above 6 mg L^{-1}). Water quality parameters were monitored daily and adjusted when necessary. Mortality was monitored daily. Diets were randomly assigned to triplicate groups of 97 fish/tank (IBW: 33.4 $\pm$ 4.1 g) that were fed to satiation three times a day for 2 weeks starting at a 1.5% biomass.

4.5. Experimental Procedures

To examine the influence that *C. vulgaris* biomass and protein-rich extract supplementation may have on the health status (trial 1) and the inflammatory response against bacteria (inactivated Phdp i.p. injection; trial 2), samples of blood and gut were collected at 1 and 2 weeks (Trial 1) and after 2 weeks of feeding at 0 h, 24 h and 48 h post-injection (Trial 2).

4.5.1. Health Status (Experiment One)

After 1 and 2 weeks, 12 fish/treatment were weighed and sampled for tissues (blood, head-kidney, liver and gut), after being sacrificed with a 2-phenoxyethanol lethal dose (0.5 mL L^{-1}) [55]. Blood was collected from the caudal vein using heparinised syringes and centrifuged at $10,000\times g$ for 10 min at 4 $^\circ$C to obtain plasma samples. Plasma and tissue samples were immediately frozen in liquid nitrogen and stored at $-80\ ^\circ$C until further analysis.

4.5.2. Inflammatory Response (Experiment Two)

At 2 weeks, 24 fish/treatment were subjected to an inflammatory insult by intraperitoneal (i.p.) injection of heat-inactivated Phdp (see Section 2.2) and immediately transferred to a similar recirculation system in triplicates. After 24 and 48 h post-injection (time-course), 9 fish/treatment were sampled as described above.

4.6. Haematological Procedures

The haematological profile consisted of total white (WBC) and red (RBC) blood cells counts. To determine WBC and RBC concentration, whole blood was diluted 1/20 and 1/200, respectively, in HBSS with heparin (30 U mL^{-1}) and cell counts were done in a Neubauer chamber. Blood smears were prepared from peripheral blood, air-dried and stained with Wright's stain (Haemacolor; Merck, Darmstadt, Germany), after fixation for 1 min with formol–ethanol (10% formaldehyde in ethanol). Neutrophils were labelled by detecting peroxidase activity revealed by Antonow's technique described in Afonso et al. [56].

The slides were examined under oil immersion (1000×), and at least 200 leucocytes were counted and classified as thrombocytes, lymphocytes, monocytes and neutrophils. The relative percentage and absolute value ($\times 10^4$ mL^{-1}) of each cell type was calculated.

4.7. Innate Humoral Parameters

4.7.1. Antiprotease Activity

The antiprotease activity was determined as described by Ellis et al. [57], with some modifications. Briefly, 10 µL of plasma were incubated with the same volume of trypsin solution (5 mg mL^{-1} in NaHCO$_3$, 5 mg mL^{-1}, pH 8.3) for 10 min at 22 °C. After incubation, 100 µL of phosphate buffer (NaH$_2$PO$_4$, 13.9 mg mL^{-1}, pH 7.0) and 125 µL of azocasein solution (20 mg mL^{-1} in NaHCO$_3$, 5 mg mL^{-1}, pH 8.3) were added and incubated for 1 h at 22 °C. Finally, 250 µL of trichloroacetic acid were added to the reaction mixture and incubated for 30 min at 22 °C. The mixture was centrifuged at 10,000× g for 5 min at room temperature. Afterwards, 100 µL of the supernatant was transferred to a 96 well-plate and mixed with 100 µL of NaOH (40 mg mL^{-1}). The OD was read at 450 nm in a Synergy HT microplate reader (Biotek, Winooski, VT, USA). Phosphate buffer instead of plasma and trypsin served as blank, whereas the reference sample was phosphate buffer instead of plasma. The sample inhibition percentage of trypsin activity was calculated as follows: 100 − ((sample absorbance/Reference absorbance) × 100). All analyses were conducted in duplicates.

4.7.2. Peroxidase Activity

Total peroxidase activity in plasma and intestine was measured, following the procedure described by Quade and Roth [58]. Briefly, 10 µL of plasma and 5 µL of intestine homogenate were diluted with 140 and 145 µL, respectively, of HBSS without Ca^{2+} and Mg^{2+} in 96-well plates. Then, 50 µL of 20 mM 3,3′,5,5′-tetramethylbenzidine hydrochloride (TMB; Sigma-Aldrich®, Merck, Darmstadt, Germany) and 50 µL of 5 mM H$_2$O$_2$ were added to the wells. The reaction was stopped after 2 min by adding 50 µL of H$_2$SO$_4$ (2 M) and the optical density (OD) was read at 450 nm in a Synergy HT microplate reader (Biotek, Winooski, VT, USA). Wells without plasma or mucus were used as blanks. The peroxidase activity (U mL^{-1} tissue) was determined, defining that one unit of peroxidase produces an absorbance change of 1 OD.

4.7.3. Nitric Oxide (NO) Production

NO production was measured in plasma (1:10 sample dilution) and intestine (1:5 sample dilution) samples. Total nitrite and nitrate concentrations in the sample were assessed using the Nitrite/Nitrate colorimetric method kit (Roche, Basel, Switzerland) adapted to microplates. Nitrite concentration was calculated by comparison with a sodium nitrite standard curve. Since nitrite and nitrate are endogenously produced as oxidative metabolites of the NO molecule, these compounds are considered as indicative of NO production.

4.8. Analysis of Oxidative Stress Biomarkers

Intestine samples were homogenised (1:10) in phosphate buffer 0.1 M (pH 7.4), using Precellys evolution tissue lyser homogenizer (Bertin Instruments, Montigny-le-Bretonneux, France).

4.8.1. Lipid Peroxidation (LPO)

One aliquot of tissue homogenate was used to determine the extent of endogenous LPO by measuring thiobarbituric acid-reactive species (TBARS) as suggested by Bird and Draper [59]. To prevent artifactual lipid peroxidation, butylhydroxytoluene (BHT 0.2 mM) was added to the aliquot. Briefly, 1 mL of 100% trichloroacetic acid and 1 mL of 0.73% thiobarbituric acid solution (in Tris–HCl 60 mM pH 7.4 with DTPA 0.1 mM) were added to 0.2 mL of intestine homogenate. After incubation at 100 °C for 60 min, the solution was centrifuged at 12,000× g for 5 min and LPO levels were determined at 535 nm.

4.8.2. Total Protein Quantification

The remaining tissue homogenate was centrifuged for 20 min at 12,000 rpm (4 °C) to obtain the post-mitochondrial supernatant fraction (PMS). Total proteins in homogenates were measured by using Pierce™ BCA Protein Assay Kit, as described by the manufacturer (ThermoFisher Scientific, Waltham, MA, USA).

4.8.3. Catalase (CAT)

CAT activity was determined in PMS by measuring substrate (H_2O_2) consumption at 240 nm according to Claiborne [60] adapted to microplate. Briefly, in a microplate well, 0.140 mL of phosphate buffer (0.05 M pH 7.0) and a 0.150 mL H_2O_2 solution (30 mM in phosphate buffer 0.05 M pH 7.0) were added to 0.01 mL of intestine PMS (0.7 mg mL^{-1} total protein). Enzymatic activity was determined in a microplate reader (BioTek Synergy HT, Winooski, VT, USA), reading the optical density at 240 nm for 2 min every 15 s interval.

4.8.4. Superoxide Dismutase (SOD)

SOD activity was measured according to Flohé and Otting [61], adapted to microplate by Lima, et al. [62]. Briefly, in a microplate well, 0.2 mL of the reaction solution [1 part xanthine solution 0.7 mM (in NaOH 1 mM) and 10 parts cytochrome c solution 0.03 mM (in phosphate buffer 50 mM pH 7.8 with 1 mM Na-EDTA)] was added to 0.05 mL of intestine PMS (0.25 mg mL^{-1} total protein). Optical density was measured at 550 nm in a microplate reader (BioTek Synergy HT, Winooski, VT, USA) every 20 s interval for 3 min at 25 °C.

4.9. Gene Expression

RNA isolation from target tissue (anterior gut) and cDNA synthesis was conducted with NZY Total RNA Isolation kit and NZY first-strand cDNA synthesis kit (NZYTech, Lisbon, Portugal), following manufacturer's specifications. Real-time quantitative PCR was carried out on a CFX384 Touch Real-Time PCR system (Bio-Rad Laboratories, Hercules, CA, USA). Genes comprised in the assay were selected for their involvement in gut integrity, health and immunity (Table 10). Specific primer pair sequences are listed in Table S1. Controls of general PCR performance were included on each array. Briefly, RT reactions were diluted to obtain the equivalent concentration of 20 ng of total input RNA which were used in a 10 μL volume for each PCR reaction. PCR wells contained a 2× SYBR Green Master Mix (Bio-Rad Laboratories, Hercules, CA, USA) and specific primers were used to obtain amplicons 50–250 bp in length. The program used for PCR amplification included an initial denaturation step at 95 °C for 10 min, followed by 40 cycles of 95 °C denaturation for 15 s, with primer annealing and extension temperature (Table S1) for 1 min. The efficiency of PCR reactions was always higher than 90%, and negative controls without sample templates were routinely performed for each primer set. The specificity of reactions was verified by analysis of melting curves (ramping rates of 0.5 °C/10 s over a temperature range of 55–95 °C). Fluorescence data acquired during the PCR extension phase were normalised using the Pfaffl [63] method. The geometric mean of two carefully selected housekeeping genes (elongation factor 1-α (ef1α) and ribosomal protein S18 (rps18)) was used as the normalisation factor to normalise the expression of target genes. For comparing the mRNA expression level of each gene in a given dietary treatment, all data values were in reference to the expression level of CTR fish.

Table 10. PCR-array layout for gene expression profiling of anterior gut in sea bream.

Function	Gene	Symbol	Accession Number
Intestinal epithelium protection	Mucin 2	*muc2*	JQ277710
	Mucin 13	*muc13*	JQ277713
Cytokines	Interleukin 1 beta	*il1b*	AJ277166.2
	Interleukin 34	*Il34*	JX976629.1
Pattern recognition receptors	Toll like receptor 1	*tlr1*	KF857322
Cell markers	CD8 alpha	*cd8α*	AJ878605
Antibodies	Immunoglobulin M	*igm*	AM493677
Antimicrobial defence/Iron recycling	Hepcidin	*hepc*	EF625901
Oxidative stress defences	Heat-shock protein 70	*hsp70*	DQ524995.1
	Glutathione peroxidase	*gpx*	DQ524992
	Manganese superoxide dismutase	*Sod(mn)*	JQ308833
Reference genes	Elongation factor 1α	*ef1α*	AF184170
	Ribosomal protein 18S	*rps18*	AM490061

4.10. Data Analysis

All results are expressed as mean $\pm$ standard error (mean $\pm$ SE). Residuals were tested for normality (Shapiro–Wilk's test) and homogeneity of variance (Levene's test). When residuals did not meet the assumptions, data was transformed by a Log10 or square root transformation. For gene expression data, a log2 transformation was applied to all expression values. Two-way ANOVAs were performed in data arising from both trials one and two, with "dietary treatment and time" as the fixed effects. Analysis of variance was followed by Tukey post-hoc tests. All statistical analyses were performed using the computer package SPSS 26 for WINDOWS. The level of significance used was $p \leq 0.05$ for all statistical tests.

Supplementary Materials: The following supporting information can be downloaded at: https://www.mdpi.com/article/10.3390/md20070407/s1, Table S1. Relative gene expression profiling of anterior intestine in gilthead seabream juveniles fed experimental diets.; Figure S1. Protein/peptide profile of *C. vulgaris* hydrolysate, showing the main molecular weight ranges, the area of the main peak, and the localization of all the 42 identified peaks.

Author Contributions: Conceptualization, B.R., J.D., L.C., E.M. and B.C.; data curation, B.R.; formal analysis, B.R. and L.R.-P.; funding acquisition, J.D., L.C. and B.C.; investigation, B.R., L.R.-P. and S.A.C.; project administration, J.D. and B.C.; resources, M.P., J.L.d.S., J.D., E.M. and B.C.; supervision, J.D., L.C. and B.C.; writing—original draft, B.R.; writing—review and editing, L.R.-P., S.A.C., M.P., J.L.d.S., J.D., L.C., E.M. and B.C. All authors have read and agreed to the published version of the manuscript.

Funding: This work was funded by Compete 2020, Lisboa 2020, Algarve 2020, Portugal 2020, and the European Union through FEDER in the framework of VALORMAR project (POCI-01-0247-FEDER-024517) and by national funds through the Foundation for Science and Technology (FCT) within the scope of UIDB/50016/2020, UIDB/04423/2020, and UIDP/04423/2020. The views expressed in this work are the sole responsibility of the authors. B. Reis was supported by FCT, Soja de Portugal, SA, and Sparos Lda., through the grant PD/BDE/129262/2017. S.A. Cunha and B. Costas were supported by FCT, through grants SFRH/BD/144155/2019 and 2020.00290.CEECIND, respectively.

Institutional Review Board Statement: The experiment was carried out in compliance with the Guidelines of the European Union Council (Directive 2010/63/EU) and Portuguese legislation for the use of laboratory animals. CIIMAR facilities and their staff are certified to house and to conduct experiments with live animals (Group-C licences by the Direção Geral de Alimentação e Veterinária (DGAV), Ministério da Agricultura, Florestas e Desenvolvimento Rural, Portugal). The protocol was approved by the CIIMAR Animal Welfare Committee in 29/04/2020 with the reference 0421/000/000/2020 from DGAV.

Informed Consent Statement: Not applicable.

Data Availability Statement: Not applicable.

Conflicts of Interest: The authors declare that they have no known competing financial interests or personal relationships that could have appeared to influence the work reported in this paper.

References

1. Meena, D.K.; Das, P.; Kumar, S.; Mandal, S.C.; Prusty, A.K.; Singh, S.K.; Akhtar, M.S.; Behera, B.K.; Kumar, K.; Pal, A.K.; et al. Beta-glucan: An ideal immunostimulant in aquaculture (a review). *Fish Physiol. Biochem.* **2013**, *39*, 431–457. [CrossRef] [PubMed]
2. World Health Organization; Food and Agriculture Organization of the United Nations; International Office of Epizootics. *Report of a Joint FAO/OIE/WHO Expert Consultation on Antimicrobial Use in Aquaculture and Antimicrobial Resistance, Seoul, Republic of Korea, 13–16 June 2006*; World Health Organization: Geneva, Switzerland, 2006.
3. Credence Research. Algae Products Market by Type (Spirulina, Chlorella, Astaxanthin, Beta Carotene, Hydrocolloids), By Source (Brown, Blue—Green, Green, Red, Others), By Application (Nutraceuticals, Food & Feed Supplements, Pharmaceuticals, Paints & Colorants, Chemicals, Fuels, Others)—Growth, Share, Opportunities & Competitive Analysis, 2019–2027. Available online: https://www.credenceresearch.com/report/algae-products-market (accessed on 20 February 2021).
4. Ahmad, M.T.; Shariff, M.; Yusoff, F.M.; Goh, Y.M.; Banerjee, S. Applications of microalga *Chlorella vulgaris* in aquaculture. *Rev. Aquac.* **2020**, *12*, 328–346. [CrossRef]
5. Ru, I.T.K.; Sung, Y.Y.; Jusoh, M.; Wahid, M.E.A.; Nagappan, T. *Chlorella vulgaris*: A perspective on its potential for combining high biomass with high value bioproducts. *Appl. Phycol.* **2020**, *1*, 2–11. [CrossRef]
6. Cunha, S.A.; Pintado, M.E. Bioactive peptides derived from marine sources: Biological and functional properties. *Trends Food Sci. Technol.* **2022**, *119*, 348–370. [CrossRef]
7. Tomaselli, L. The Microalgal Cell. In *Handbook of Microalgal Culture: Biotechnology and Applied Phycology*; Richmond, A., Ed.; Blackwell Science Ltd.: Oxford, UK, 2004.
8. Borowitzka, M.A. Biology of Microalgae. In *Microalgae in Health and Disease Prevention*; Levine, I., Fleurence, J., Eds.; Academic Press: London, UK, 2018; pp. 23–72.
9. Plaza, M.; Herrero, M.; Cifuentes, A.; Ibáñez, E. Innovative Natural Functional Ingredients from Microalgae. *J. Agric. Food Chem.* **2009**, *57*, 7159–7170. [CrossRef]
10. Cuellar-Bermudez, S.P.; Aguilar-Hernandez, I.; Cardenas-Chavez, D.L.; Ornelas-Soto, N.; Romero-Ogawa, M.A.; Parra-Saldivar, R. Extraction and purification of high-value metabolites from microalgae: Essential lipids, astaxanthin and phycobiliproteins. *Microb. Biotechnol.* **2015**, *8*, 190–209. [CrossRef]
11. Rahman, M.M.; Khosravi, S.; Chang, K.H.; Lee, S.-M. Effects of Dietary Inclusion of Astaxanthin on Growth, Muscle Pigmentation and Antioxidant Capacity of Juvenile Rainbow Trout (*Oncorhynchus mykiss*). *Prev. Nutr. Food Sci.* **2016**, *21*, 281–288. [CrossRef]
12. Chew, B.P.; Park, J.S. Carotenoid action on the immune response. *J. Nutr.* **2004**, *134*, 257s–261s. [CrossRef]
13. Bai, S.; Koo, J.-W.; Kim, K.; Kim, S.-G. Effects of Chlorella powder as a feed additive on growth performance in juvenile Korean rockfish, *Sebastes schlegeli* (Hilgendorf). *Aquac. Res.* **2001**, *32*, 92–98. [CrossRef]
14. Rahimnejad, S.; Lee, S.-M.; Park, H.-G.; Choi, J. Effects of Dietary Inclusion of *Chlorella vulgaris* on Growth, Blood Biochemical Parameters, and Antioxidant Enzyme Activity in Olive Flounder, Paralichthys olivaceus. *J. World Aquac. Soc.* **2017**, *48*, 103–112. [CrossRef]
15. Pakravan, S.; Akbarzadeh, A.; Sajjadi, M.M.; Hajimoradloo, A.; Noori, F. *Chlorella vulgaris* meal improved growth performance, digestive enzyme activities, fatty acid composition and tolerance of hypoxia and ammonia stress in juvenile Pacific white shrimp *Litopenaeus vannamei*. *Aquac. Nutr.* **2018**, *24*, 594–604. [CrossRef]
16. Zahran, E.; Risha, E. Modulatory role of dietary *Chlorella vulgaris* powder against arsenic-induced immunotoxicity and oxidative stress in Nile tilapia (*Oreochromis niloticus*). *Fish Shellfish Immunol.* **2014**, *41*, 654–662. [CrossRef]
17. Castro, C.; Coutinho, F.; Iglesias, P.; Oliva-Teles, A.; Couto, A. *Chlorella sp.* and *Nannochloropsis sp.* Inclusion in Plant-Based Diets Modulate the Intestine and Liver Antioxidant Mechanisms of European Sea Bass Juveniles. *Front. Vet. Sci.* **2020**, *7*, 607575. [CrossRef]
18. Zhang, Q.; Qiu, M.; Xu, W.; Gao, Z.; Shao, R.; Qi, Z. Effects of Dietary Administration of Chlorella on the Immune Status of Gibel Carp, *Carassius Auratus Gibelio*. *Ital. J. Anim. Sci.* **2014**, *13*, 3168. [CrossRef]
19. Lupatsch, I.; Blake, C. Algae alternative: Chlorella studied as protein source in tilapia feeds. *Glob. Aquac. Advocate* **2013**, *16*, 78–79.
20. Xu, W.; Gao, Z.; Qi, Z.; Qiu, M.; Peng, J.; Shao, R. Effect of Dietary Chlorella on the Growth Performance and Physiological Parameters of Gibel carp, *Carassius auratus gibelio*. *Turk. J. Fish. Aquat. Sci.* **2014**, *14*, 53–57. [CrossRef]
21. Tibbetts, S.M.; Mann, J.; Dumas, A. Apparent digestibility of nutrients, energy, essential amino acids and fatty acids of juvenile Atlantic salmon (*Salmo salar* L.) diets containing whole-cell or cell-ruptured *Chlorella vulgaris* meals at five dietary inclusion levels. *Aquaculture* **2017**, *481*, 25–39. [CrossRef]
22. Teuling, E.; Wierenga, P.A.; Agboola, J.O.; Gruppen, H.; Schrama, J.W. Cell wall disruption increases bioavailability of *Nannochloropsis gaditana* nutrients for juvenile Nile tilapia (*Oreochromis niloticus*). *Aquaculture* **2019**, *499*, 269–282. [CrossRef]
23. Valente, L.M.P.; Batista, S.; Ribeiro, C.; Pereira, R.; Oliveira, B.; Garrido, I.; Baião, L.F.; Tulli, F.; Messina, M.; Pierre, R.; et al. Physical processing or supplementation of feeds with phytogenic compounds, alginate oligosaccharide or nucleotides as methods

to improve the utilization of *Gracilaria gracilis* by juvenile European seabass (*Dicentrarchus labrax*). *Aquaculture* **2021**, *530*, 735914. [CrossRef]

24. Wang, X.; Zhang, X. Optimal extraction and hydrolysis of *Chlorella pyrenoidosa* proteins. *Bioresour. Technol.* **2012**, *126*, 307–313. [CrossRef]

25. Kose, A.; Oncel, S.S. Properties of microalgal enzymatic protein hydrolysates: Biochemical composition, protein distribution and FTIR characteristics. *Biotechnol. Rep.* **2015**, *6*, 137–143. [CrossRef] [PubMed]

26. Siddik, M.A.B.; Howieson, J.; Fotedar, R.; Partridge, G.J. Enzymatic fish protein hydrolysates in finfish aquaculture: A review. *Rev. Aquac.* **2021**, *13*, 406–430. [CrossRef]

27. Kotzamanis, Y.P.; Gisbert, E.; Gatesoupe, F.J.; Zambonino Infante, J.; Cahu, C. Effects of different dietary levels of fish protein hydrolysates on growth, digestive enzymes, gut microbiota, and resistance to *Vibrio anguillarum* in European sea bass (*Dicentrarchus labrax*) larvae. *Comp. Biochem. Physiol. A Mol. Integr. Physiol.* **2007**, *147*, 205–214. [CrossRef] [PubMed]

28. Leduc, A.; Zatylny-Gaudin, C.; Robert, M.; Corre, E.; Corguille, G.L.; Castel, H.; Lefevre-Scelles, A.; Fournier, V.; Gisbert, E.; Andree, K.B.; et al. Dietary aquaculture by-product hydrolysates: Impact on the transcriptomic response of the intestinal mucosa of European seabass (*Dicentrarchus labrax*) fed low fish meal diets. *BMC Genomics* **2018**, *19*, 396. [CrossRef]

29. Siddik, M.A.B.; Howieson, J.; Fotedar, R. Beneficial effects of tuna hydrolysate in poultry by-product meal diets on growth, immune response, intestinal health and disease resistance to *Vibrio harveyi* in juvenile barramundi, *Lates calcarifer*. *Fish Shellfish Immunol.* **2019**, *89*, 61–70. [CrossRef]

30. Zheng, K.; Xu, T.; Qian, C.; Liang, M.; Wang, X. Effect of low molecular weight fish protein hydrolysate on growth performance and IGF-I expression in Japanese flounder (*Paralichthys olivaceus*) fed high plant protein diets. *Aquac. Nutr.* **2014**, *20*, 372–380. [CrossRef]

31. Ospina-Salazar, G.H.; Ríos-Durán, M.G.; Toledo-Cuevas, E.M.; Martínez-Palacios, C.A. The effects of fish hydrolysate and soy protein isolate on the growth performance, body composition and digestibility of juvenile pike silverside, *Chirostoma estor*. *Anim. Feed Sci. Technol.* **2016**, *220*, 168–179. [CrossRef]

32. Xu, H.; Mu, Y.; Zhang, Y.; Li, J.; Liang, M.; Zheng, K.; Wei, Y. Graded levels of fish protein hydrolysate in high plant diets for turbot (*Scophthalmus maximus*): Effects on growth performance and lipid accumulation. *Aquaculture* **2016**, *454*, 140–147. [CrossRef]

33. Khosravi, S.; Bui, H.T.D.; Rahimnejad, S.; Herault, M.; Fournier, V.; Kim, S.-S.; Jeong, J.-B.; Lee, K.-J. Dietary supplementation of marine protein hydrolysates in fish-meal based diets for red sea bream (*Pagrus major*) and olive flounder (*Paralichthys olivaceus*). *Aquaculture* **2015**, *435*, 371–376. [CrossRef]

34. Bui, H.T.D.; Khosravi, S.; Fournier, V.; Herault, M.; Lee, K.-J. Growth performance, feed utilization, innate immunity, digestibility and disease resistance of juvenile red seabream (*Pagrus major*) fed diets supplemented with protein hydrolysates. *Aquaculture* **2014**, *418–419*, 11–16. [CrossRef]

35. Chaklader, M.R.; Fotedar, R.; Howieson, J.; Siddik, M.A.B.; Foysal, M.J. The ameliorative effects of various fish protein hydrolysates in poultry by-product meal based diets on muscle quality, serum biochemistry and immunity in juvenile barramundi, *Lates calcarifer*. *Fish Shellfish Immunol.* **2020**, *104*, 567–578. [CrossRef]

36. Sedighi, M.; Jalili, H.; Ranaei-Siadat, S.-O.; Amrane, A. Potential Health Effects of Enzymatic Protein Hydrolysates from *Chlorella vulgaris*. *Appl. Food Biotechnol.* **2016**, *3*, 160–169. [CrossRef]

37. Sheih, I.C.; Wu, T.-K.; Fang, T.J. Antioxidant properties of a new antioxidative peptide from algae protein waste hydrolysate in different oxidation systems. *Bioresour. Technol.* **2009**, *100*, 3419–3425. [CrossRef]

38. Clemente, A.; Vioque, J.; Sánchez-Vioque, R.; Pedroche, J.; Bautista, J.; Millán, F. Protein quality of chickpea (*Cicer arietinum* L.) protein hydrolysates. *Food Chem.* **1999**, *67*, 269–274. [CrossRef]

39. Kang, H.K.; Salim, H.M.; Akter, N.; Kim, D.W.; Kim, J.H.; Bang, H.T.; Kim, M.J.; Na, J.C.; Hwangbo, J.; Choi, H.C.; et al. Effect of various forms of dietary Chlorella supplementation on growth performance, immune characteristics, and intestinal microflora population of broiler chickens. *J. Appl. Poult. Res.* **2013**, *22*, 100–108. [CrossRef]

40. Bøgwald, J.; Dalmo, R.O.Y.; McQueen Leifson, R.; Stenberg, E.; Gildberg, A. The stimulatory effect of a muscle protein hydrolysate from Atlantic cod, *Gadus morhua* L., on Atlantic salmon, *Salmo salar* L.; head kidney leucocytes. *Fish Shellfish Immunol.* **1996**, *6*, 3–16. [CrossRef]

41. Cunha, S.A.; Coscueta, E.R.; Nova, P.; Silva, J.L.; Pintado, M.M. Bioactive Hydrolysates from Chlorella vulgaris: Optimal Process and Bioactive Properties. *Molecules* **2022**, *27*, 2505. [CrossRef]

42. Gildberg, A.; Bøgwald, J.; Johansen, A.; Stenberg, E. Isolation of acid peptide fractions from a fish protein hydrolysate with strong stimulatory effect on atlantic salmon (*Salmo salar*) head kidney leucocytes. *Comp. Biochem. Physiol. B Biochem. Mol. Biol.* **1996**, *114*, 97–101. [CrossRef]

43. Murray, A.L.; Pascho, R.J.; Alcorn, S.W.; Fairgrieve, W.T.; Shearer, K.D.; Roley, D. Effects of various feed supplements containing fish protein hydrolysate or fish processing by-products on the innate immune functions of juvenile coho salmon (*Oncorhynchus kisutch*). *Aquaculture* **2003**, *220*, 643–653. [CrossRef]

44. Zheng, K.; Liang, M.; Yao, H.; Wang, J.; Chang, Q. Effect of size-fractionated fish protein hydrolysate on growth and feed utilization of turbot (*Scophthalmus maximus* L.). *Aquac. Res.* **2013**, *44*, 895–902. [CrossRef]

45. Botebol, H.; Lesuisse, E.; Šuták, R.; Six, C.; Lozano, J.-C.; Schatt, P.; Vergé, V.; Kirilovsky, A.; Morrissey, J.; Léger, T.; et al. Central role for ferritin in the day/night regulation of iron homeostasis in marine phytoplankton. *Proc. Natl. Acad. Sci. USA* **2015**, *112*, 14652. [CrossRef] [PubMed]

46. Dirks, R.C.; Faiman, M.D.; Huyser, E.S. The role of lipid, free radical initiator, and oxygen on the kinetics of lipid peroxidation. *Toxicol. Appl. Pharmacol.* **1982**, *63*, 21–28. [CrossRef]

47. Shibata, S.; Natori, Y.; Nishihara, T.; Tomisaka, K.; Matsumoto, K.; Sansawa, H.; Nguyen, V.C. Antioxidant and anti-cataract effects of *Chlorella* on rats with streptozotocin-induced diabetes. *J. Nutr. Sci. Vitaminol.* **2003**, *49*, 334–339. [CrossRef] [PubMed]

48. Wang, H.-M.; Pan, J.-L.; Chen, C.-Y.; Chiu, C.-C.; Yang, M.-H.; Chang, H.-W.; Chang, J.-S. Identification of anti-lung cancer extract from *Chlorella vulgaris* C-C by antioxidant property using supercritical carbon dioxide extraction. *Process Biochem.* **2010**, *45*, 1865–1872. [CrossRef]

49. Circu, M.L.; Aw, T.Y. Intestinal redox biology and oxidative stress. *Semin. Cell Dev. Biol.* **2012**, *23*, 729–737. [CrossRef]

50. Yu, G.; Liu, Y.; Ou, W.; Dai, J.; Ai, Q.; Zhang, W.; Mai, K.; Zhang, Y. The protective role of daidzein in intestinal health of turbot (*Scophthalmus maximus* L.) fed soybean meal-based diets. *Sci. Rep.* **2021**, *11*, 3352. [CrossRef]

51. Jorge, S.S.; Enes, P.; Serra, C.R.; Castro, C.; Iglesias, P.; Oliva Teles, A.; Couto, A. Short-term supplementation of gilthead seabream (*Sparus aurata*) diets with *Nannochloropsis gaditana* modulates intestinal microbiota without affecting intestinal morphology and function. *Aquac. Nutr.* **2019**, *25*, 1388–1398. [CrossRef]

52. Grammes, F.; Reveco, F.E.; Romarheim, O.H.; Landsverk, T.; Mydland, L.T.; Øverland, M. *Candida utilis* and *Chlorella vulgaris* Counteract Intestinal Inflammation in Atlantic Salmon (*Salmo salar* L.). *PLoS ONE* **2013**, *8*, e83213. [CrossRef]

53. Bravo-Tello, K.; Ehrenfeld, N.; Solís, C.J.; Ulloa, P.E.; Hedrera, M.; Pizarro-Guajardo, M.; Paredes-Sabja, D.; Feijóo, C.G. Effect of microalgae on intestinal inflammation triggered by soybean meal and bacterial infection in zebrafish. *PLoS ONE* **2017**, *12*, e0187696. [CrossRef]

54. Silver, J.T.; Noble, E.G. Regulation of survival gene hsp70. *Cell Stress Chaperones* **2012**, *17*, 1–9. [CrossRef]

55. Mylonas, C.C.; Cardinaletti, G.; Sigelaki, I.; Polzonetti-Magni, A. Comparative efficacy of clove oil and 2-phenoxyethanol as anesthetics in the aquaculture of European sea bass (*Dicentrarchus labrax*) and gilthead sea bream (*Sparus aurata*) at different temperatures. *Aquaculture* **2005**, *246*, 467–481. [CrossRef]

56. Afonso, A.; Ellis, A.E.; Silva, M.T. The leucocyte population of the unstimulated peritoneal cavity of rainbow trout (*Oncorhynchus mykiss*). *Fish Shellfish Immunol.* **1997**, *7*, 335–348. [CrossRef]

57. Ellis, A.E.; Cavaco, A.; Petrie, A.; Lockhart, K.; Snow, M.; Collet, B. Histology, immunocytochemistry and qRT PCR analysis of Atlantic salmon, *Salmo salar* L.; post-smolts following infection with infectious pancreatic necrosis virus (IPNV). *J. Fish Dis.* **2010**, *33*, 803–818. [CrossRef]

58. Quade, M.J.; Roth, J.A. A rapid, direct assay to measure degranulation of bovine neutrophil primary granules. *Vet Immunol. Immunopathol.* **1997**, *58*, 239–248. [CrossRef]

59. Bird, R.P.; Draper, H.H. Comparative studies on different methods of malonaldehyde determination. *Methods Enzymol.* **1984**, *105*, 299–305. [CrossRef]

60. Claiborne, A. Catalase activity. In *CRC Handbook of Methods for Oxygen Radical Research*; Greenwald, R.A., Ed.; CRC Press: Boca Raton, FL, USA, 1985; pp. 283–284.

61. Flohé, L.; Otting, F. Superoxide dismutase assays. *Methods Enzymol.* **1984**, *105*, 93–104. [CrossRef]

62. Lima, I.; Moreira, S.M.; Osten, J.R.-V.; Soares, A.M.V.M.; Guilhermino, L. Biochemical responses of the marine mussel *Mytilus galloprovincialis* to petrochemical environmental contamination along the North-western coast of Portugal. *Chemosphere* **2007**, *66*, 1230–1242. [CrossRef]

63. Pfaffl, M.W. A new mathematical model for relative quantification in real-time RT-PCR. *Nucleic Acids Res.* **2001**, *29*, e45. [CrossRef]

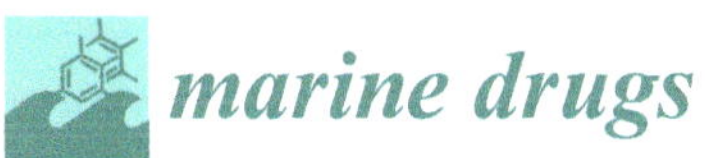

marine drugs

Article

Astaxanthin Confers a Significant Attenuation of Hippocampal Neuronal Loss Induced by Severe Ischemia-Reperfusion Injury in Gerbils by Reducing Oxidative Stress

Joon Ha Park [1,†], Tae-Kyeong Lee [2,†], Dae Won Kim [3], Ji Hyeon Ahn [4], Choong-Hyun Lee [5], Jong-Dai Kim [6], Myoung Cheol Shin [7], Jun Hwi Cho [7], Jae-Chul Lee [8], Moo-Ho Won [8,*] and Soo Young Choi [9,*]

[1] Department of Anatomy, College of Korean Medicine, Dongguk University, Gyeongju 38066, Korea; jh-park@dongguk.ac.kr

[2] Department of Food Science and Nutrition, Hallym University, Chuncheon 24252, Korea; tk_lee@hallym.ac.kr

[3] Department of Biochemistry and Molecular Biology, Research Institute of Oral Sciences, College of Dentistry, Gangnung-Wonju National University, Gangneung 25457, Korea; kimdw@gwnu.ac.kr

[4] Department of Physical Therapy, College of Health Science, Youngsan University, Yangsan 50510, Korea; jh-ahn@ysu.ac.kr

[5] Department of Pharmacy, College of Pharmacy, Dankook University, Cheonan 31116, Korea; anaphy@dankook.ac.kr

[6] Division of Food Biotechnology, School of Biotechnology, Kangwon National University, Chuncheon 24341, Korea; jongdai@kangwon.ac.kr

[7] Department of Emergency Medicine, Kangwon National University Hospital, School of Medicine, Kangwon National University, Chuncheon 24289, Korea; dr10126@naver.com (M.C.S.); cjhemd@kangwon.ac.kr (J.H.C.)

[8] Department of Neurobiology, School of Medicine, Kangwon National University, Chuncheon 24341, Korea; anajclee@kangwon.ac.kr

[9] Department of Biomedical Science and Research Institute for Bioscience and Biotechnology, Hallym University, Chuncheon 24252, Korea

* Correspondence: mhwon@kangwon.ac.kr (M.-H.W.); sychoi@hallym.ac.kr (S.Y.C.); Tel.: +82-33-250-8891 (M.-H.W.); +82-33-248-2112 (S.Y.C.); Fax: +82-33-256-1614 (M.-H.W.); +82-33-241-1463 (S.Y.C.)

† These authors contributed equally to this work.

Citation: Park, J.H.; Lee, T.-K.; Kim, D.W.; Ahn, J.H.; Lee, C.-H.; Kim, J.-D.; Shin, M.C.; Cho, J.H.; Lee, J.-C.; Won, M.-H.; et al. Astaxanthin Confers a Significant Attenuation of Hippocampal Neuronal Loss Induced by Severe Ischemia-Reperfusion Injury in Gerbils by Reducing Oxidative Stress. *Mar. Drugs* **2022**, *20*, 267. https://doi.org/10.3390/md20040267

Academic Editors: Donatella Degl'Innocenti and Marzia Vasarri

Received: 22 March 2022
Accepted: 13 April 2022
Published: 14 April 2022

Publisher's Note: MDPI stays neutral with regard to jurisdictional claims in published maps and institutional affiliations.

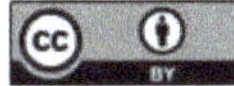

Abstract: Astaxanthin is a powerful biological antioxidant and is naturally generated in a great variety of living organisms. Some studies have demonstrated the neuroprotective effects of ATX against ischemic brain injury in experimental animals. However, it is still unknown whether astaxanthin displays neuroprotective effects against severe ischemic brain injury induced by longer (severe) transient ischemia in the forebrain. The purpose of this study was to evaluate the neuroprotective effects of astaxanthin and its antioxidant activity in the hippocampus of gerbils subjected to 15-min transient forebrain ischemia, which led to the massive loss (death) of pyramidal cells located in hippocampal cornu Ammonis 1-3 (CA1-3) subfields. Astaxanthin (100 mg/kg) was administered once daily for three days before the induction of transient ischemia. Treatment with astaxanthin significantly attenuated the ischemia-induced loss of pyramidal cells in CA1-3. In addition, treatment with astaxanthin significantly reduced ischemia-induced oxidative DNA damage and lipid peroxidation in CA1-3 pyramidal cells. Moreover, the expression of the antioxidant enzymes superoxide dismutase (SOD1 and SOD2) in CA1-3 pyramidal cells were gradually and significantly reduced after ischemia. However, in astaxanthin-treated gerbils, the expression of SOD1 and SOD2 was significantly high compared to in-vehicle-treated gerbils before and after ischemia induction. Collectively, these findings indicate that pretreatment with astaxanthin could attenuate severe ischemic brain injury induced by 15-min transient forebrain ischemia, which may be closely associated with the decrease in oxidative stress due to astaxanthin pretreatment.

Keywords: antioxidant enzymes; DNA damage; ischemia and reperfusion; lipid peroxidation; lipid-soluble carotenoid; neuroprotection

---

1. Introduction

Brains are very sensitive and vulnerable to disruption of the blood supply. Transient cerebral ischemia is a medical emergency that results from the temporary cessation of the blood supply to the brain, which results in irrecoverable neuronal damage in various brain regions [1,2]. Compared to other brain regions, the hippocampus is the region most vulnerable to ischemic injury, where neuronal loss (death) in the hippocampal CA1 occurs a few days after five minutes of transient forebrain ischemia [3,4]. The extent and time of neuronal death in the hippocampus are closely correlated with the duration of transient ischemia [5–7]. The diverse mechanisms of hippocampal neuronal death following transient ischemia (ischemia and reperfusion, IR) have been addressed, and, among the mechanisms, oxidative stress caused by the overgeneration of reactive oxygen species (ROS) following IR is well understood [8,9]. Hence, antioxidant strategies to improve cellular defenses against oxidative stress in IR injury have been proposed as useful therapeutic approaches [10,11]

Astaxanthin (ATX), a lipid-soluble carotenoid, is a powerful biological antioxidant and exists widely in natural organisms, including marine organisms, green plants, and microorganisms [12]. It exerts a broad spectrum of pharmacological effects, such as anticoagulant, anti-inflammatory, and antioxidant activities with the characteristic of low toxicity [13–15]. ATX has been reported to have higher antioxidant activity than a range of carotenoids including α-carotene, β-carotene, lycopene, and lutein [16]. In addition, ATX can cross the blood-brain barrier (BBB) and accumulate in the brain, where it can potentially provide a beneficial effect [17]. Due to these advantages, ATX has been regarded as a promising therapeutic agent for neurological diseases [18].

ATX has been demonstrated to exert neuroprotective effects via antioxidant activity in experimental animal models of cerebral ischemia. Zhang et al. (2020) showed that pretreatment with ATX protected the SH-SY5Y neuronal cells from oxygen and glucose deprivation-induced oxidative damage [19], and Pan et al. (2017) showed that pretreatment with ATX significantly reduced infarction volume in rat brains after transient focal brain ischemia, via activation of the antioxidant defense pathway [20]. Pretreatment with ATX was also reported to protect hippocampal neurons from repeated IR-induced brain injury in mice, suggesting that the effect might be related to the alleviation of oxidative stress [21]. Furthermore, it has been demonstrated that treatment with ATX significantly reduces brain injury following transient focal cerebral ischemia induced by middle cerebral artery occlusion in rats via antioxidant efficacy [22,23]. In addition, treatment with ATX ameliorates neuronal loss in the spinal cord following IR in rats via activation of the PI3K/Akt/GSK-3 beta pathway [24].

However, to the best of our knowledge, the neuroprotective effects of ATX against severe IR injury in the forebrain induced by a long period of transient ischemia have not been explored yet, and it is unclear whether ATX can attenuate severe IR injury in the forebrain by antioxidative activity. Thus, the aim of this experiment was to investigate the neuroprotective effects of ATX in a gerbil model of 15-min transient forebrain ischemia which results in massive neuronal loss (death) in the hippocampal CA1-3 [7,25]. In addition, we examined whether the neuroprotective effects were closely associated with the potent antioxidant activity of ATX.

2. Results

2.1. Neuroprotection by ATX

2.1.1. Findings by Nissl Staining

In the vehicle-sham group, intact cells stained with cresyl violet (CV), which have intact Nissl substance (aggregation of rough endoplasmic reticulum) in the cytoplasm, were distinctly observed in the stratum pyramidale (SP) in the hippocampal proper (CA1-CA3) (Figure 1(Ba)). In the vehicle-IR group, CV stainability at one day after IR was not significantly altered compared with the vehicle-sham group (Figure 1(Bb)). However, at two days after IR, CV stainability was decreased in the SP of CA1 (Figure 1(Bc)), and, at five days after IR, a significant loss of CV stainability was observed in the SP of CA1-3

(Figure 1(Bd)). In the ATX-sham group, CV stainability in the SP of CA1-3 was not different from that of the vehicle-sham group (Figure 1(Be)). In the ATX-IR group, a significant change in CV stainability was not observed until two days after IR (Figure 1(Bf,Bg)), and, at five days after IR, CV stainability was weak in the SP of CA1 alone (Figure 1(Bh)). This finding means that severe IR damages Nissl substance, and ATX could protect it from IR injury.

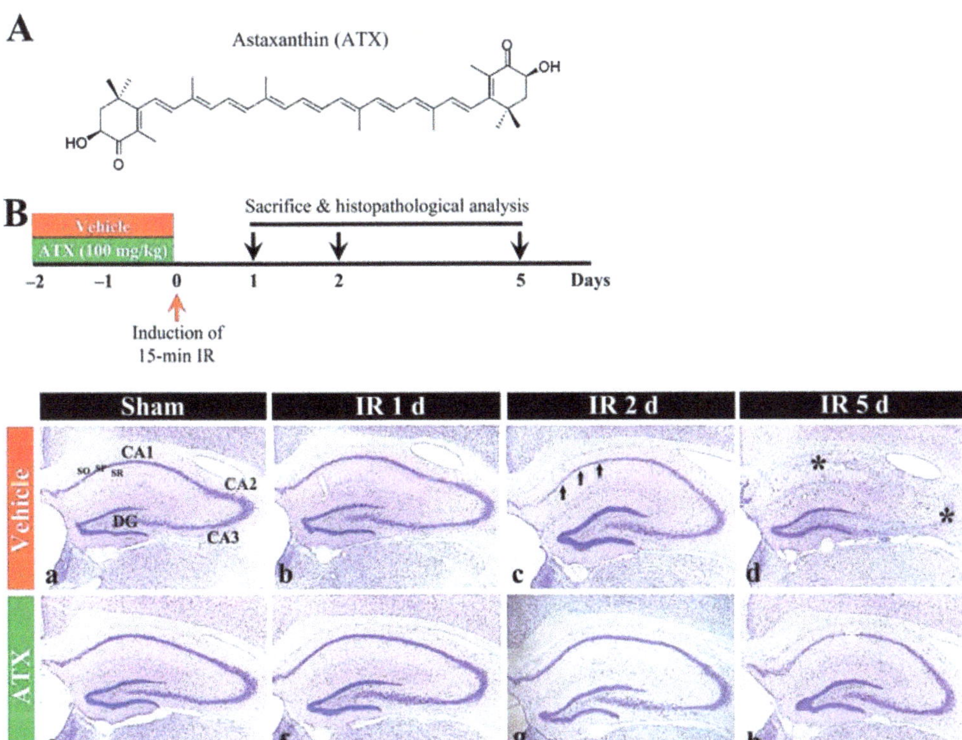

Figure 1. (**A**) The chemical structure of ATX and experimental procedure. ATX is dissolved in saline and orally administered once a day for three days before IR induction. The gerbils are sacrificed on day 1, 2 and 5 after IR; (**B**) Representative photographs of Nissl staining in the hippocampus (CA1-3) of the vehicle-treated (upper low) and ATX-treated (lower low) groups in sham (**a,e**), and on day 1 (**b,f**), day 2 (**c,g**), and day 5 (**d,h**) after IR. In the vehicle-IR group, CV stainability in the SP of CA1 (arrows in (**c**)) is pale at two days after IR, and, at five days after IR, very pale CV stainability is shown in the SP of CA1-3 (black asterisks in (**d**)). In the ATX-IR group, pale CV stainability is shown only in the SP of CA1 (white asterisk in (**h**)) at five days after IR. DG, dentate gyrus; SO, stratum oriens; SR, stratum radiatum. Scale bar = 400 μm.

2.1.2. Findings by Neuronal Nuclei (NeuN, a Marker for Mature Neurons) Immunohistochemistry

In the vehicle-sham group, cells in the SP (named pyramidal cells or neurons) of CA1-3 were shown to have clear NeuN immunoreactivity (Figure 2(Aa,Ca)). In the vehicle-IR group, NeuN immunostained cells (NeuN-pyramidal cells) of CA1-3 at one day after IR were not altered in morphology and numbers (Figure 2(Ab,B,Cb,D)). However, NeuN-pyramidal cells of CA1-3 were significantly decreased (67% of the vehicle sham group) in numbers at two days after IR (Figure 2(Ac,B,Cc,D)), and, at five days after IR, a massive loss (27% of the vehicle-sham group) of NeuN-pyramidal cells of CA1-3 were observed, showing that the number in CA1 and CA2/3 was 9 and 35 cells/300 μm^2, respectively

(Figure 2(Ad,B,Cd,D)). In the ATX-sham group, NeuN-pyramidal cells in CA1-3 were not different in numbers and morphology from the vehicle-sham group (Figure 2(Ae,B,Ce,D)). In the ATX-IR group, NeuN-pyramidal cells were not significantly changed until two days after IR (Figure 2(Ae,Af,B,Cf,Cg,D)), and, at five days after IR, NeuN-pyramidal cells of CA1-3 were decreased in numbers, but the number in CA1 and CA2/3 was higher (603% and 268% of the vehicle-IR group) than the vehicle-IR group, showing that the number in CA1 and CA2/3 was 51 and 92 cells/300 μm^2, respectively (Figure 2(Ah,B,Ch,D)). This finding means that severe IR damages the NeuN protein located in the nucleus, and ATX could protect it from IR injury.

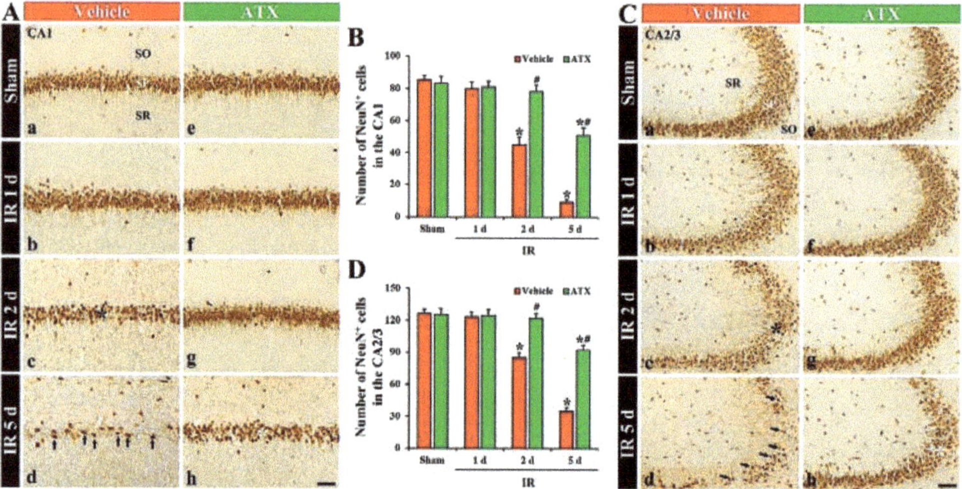

Figure 2. (**A**,**C**) Representative photographs of NeuN immunohistochemistry in CA1 (**A**) and CA2/3 (**C**) of the vehicle-treated (left column) and ATX-treated (right column) groups in sham (**Aa,Ca,Ae,Ce**), and on day 1 (**Ab,Cb,Af,Cf**), day 2 (**Ac,Cc,Ag,Cg**), and day 5 (**Ad,Cd,Ah,Ch**) after IR. In the vehicle-IR group, a loss of NeuN-cells (black asterisks in (**Ac,Cc**)) in the SP of CA1-3 is observed on day 2 after IR. At five days after IR, NeuN-pyramidal cells of CA1-3 (arrows in (**Ad,Cd**)) are markedly decreased; however, in the ATX-IR group, many NeuN-pyramidal cells (white asterisks in (**Ah,Ch**)) are shown. Scale bar = 60 μm; (**B**,**D**) Mean numbers of NeuN-pyramidal cells in CA1 (**B**) and CA2/3 (**D**). The bars indicate the means ± SEM (*n* = 7, respectively; * *p* < 0.05 vs. corresponding sham group, # *p* < 0.05 vs. vehicle-IR group).

2.1.3. Findings by Fluoro-Jade B (FJB) Histofluorescence

In the vehicle-sham and ATX-sham groups, no FJB-stained cells (FJB-cells), which are degenerating or dead cells, were detected in CA1-3 (Figure 3(Aa,Ae,Ca,Ce)). In the vehicle-IR group, FJB-pyramidal cells in CA1-3 were observed from two days after IR (Figure 3(Ab,Ac,B,Cb,Cc,D)), and FJB-pyramidal cells of CA1-3 were dramatically increased at five days after IR; the number of FJB-pyramidal cells in CA1 and CA2/3 was 63 and 67 cells/300 μm^2, respectively (Figure 3(Ad,B,Cd,D)). In the ATX-IR group, FJB-pyramidal cells in CA1-3 were not found until two days after IR (Figure 3(Af,Ag,B,Cf,Cg,D)). At five days after IR, many FJB-pyramidal cells were detected in CA1 and CA2/3 (26 and 13 cells/300 μm^2, respectively), but the number was significantly low (41% in CA1 and 19% in CA2/3 of vehicle-IR group) when compared with the vehicle-IR group (Figure 3(Ah,B,Ch,D)). This finding means that the pyramidal cells in CA1-3 were lost (dead) after severe IR, and ATX could attenuate the death of pyramidal cells induced by severe IR.

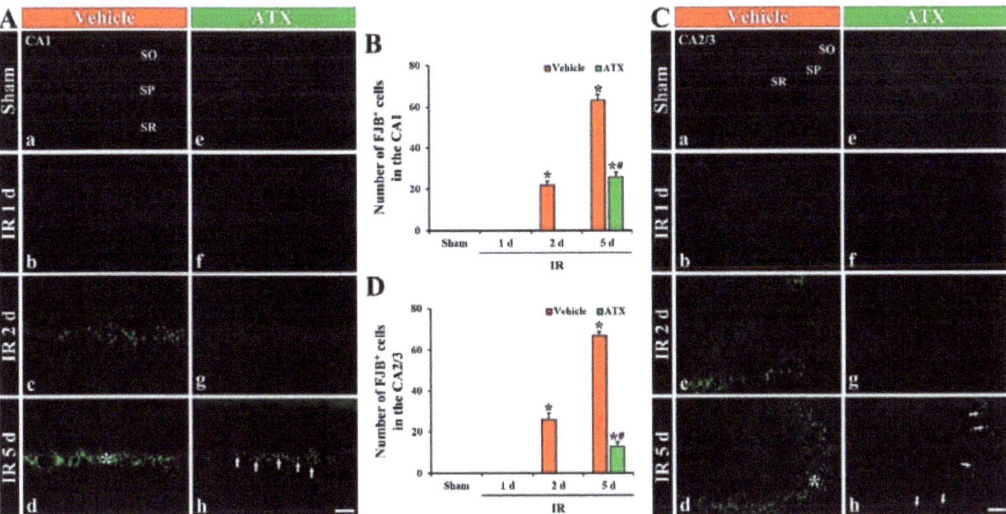

Figure 3. (**A**,**C**) Representative photographs of FJB staining in CA1 (**A**) and CA2/3 (**C**) of the vehicle-treated (left column) and ATX-treated (right column) groups in sham (**Aa**,**Ca**,**Ae**,**Ce**), and on day 1 (**Ab**,**Cb**,**Af**,**Cf**), day 2 (**Ac**,**Cc**,**Ag**,**Cg**), and day 5 (**Ad**,**Cd**,**Ah**,**Ch**) after IR. In the vehicle-IR group, FJB-pyramidal cells are detected in the SP of CA1-3 from two days after IR, and, at five days after IR, FJB-pyramidal cells (white asterisks in (**Ad**,**Cd**)) are significantly increased. However, in the ATX-IR group, decreased FJB-pyramidal cells (arrows in (**Ah**,**Ch**)) are observed in CA1-3 only at five days after IR. Scale bar = 60 µm; (**B**,**D**) Mean numbers of FJB- pyramidal cells in CA1 (**B**) and CA2/3 (**D**). The bars indicate the means ± SEM (n = 7, respectively; * $p < 0.05$ vs. corresponding sham group, # $p < 0.05$ vs. vehicle-IR group).

2.2. Attenuation of Oxidative DNA Damage and Lipid Peroxidation by ATX

2.2.1. 8-Hydroxydeoxyguanosine (8OHdG a Marker of Oxidative DNA Damage) Immunoreactivity

In the vehicle-sham group, 8OHdG immunoreactivity was weakly shown in the intact pyramidal cells of CA1-3 (Figure 4(Aa,Ca)). In the vehicle-IR group, 8OHdG immunoreactivity in the CA1 and 2/3 pyramidal cells was significantly increased (331% and 310% of the vehicle-sham group, respectively) at one day after IR (Figure 4(Ab,B,Cb,D)). At two days after IR, 8OHdG immunoreactivity in the CA1-3 pyramidal cells was decreased; at this point in time, many of the CA1-3 pyramidal cells were lost (dead) (Figure 4(Ac,B,Cc,D)). At five days after IR, 8OHdG immunoreactivity in the CA1-3 pyramidal cells was more significantly decreased: at this time, an extensive loss of the CA1-3 pyramidal cells occurred (Figure 4(Ad,B,Cd,D)). In the ATX-sham group, 8OHdG immunoreactivity in the pyramidal cells of CA1-3 was not different from that shown in the vehicle-sham group (Figure 4(Ae,B,Ce,D)). In the ATX-IR group, 8OHdG immunoreactivity in the CA1 and CA2/3 pyramidal cells was increased (278% and 226% of the ATX-sham group, respectively) at one day after IR, but the immunoreactivity was significantly lower (82% and 72% of the vehicle-IR group, respectively) than that in the vehicle-IR group (Figure 4(Af,B,Cf,D)). Thereafter, 8OHdG immunoreactivity in the CA1-3 pyramidal cells was slightly and gradually decreased with time (Figure 4(Ag,Ah,B,Cg,Ch,D)). This finding means that damage of DNA in the pyramidal cells of CA1-3 was significant at one day after severe IR, and ATX could attenuate the DNA damage induced by severe IR.

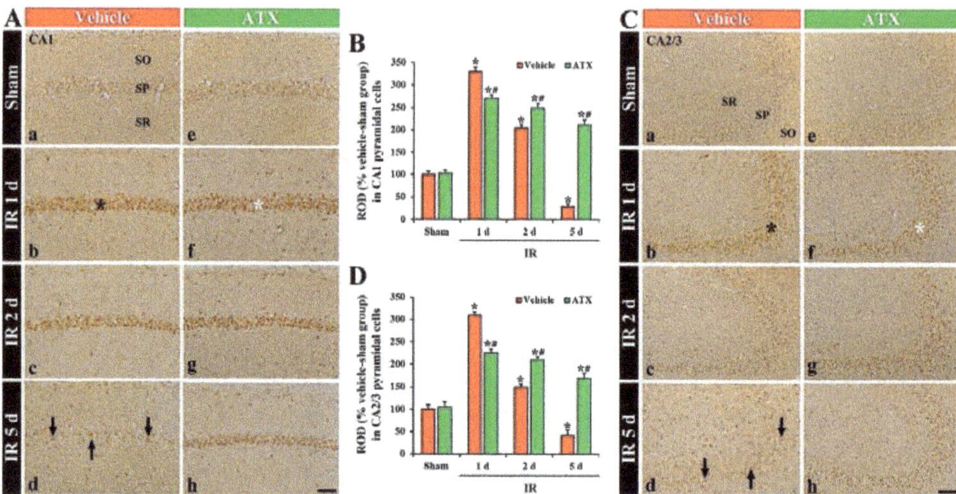

Figure 4. (**A,C**) Representative photographs of 8OHdG immunohistochemistry in CA1 (**A**) and CA2/3 (**C**) of the vehicle-treated (left column) and ATX-treated (right column) groups in sham (**Aa,Ca,Ae,Ce**), and on day 1 (**Ab,Cb,Af,Cf**), day 2 (**Ac,Cc,Ag,Cg**), and day 5 (**Ad,Cd,Ah,Ch**) after IR. In the vehicle-IR group, 8OHdG immunoreactivity in CA1-3 pyramidal cells (black asterisks in (**Ab,Cb**)) is significantly increased at one day after IR. However, in the ATX-IR group, 8OHdG immunoreactivity in CA1-3 pyramidal cells (white asterisks in (**Af,Cf**)) at one day after IR is significantly low when compared with the vehicle-IR group. Note that, at five days after IR, 8OHdG immunoreactivity is very weak (arrows in (**Ad,Cd**)) in the vehicle-IR group due to death of pyramidal cells. Scale bar = 60 μm; (**B,D**) ROD of 8OHdG immunoreactivity in CA1 (**B**) and CA2/3 (**D**). The bars indicate the means ± SEM ($n = 7$, respectively; * $p < 0.05$ vs. corresponding sham group, # $p < 0.05$ vs. vehicle-IR group).

2.2.2. 4-Hydroxy-2-Nonenal (4HNE, a Marker for Lipid Peroxidation) Immunoreactivity

In the vehicle-sham group, 4HNE immunoreactivity was weakly found in the intact CA1-3 pyramidal cells (Figure 5(Aa,Ca)). In the vehicle-IR group, 4HNE immunoreactivity in the pyramidal cells of CA1 and CA2/3 was significantly increased (296% and 305% of the vehicle-IR group, respectively) at one day after IR (Figure 5(Ab,B,Cb,D)). At two days after IR, 4HNE immunoreactivity in the CA1-3 pyramidal cells was decreased compared to that shown in the vehicle-IR group at one day after IR; at this time, many of the CA1-3 pyramidal cells died (Figure 5(Ac,B,Cc,D)). At five days after IR, 4HNE immunoreactivity was very low due to a massive loss of the CA1-3 pyramidal cells (Figure 5(Ad,B,C,D)). In the ATX-sham group, 4HNE immunoreactivity in the CA1-3 pyramidal cells was similar to the vehicle-sham group (Figure 5(Ae,B,Ce,D)). In the ATX-IR group, 4HNE immunoreactivity in CA1 and CA2/3 pyramidal cells was also increased (214% and 221% of ATX-sham group, respectively) at one day after IR, but the immunoreactivity was significantly lower than that in the vehicle-IR group (Figure 5(Af,B,Cf,D)). Thereafter, 4HNE immunoreactivity in the CA1-3 pyramidal cells was gradually and slightly decreased with time due to the attenuation of IR-induced neuronal loss (Figure 5(Ag,Ah,B,Cg,Ch,D)). This finding means that lipid peroxidation in the pyramidal cells of CA1-3 was significantly increased at one day after severe IR, and ATX could attenuate the lipid peroxidation induced by severe IR.

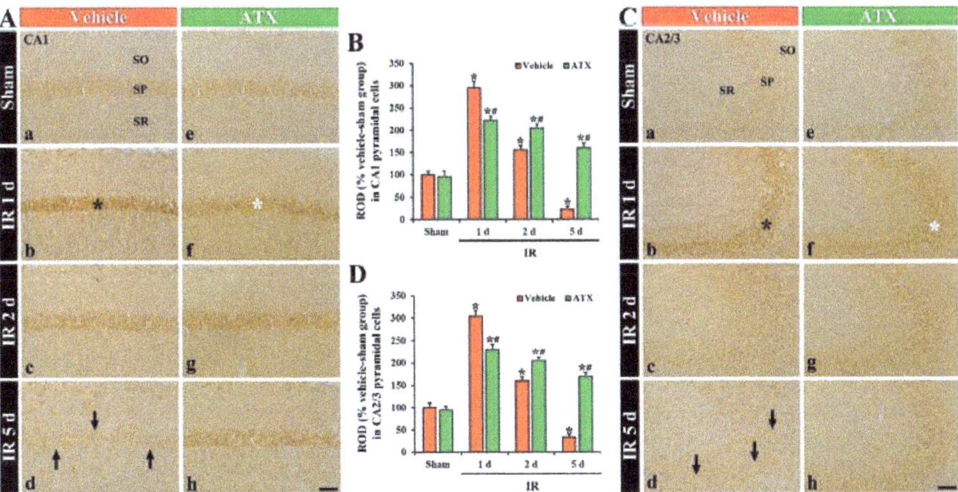

Figure 5. (**A,C**) Representative photographs of 4HNE immunohistochemistry in CA1 (**A**) and CA2/3 (**C**) of the vehicle-treated (left column) and ATX-treated (right column) groups in sham (**Aa,Ca,Ae,Ce**), and on day 1 (**Ab,Cb,Af,Cf**), day 2 (**Ac,Cc,Ag,Cg**), and day 5 (**Ad,Cd,Ah,Ch**) after IR. Black asterisks (in (**Ab,Cb**)) indicate that, in the vehicle-IR group, 4HNE immunoreactivity is significantly increased in CA1-3 pyramidal cells at one day after IR. However, in the ATX-IR group, 4HNE immunoreactivity in CA1-3 pyramidal cells (white asterisks in (**Af,Cf**)) at 1 day after IR is significantly low when compared with in the vehicle-IR group. Note that, at five days after IR, 4HNE immunoreactivity is very weak (arrows in Ad and Cd) in the vehicle-IR group due to death of pyramidal cells. Scale bar = 60 µm; (**B,D**) ROD of 4HNE immunoreactivity in CA1 (**B**) and CA2/3 (**D**). The bars indicate the means ± SEM (n = 7, respectively; * $p < 0.05$ vs. corresponding sham group, # $p < 0.05$ vs. vehicle-IR group).

2.3. Increase of SOD1 and SOD2 Expressions by ATX

2.3.1. SOD1 Immunoreactivity

SOD1 immunoreactivity, in the vehicle-sham group, was shown in the pyramidal cells of CA1 and CA2/3 (Figure 6(Aa,Ca)). In the vehicle-IR group, SOD1 immunoreactivity in the CA1 and CA2/3 pyramidal cells was significantly decreased (69% and 71% of vehicle-sham group, respectively) on day 1 after IR (Figure 6(Ab,B,Cb,D)). On day 2 after IR, SOD1 immunoreactivity in the CA1-3 pyramidal cells was further decreased (Figure 6(Ac,B,Cc,D)), and, on day 5 after IR, SOD1 immunoreactivity was very low (56% and 21% of the vehicle-sham group, respectively) (Figure 6(Ad,B,Cd,D)) due to an extensive loss of CA1-3 pyramidal cells. In the ATX-sham group, SOD1 immunoreactivity in the CA1 and CA2/3 pyramidal cells was significantly higher (144% and 155% of the vehicle-sham group, respectively) than the vehicle-sham group (Figure 6(Ae,B,Ce,D)). In the ATX IR group, SOD1 immunoreactivity in CA1 and CA2/3 pyramidal cells was also decreased with time, but each immunoreactivity was significantly high (on day 5 after IR, 378% and 382% of the vehicle-IR group, respectively) when compared with the ATX-IP group (Figure 6(Af–Ah,B,Cf–Ch,D)). This finding means that SOD1 in the CA1-3 pyramidal cells was significantly decreased with time after severe IR, and ATX could attenuate the decrease of SOD1 induced by severe IR.

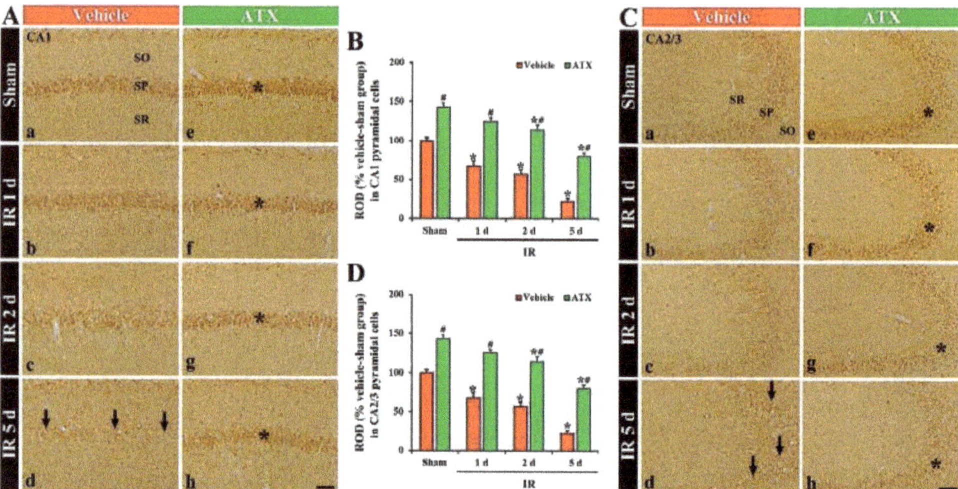

Figure 6. (**A,C**) Representative photographs of SOD1 immunohistochemistry in CA1 (**A**) and CA2/3 (**C**) of the vehicle-treated (left column) and ATX-treated (right column) groups in sham (**Aa,Ca,Ae,Ce**), and on day 1 (**Ab,Cb,Af,Cf**), day 2 (**Ac,Cc,Ag,Cg**), and day 5 (**Ad,Cd,Ah,Ch**) after IR. In the vehicle-IR group, SOD1 immunoreactivity in CA1-3 pyramidal cells is decreased with time after IR, and very low (arrows in (**Ad,Cd**)) on day 5 after IR. In the ATX-sham group, SOD1 immunoreactivity in CA1-3 pyramidal cells is significantly higher (asterisk in (**Ae,Ce**)) than in the vehicle-sham group. In the ATX-IR group, SOD1 immunoreactivity in CA1-3 pyramidal cells is decreased with time, but the immunoreactivity is significantly high (asterisks in (**Af–Ah,Cf–Ch**)) as compared with the vehicle-IR group. Scale bar = 60 μm; (**B,D**) ROD of SOD1 immunoreactivity in CA1 (**B**) and CA2/3 (**D**). The bars indicate the means ± SEM ($n = 7$, respectively; * $p < 0.05$ vs. corresponding sham group, # $p < 0.05$ vs. vehicle-IR group).

2.3.2. SOD2 Immunoreactivity

SOD2 immunoreactivity, in the vehicle-sham group, was mainly shown in the CA1 and CA2/3 pyramidal cells (Figure 7(Aa,Ca)). In the vehicle-IR group, a significant decrease of SOD2 immunoreactivity in the CA1 and CA2/3 pyramidal cells (65% and 68% of the vehicle-sham group, respectively) was observed at one day after IR (Figure 7(Ab,B,Cb,D)). At two days after IR, SOD2 immunoreactivity in the CA1-3 pyramidal cells was more decreased (Figure 7(Ac,B,Cc,D)), and, at five days after IR, SOD2 immunoreactivity in the CA1-3 pyramidal cells was very low (51% and 18% of the vehicle-sham group, respectively) due to an extensive loss of pyramidal cells (Figure 7(Ad,B,Cd,D)). In the ATX-sham group, SOD2 immunoreactivity in the CA1 and CA2/3 pyramidal cells was significantly higher (205% and 196% of the vehicle-sham group, respectively) when compared with the vehicle-sham group (Figure 7(Ae,B,Ce,D)). In the ATX-IR group, SOD2 immunoreactivity in the CA1-3 pyramidal cells was also decreased with time, but each immunoreactivity was significantly high when compared with the vehicle-IR group (Figure 7(Af–Ah,B,Cf–Ch,D)). This finding means that SOD2 in CA1-3 pyramidal cells was also significantly decreased with time after severe IR, and ATX could attenuate the decrease of SOD2 induced by severe IR.

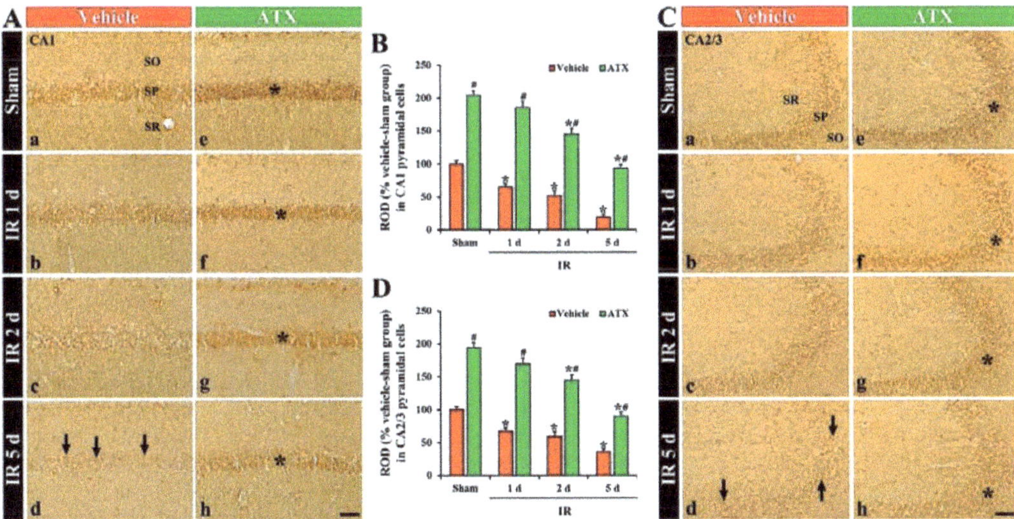

Figure 7. (**A**,**C**) Representative photographs of SOD2 immunohistochemistry in CA1 (**A**) and CA2/3 (**C**) of the vehicle-treated (left column) and ATX-treated (right column) groups in sham (**Aa,Ca,Ae,Ce**), and on day 1 (**Ab,Cb,Af,Cf**), day 2 (**Ac,Cc,Ag,Cg**), and day 5 (**Ad,Cd,Ah,Ch**) after IR. SOD1 immunoreactivity, in the vehicle-IR group, is decreased in CA1-3 pyramidal cells with time after IR, and very low (arrows in (**Ad,Cd**)) at five days after IR. In the ATX-sham group, SOD1 immunoreactivity in CA1-3 pyramidal cells is significantly higher (asterisk in (**Ae,Ce**)) than the vehicle-sham group. SOD1 immunoreactivity in CA1-3 pyramidal cells of the ATX-IR group is decreased with time, but the immunoreactivity is significantly high (asterisks in (**Af–Ah,Cf–Ch**)) when compared with the vehicle-IR group. Scale bar = 60 μm; (**B**,**D**) ROD of SOD2 immunoreactivity in CA1 (**B**) and CA2/3 (**D**). The bars indicate the means ± SEM ($n = 7$, respectively; * $p < 0.05$ vs. corresponding sham group, # $p < 0.05$ vs. vehicle-IR group).

3. Discussion

The degree of hippocampal neuronal death following IR injury varies according to the ischemic duration. It has been demonstrated that the selective death of pyramidal cells in hippocampal CA1 occurs four to five days after five minutes of transient ischemia in the forebrain of gerbils [4,26]. We reported that the death of pyramidal cells in CA1-3 of gerbils subjected to 15 min of transient ischemia was observed from two days post-ischemia, indicating that a longer period of transient ischemia could evoke the acceleration and aggravation of pyramidal cell death in the hippocampus [7,25]. In this study, we examined the neuroprotective effects of ATX in CA1-3 of gerbils subjected to transient ischemia for 15 min using Nissl staining, NeuN immunohistochemistry, and FJB histofluorescence staining, and found that pretreatment with ATX significantly alleviated ischemia induced pyramidal cell death in CA1-3. We believe that this finding was the first showing that ATX elicited strong neuroprotection against severe IR injury in the gerbil hippocampus. In rats, global cerebral ischemia for 10 min induced pyramidal cell death in CA1 alone, which might be a phenomenon of mild IR injury in the hippocampus compared to severe IR injury in the hippocampus, and the administration of ATX significantly reduced the selective death [27]. To the best of our knowledge, it is impossible to develop a rat model of severe IR injury in the hippocampus by occluding four vessels (two common carotid arteries and two vertebral arteries) for 15 min or more because rats subjected to this ischemic injury die a few days later due to failure of the brainstem which receives arterial blood supply from the vertebral arteries [28,29]. However, as described in the Materials and Methods Section, a gerbil model of severe IR injury in the hippocampus can be developed, because gerbils with severe IR injury induced by the ligation of two common carotid arteries (not two vertebral arteries) survive a long time without brainstem failure [6,7]. Regarding the anatomy of the circle of Willis in rats and gerbils, rats have a perfect circle of Willis, whereas gerbils have an incomplete circle of Willis so that there is a lack of posterior communicating arteries [7,30]. These anatomical characteristics helped us to develop a gerbil model of severe IR injury in the forebrain. Many years ago, Jarrott and Dommer (1980) reported that a mortality rate of 100% was obtained if the occlusion of bilateral common carotid arteries was maintained for 60 min in gerbils weighing 45–55 g [31].

Oxidative stress is a phenomenon induced by an imbalance between the production and accumulation of ROS in cells and/or tissues and the ability of a system to detoxify the reactive products [32]. When the production of ROS increases, harmful effects are exerted on important structures in cells such as proteins, lipids, and nucleic acids [33]. In ischemic insults to the brain, oxidative stress has also been considered to be a major factor to overcome following ischemic brain injury. Many preclinical studies have demonstrated that oxidative stress following ROS accumulation during IR irreversibly damaged cellular biomolecules, including lipids, proteins, and DNA, and led to neuronal death [8,10]. In particular, early during IR, due to an elevated oxygen supply, large quantities of oxygen radicals increase rapidly in the ischemic lesions and DNA damage occurs [34]. Lipid peroxidation can be described as a process under which oxidants including ROS attack lipids containing carbon–carbon double bond(s) [35]. In this respect, various substances reducing oxidative stress have been demonstrated to attenuate ischemic brain injury following IR injury [36–38]. In this study, the immunoreactivity of 8OHdG (an oxidative DNA adduct) in CA1-3 pyramidal cells was significantly enhanced on day 1 after IR (before the time of IR-induced loss of CA1-3 pyramidal cells), but it was significantly reduced by ATX treatment. Resveratrol, which is a naturally occurring polyphenolic compound and elicits a variety of biological and pharmacological functions, including anti-oxidant and anti-inflammatory properties, protected HT22 cells from oxygen-glucose deprivation and reoxygenation-induced injuries by reducing DNA damage (decreases in 8OHdG levels) [39]. In addition, we found that the immunoreactivity of 4HNE (an end-product of lipid peroxidation) in CA1-3 pyramidal cells was significantly increased on day 1 after IR. However, ATX significantly decreased 4HNE immunoreactivity. These results indicate that pretreatment with ATX mitigated severe IR-induced oxidative stress in CA1-3 pyramidal cells, which may be closely associated with ATX-mediated neuroprotection against severe IR injury.

The antioxidant defense system neutralizes or scavenges ROS and plays a protective role against ischemic brain injury [11,40]. One of the key enzymes in the antioxidant defense system is SOD, which acts first to defend against the harmful effects of oxidative stress. Targeting SOD expression has shown substantial success in animal models of transient brain ischemia. Sugawara et al. (2002) showed that IR-induced superoxide production and the selective death of CA1 pyramidal cells were significantly decreased in transgenic rats overexpressing SOD1 [41]. Keller et al. (1998) also found that lipid peroxidation, protein nitration, and brain infarction following transient focal cerebral ischemia were significantly reduced in transgenic mice overexpressing SOD2 [42]. Moreover, we reported that the increased expression of SOD1 and SOD2 in CA1 pyramidal cells following pretreatment with natural antioxidants derived from plant materials, such as quercetin and chlorogenic acid, contributed to the protection of CA1 pyramidal cells against IR injury in gerbils [43,44]. In this study, SOD1 and SOD2 immunoreactivity in the CA1-3 pyramidal cells of both the vehicle-IR and ATX-IR groups were gradually decreased with time after severe IR, but, in the ATX-IR group, SOD1 and SOD2 immunoreactivity were significantly high compared to the vehicle-IR group. These results suggest that SOD1 and SOD2 in CA1-3 pyramidal cells were increased by ATX pretreatment and these increases could contribute to the neuroprotection against oxidative stress following severe IR.

Collectively, this study showed that pretreatment with ATX attenuated the massive loss (death) of CA1-3 pyramidal cells in gerbil hippocampi following severe IR injury induced by

15-min transient forebrain ischemia, and the pretreatment with ATX significantly enhanced the expressions of SOD1 and 2 in the CA1-3 pyramidal cells before IR and reduced oxidative stress in pyramidal cells following severe IR. These findings suggest that ATX can be used as a potential dietary supplement to prevent the progression of severe IR injury in brains. However, we need an in-depth study on the mechanism of the neuroprotective effect of ATX. For instance, examination of changes in antioxidant markers such as nuclear factor erythroid 2-related factor 2 (Nrf2) should be conducted to demonstrate the antioxidant defense of ATX against IR. Moreover, since IR injury in gerbils triggers delayed neuronal death in the hippocampus, examination of behavioral changes needs to be carried out to demonstrate the amelioration of IR-induced cognitive decline by treatment with ATX.

4. Materials and Methods

4.1. Animals

The protocol of all experiments was approved (approval no., KW-2000113-1) on 13 January 2020 by the Ethics Committee of Kangwon National University (Chuncheon, Gangwon, Korea). Animal suffering during the whole experiments was minimized. Six-month male gerbils (*Meriones unguiculatus*), weighing 70–80 g, were used. The gerbils originated from Charles River Laboratories International, Inc. (Wilmington, MA, USA). The gerbils were housed in pathogen-free environment under standard condition at a controlled temperature (about 24 °C) and humidity (about 60%) on a 12:12 h light–dark cycle.

4.2. Groups and Treatment of ATX

The gerbils were blindly and randomly divided into four groups: (1) vehicle treated and sham operated group (sham group, $n = 14$), which was treated with vehicle (saline) and received sham IR; (2) vehicle-treated and IR-operated group (IR group, $n = 21$), which was treated with saline and received IR; (3) ATX-treated and sham-operated group (ATX-sham group, $n = 14$), which was treated with ATX and received sham; (4) ATX-IR group ($n = 21$), which was treated with ATX and received IR.

The chemical structure of ATX (SML0982; Sigma-Aldrich, St. Louis, MO, USA) and the plan schedule of the experiment are shown in Figure 1A. ATX (100 mg/kg) was dissolved in saline and injected intraperitoneally once a day for three consecutive days before IR. The dosage and duration of ATX treatment were selected based on a recent study showing that pretreatment with 100 mg/kg of ATX provided robust neuroprotection against transient focal cerebral ischemia-induced brain injury in rats [45].

The gerbils ($n = 7$, respectively) in the IR groups on day 1, day 2, and day 5 after IR, and the ones ($n = 7$, respectively) in the sham groups were sacrificed at 0 h and five days after IR to reduce the numbers

4.3. Induction of Severe IR Injury

Severe IR injury in the hippocampus was induced as follows. As described in a previous study [6], in brief, the gerbils were anesthetized with 2.5% isoflurane (4 L/min; JW Pharmaceutical Corporation, Seoul, Korea). Midline cervical incision was executed in the neck, and bilateral common carotid arteries, which supply arterial blood to the brain, were isolated from the carotid sheath and ligated with clips (Fine Science Tools, Foster City, CA, USA) for 15 min to develop severe IR injury in the forebrain, which contains the hippocampus. The complete stop of the blood supply was confirmed by the right and left central arteries located in the retinae using HEINE K180 ophthalmoscope (Heine Optotechnik, Herrsching, Germany). The clips were removed to restore the blood supply and the incision region was sutured. Body temperatures were controlled at normothermia (37 ± 0.5 °C) using a heating lamp (Harvard Apparatus, Holliston, MA, USA) and TR-100 rectal temperature probe (Fine Science Tools, Foster City, CA, USA). The gerbils of all sham groups received identical surgery without the ligation of the arteries. After the sham and IR operation, the gerbils were housed in adequate rooms (about 24 °C of temperature and about 55% of relative humidity).

4.4. Preparation of Histological Sections

Brain sections containing the hippocampus were prepared in the usual way. In brief, the gerbils were deeply anesthetized with urethane (1.5 g/kg, intraperitoneal injection). Under the deep anesthesia, the gerbils were rinsed by transcardial perfusion of 50 mM phosphate-buffered saline (pH 7.4) and fixed with 4% paraformaldehyde. Thereafter, the fixed brains were obtained from the skulls and more fixed in the 4% paraformaldehyde overnight and soaked in 25% sucrose for cryoprotection. Thereafter, coronal sections of 30-μm thickness were made using SM2010 R sliding microtome (Leica Biosystems, Wetzlar, Germany).

4.5. Nissl Staining

Nissl staining is a widely used method to study the morphology and pathology of neural tissue. To examine IR injury in the gerbil hippocampus, Nissl staining was performed in the usual way. Briefly, the sections were submerged in 0.1% CV acetate solution for 20 min at room temperature. These sections were briefly washed in distilled water, dehydrated in graded ethanol and then cleared in xylene. Lastly, they were mounted with Canada balsam (Sigma-Aldrich).

4.6. FJB Staining

FJB stains all degenerating neurons regardless of specific insult or mechanism of cell death. FJB staining was performed, as described previously [37]. In short, the sections were soaked in 0.06% potassium permanganate and incubated in 0.0004% FJB (Cell Signaling Technology, Beverly, MA, USA). Thereafter, these sections were washed and put on a hot plate (about 50 °C) for the reaction of FJB. Finally, the sections were cleared in xylene and coverslipped with DPX (Thermo Fisher Scientific, Waltham, MA, USA).

4.7. Immunohistochemistry

Immunohistochemistry was conducted in the usual way to evaluate neuronal damage using NeuN antibody, and to examine oxidative stress using 8OHdG antibody, 4HNE antibody, and endogenous antioxidant (SOD1 and SOD2) antibodies (Table 1). In brief, the sections were reacted with 0.3% hydrogen peroxide and subsequently immersed in 5% normal horse serum at room temperature. After washing, these sections were incubated in each primary antibody solution overnight at 4 °C. Subsequently, the sections were exposed to corresponding secondary antibody, as shown in Table 1, for two hours at room temperature and to avidin-biotin complex (diluted 1:200, Vector) for one hour at room temperature. These sections were then visualized using 0.06% 3,3′-diaminobenzidine tetrahydrochloride (Sigma-Aldrich Co., St. Louis, MO, USA) for one minute, and the immunoreactions were checked. Finally, they were mounted onto gelatin-coated slides and were sealed with mounting medium.

Table 1. Primary and secondary antibodies for immunohistochemical staining.

Primary Antibodies	Dilutions	Suppliers
Mouse anti-neuronal nuclei (NeuN)	1:1000	Chemicon, Temecula, CA, USA
Goat anti-8-hydroxydeoxyguanosine (8OHdG)	1:500	Millipore, Billerica, MA, USA
Mouse 4-hydroxy-2-nonenal (4HNE)	1:800	Alexis Biochemicals, San Diego, CA, USA
Sheep anti-Cu, Zn-superoxide dismutase (SOD1)	1:800	Calbiochem, La Jolla, CA, USA
Sheep anti-Mn-superoxide dismutase (SOD2)	1:800	Calbiochem, La Jolla, CA, USA
Secondary Antibodies	**Dilutions**	**Suppliers**
Biotinylated horse anti-mouse IgG	1:250	Vector Laboratories Inc., Burlingame, CA, USA
Biotinylated horse anti-goat IgG	1:250	Vector Laboratories Inc., Burlingame, CA, USA
Biotinylated rabbit anti-sheep IgG	1:250	Vector Laboratories Inc., Burlingame, CA, USA

4.8. Analyses of Data

For quantitative analysis of IR-induced neuronal death, nine sections per animal were selected at the corresponding levels using the brain atlas of gerbil [46]. In short, as described previously [47], the digital images of NeuN- and FJB-stained cells were taken using a light microscope (BX53, Olympus, Tokyo, Japan) and an epifluorescent microscope (Carl Zeiss, Göttingen, Germany), respectively. The cell count was evaluated using Optimas 6.5 (an image analyzing system; CyberMetrics, Scottsdale, AZ, USA).

To quantitatively analyze the changes in 8OHdG, 4HNE, SOD1, and SOD2 immunoreactivities, a relative optical density (ROD) was applied. As described previously [48], in short, the digital image of immunostained structure was obtained using BX53 light microscope. The obtained image was converted into grey scale image (from black to white). The grey image was calculated by using Image J software (version 1.46) of the National Institutes of Health (Bethesda, Maryland, MD, USA).

4.9. Statistical Analyses

Statistical analyses were performed with aid of GraphPad Prism (version 5.0) (GraphPad Software, La Jolla, CA, USA). The differences of the means among the groups were statistically analyzed by two-way analysis of variance (ANOVA) tests with post hoc Bonferroni's multiple comparison tests to elucidate IR-related differences among the groups. Data were presented as the means $\pm$ standard errors of the mean (SEM), and statistical significance was designated when p value was less than 0.05.

Author Contributions: Conceptualization, M.-H.W. and S.Y.C.; Methodology, D.W.K. and J.H.A.; Software, M.C.S. and J.-C.L.; Validation, T.-K.L. and C.-H.L.; Investigation, J.H.P. and T.-K.L.; Data Curation, J.H.P. and J.-D.K.; Writing—Original Draft Preparation, J.H.P. and T.-K.L.; Writing—Review & Editing, M.-H.W.; Supervision, J.H.C. and M.-H.W.; Project Administration, S.Y.C.; Funding Acquisition, J.H.P., J.-D.K. and S.Y.C. All authors have read and agreed to the published version of the manuscript.

Funding: This research was supported by Basic Science Research Program through the National Research Foundation of Korea (NRF) funded by the Ministry of Education (NRF-2019R1A6A1A11036849, NRF-2020R1I1A3060735 and NRF-2020R1F1A1062633).

Institutional Review Board Statement: The protocol of all experiments was approved (approval no., KW-2000113-1) on 13 January 2020 by the Ethics Committee of Kangwon National University (Chuncheon, Gangwon, Korea).

Informed Consent Statement: Not applicable.

Data Availability Statement: The data presented in this study are available on request from the corresponding author.

Acknowledgments: The authors would like to appreciate Hyun Sook Kim and Seung Uk Lee for their technical help in this study.

Conflicts of Interest: The authors declare that they have no conflict of interest.

Abbreviations

4HNE	4-hydroxy-2-nonenal
8OHdG	8-hydroxydeoxyguanosine
ATX	astaxanthin
CA	cornu Ammonis
CV	cresyl violet
DG	dentate gyrus
FJB	Fluoro-Jade B
IR	ischemia and reperfusion
NeuN	neuronal nuclei
ROD	relative optical density
ROS	reactive oxygen species
SOD	superoxide dismutase
SO	stratum oriens
SP	stratum pyramidale
SR	stratum radiatum

References

1. Kawai, K.; Nitecka, L.; Ruetzler, C.A.; Nagashima, G.; Joo, F.; Mies, G.; Nowak, T.S., Jr.; Saito, N.; Lohr, J.M.; Klatzo, I. Global cerebral ischemia associated with cardiac arrest in the rat: I. Dynamics of early neuronal changes. *J. Cereb. Blood Flow Metab. Off. J. Int. Soc. Cereb. Blood Flow Metab.* **1992**, *12*, 238–249. [CrossRef] [PubMed]
2. Wahul, A.B.; Joshi, P.C.; Kumar, A.; Chakravarty, S. Transient global cerebral ischemia differentially affects cortex, striatum and hippocampus in bilateral common carotid arterial occlusion (bccao) mouse model. *J. Chem. Neuroanat.* **2018**, *92*, 1–15. [CrossRef] [PubMed]
3. Globus, M.Y.; Busto, R.; Martinez, E.; Valdes, I.; Dietrich, W.D.; Ginsberg, M.D. Comparative effect of transient global ischemia on extracellular levels of glutamate, glycine, and gamma-aminobutyric acid in vulnerable and nonvulnerable brain regions in the rat. *J. Neurochem.* **1991**, *57*, 470–478. [CrossRef] [PubMed]
4. Lee, J.C.; Park, J.H.; Ahn, J.H.; Kim, I.H.; Cho, J.H.; Choi, J.H.; Yoo, K.Y.; Lee, C.H.; Hwang, I.K.; Cho, J.H.; et al. New gabaergic neurogenesis in the hippocampal ca1 region of a gerbil model of long-term survival after transient cerebral ischemic injury. *Brain Pathol.* **2016**, *26*, 581–592. [CrossRef]
5. Ahn, J.H.; Ohk, T.G.; Kim, D.W.; Kim, H.; Song, M.; Lee, T.K.; Lee, J.C.; Yang, G.E.; Shin, M.C.; Cho, J.H.; et al. Fluoro-jade b histofluorescence staining detects dentate granule cell death after repeated five-minute transient global cerebral ischemia. *Metab. Brain Dis.* **2019**, *34*, 951–956. [CrossRef]
6. Lee, C.H.; Ahn, J.H.; Lee, T.K.; Sim, H.; Lee, J.C.; Park, J.H.; Shin, M.C.; Cho, J.H.; Kim, D.W.; Won, M.H.; et al. Comparison of neuronal death, blood-brain barrier leakage and inflammatory cytokine expression in the hippocampal ca1 region following mild and severe transient forebrain ischemia in gerbils. *Neurochem. Res.* **2021**, *46*, 2852–2866. [CrossRef]
7. Lee, T.K.; Kim, H.; Song, M.; Lee, J.C.; Park, J.H.; Ahn, J.H.; Yang, G.E.; Kim, H.; Ohk, T.G.; Shin, M.C.; et al. Time-course pattern of neuronal loss and gliosis in gerbil hippocampi following mild, severe, or lethal transient global cerebral ischemia. *Neural Regen. Res.* **2019**, *14*, 1394–1403.
8. Chen, H.; Yoshioka, H.; Kim, G.S.; Jung, J.E.; Okami, N.; Sakata, H.; Maier, C.M.; Narasimhan, P.; Goeders, C.E.; Chan, P.H. Oxidative stress in ischemic brain damage: Mechanisms of cell death and potential molecular targets for neuroprotection. *Antioxid. Redox Signal.* **2011**, *14*, 1505–1517. [CrossRef]
9. Li, W.; Yang, S. Targeting oxidative stress for the treatment of ischemic stroke: Upstream and downstream therapeutic strategies. *Brain Circ.* **2016**, *2*, 153–163.
10. Kim, B.; Lee, T.K.; Park, C.W.; Kim, D.W.; Ahn, J.H.; Sim, H.; Lee, J.C.; Yang, G.E.; Kim, J.D.; Shin, M.C.; et al. Pycnogenol((r)) supplementation attenuates memory deficits and protects hippocampal ca1 pyramidal neurons via antioxidative role in a gerbil model of transient forebrain ischemia. *Nutrients* **2020**, *12*, 2477. [CrossRef]
11. Margaill, I.; Plotkine, M.; Lerouet, D. Antioxidant strategies in the treatment of stroke. *Free. Radic. Biol. Med.* **2005**, *39*, 429–443. [CrossRef] [PubMed]
12. Ambati, R.R.; Phang, S.M.; Ravi, S.; Aswathanarayana, R.G. Astaxanthin: Sources, extraction, stability, biological activities and its commercial applications—A review. *Mar. Drugs* **2014**, *12*, 128–152. [CrossRef] [PubMed]
13. Deng, Z.Y.; Shan, W.G.; Wang, S.F.; Hu, M.M.; Chen, Y. Effects of astaxanthin on blood coagulation, fibrinolysis and platelet aggregation in hyperlipidemic rats. *Pharm. Biol.* **2017**, *55*, 663–672. [CrossRef] [PubMed]
14. Farruggia, C.; Kim, M.B.; Bae, M.; Lee, Y.; Pham, T.X.; Yang, Y.; Han, M.J.; Park, Y.K.; Lee, J.Y. Astaxanthin exerts anti-inflammatory and antioxidant effects in macrophages in nrf2-dependent and independent manners. *J. Nutr. Biochem.* **2018**, *62*, 202–209. [CrossRef] [PubMed]

15. Stewart, J.S.; Lignell, A.; Pettersson, A.; Elfving, E.; Soni, M.G. Safety assessment of astaxanthin-rich microalgae biomass: Acute and subchronic toxicity studies in rats. *Food Chem. Toxicol. Int. J. Publ. Br. Ind. Biol. Res. Assoc.* **2008**, *46*, 3030–3036. [CrossRef] [PubMed]

16. Naguib, Y.M. Antioxidant activities of astaxanthin and related carotenoids. *J. Agric. Food Chem.* **2000**, *48*, 1150–1154. [CrossRef]

17. Manabe, Y.; Komatsu, T.; Seki, S.; Sugawara, T. Dietary astaxanthin can accumulate in the brain of rats. *Biosci. Biotechnol. Biochem.* **2018**, *82*, 1433–1436. [CrossRef]

18. Wu, H.; Niu, H.; Shao, A.; Wu, C.; Dixon, B.J.; Zhang, J.; Yang, S.; Wang, Y. Astaxanthin as a potential neuroprotective agent for neurological diseases. *Mar. Drugs* **2015**, *13*, 5750–5766. [CrossRef]

19. Zhang, J.; Ding, C.; Zhang, S.; Xu, Y. Neuroprotective effects of astaxanthin against oxygen and glucose deprivation damage via the pi3k/akt/gsk3beta/nrf2 signalling pathway in vitro. *J. Cell. Mol. Med.* **2020**, *24*, 8977–8985. [CrossRef]

20. Pan, L.; Zhou, Y.; Li, X.F.; Wan, Q.J.; Yu, L.H. Preventive treatment of astaxanthin provides neuroprotection through suppression of reactive oxygen species and activation of antioxidant defense pathway after stroke in rats. *Brain Res. Bull.* **2017**, *130*, 211–220. [CrossRef]

21. Xue, Y.; Qu, Z.; Fu, J.; Zhen, J.; Wang, W.; Cai, Y.; Wang, W. The protective effect of astaxanthin on learning and memory deficits and oxidative stress in a mouse model of repeated cerebral ischemia/reperfusion. *Brain Res. Bull.* **2017**, *131*, 221–228. [CrossRef] [PubMed]

22. Taheri, F.; Sattari, E.; Hormozi, M.; Ahmadvand, H.; Bigdeli, M.R.; Kordestani-Moghadam, P.; Anbari, K.; Milanizadeh, S.; Moghaddasi, M. Dose-dependent effects of astaxanthin on ischemia/reperfusion induced brain injury in mcao model rat. *Neurochem. Res.* **2022**. [CrossRef] [PubMed]

23. Cakir, E.; Cakir, U.; Tayman, C.; Turkmenoglu, T.T.; Gonel, A.; Turan, I.O. Favorable effects of astaxanthin on brain damage due to ischemia- reperfusion injury. *Comb. Chem. High Throughput Screen.* **2020**, *23*, 214–224. [CrossRef] [PubMed]

24. Fu, J.; Sun, H.; Wei, H.; Dong, M.; Zhang, Y.; Xu, W.; Fang, Y.; Zhao, J. Astaxanthin alleviates spinal cord ischemia-reperfusion injury via activation of pi3k/akt/gsk-3beta pathway in rats. *J. Orthop. Surg. Res.* **2020**, *15*, 275. [CrossRef] [PubMed]

25. Lee, J.C.; Shin, B.N.; Cho, J.H.; Lee, T.K.; Kim, I.H.; Noh, Y.; Kim, S.S.; Lee, H.A.; Kim, Y.M.; Kim, H.; et al. Brain ischemic preconditioning protects against moderate, not severe, transient global cerebral ischemic injury. *Metab. Brain Dis.* **2018**, *33*, 1193–1201. [CrossRef] [PubMed]

26. Kirino, T. Delayed neuronal death in the gerbil hippocampus following ischemia. *Brain Res.* **1982**, *239*, 57–69. [CrossRef]

27. Lee, D.H.; Lee, Y.J.; Kwon, K.H. Neuroprotective effects of astaxanthin in oxygen-glucose deprivation in sh-sy5y cells and global cerebral ischemia in rat. *J. Clin. Biochem. Nutr.* **2010**, *47*, 121–129. [CrossRef]

28. Herguido, M.J.; Carceller, F.; Roda, J.M.; Avendano, C. Hippocampal cell loss in transient global cerebral ischemia in rats: A critical assessment. *Neuroscience* **1999**, *93*, 71–80. [CrossRef]

29. Atochin, D.N.; Chernysheva, G.A.; Aliev, O.I.; Smolyakova, V.I.; Osipenko, A.N.; Logvinov, S.V.; Zhdankina, A.A.; Plotnikova, T.M.; Plotnikov, M.B. An improved three-vessel occlusion model of global cerebral ischemia in rats. *Brain Res. Bull.* **2017**, *132*, 213–221. [CrossRef]

30. Gyo, K. Experimental study of transient cochlear ischemia as a cause of sudden deafness. *World J. Otorhinolaryngol.* **2013**, *3*, 1–15. [CrossRef]

31. Jarrott, D.M.; Domer, F.R. A gerbil model of cerebral ischemia suitable for drug evaluation. *Stroke* **1980**, *11*, 203–209. [CrossRef] [PubMed]

32. Pizzino, G.; Irrera, N.; Cucinotta, M.; Pallio, G.; Mannino, F.; Arcoraci, V.; Squadrito, F.; Altavilla, D.; Bitto, A. Oxidative stress: Harms and benefits for human health. *Oxidative Med. Cell. Longev.* **2017**, *2017*, 8416763. [CrossRef] [PubMed]

33. Wu, J.Q.; Kosten, T.R.; Zhang, X.Y. Free radicals, antioxidant defense systems, and schizophrenia. *Prog. Neuro-Psychopharmacol. Biol. Psychiatry* **2013**, *46*, 200–206. [CrossRef] [PubMed]

34. Luo, H.; Huang, D.; Tang, X.; Liu, Y.; Luo, Q.; Liu, C.; Huang, H.; Chen, W.; Qi, Z. Beclin1 exerts protective effects against cerebral ischemiareperfusion injury by promoting DNA damage repair through a nonautophagydependent regulatory mechanism. *Int. J. Mol. Med.* **2022**, *49*, 1–11. [CrossRef] [PubMed]

35. Ayala, A.; Munoz, M.F.; Arguelles, S. Lipid peroxidation: Production, metabolism, and signaling mechanisms of malondialdehyde and 4-hydroxy-2-nonenal. *Oxidative Med. Cell. Longev.* **2014**, *2014*, 360438. [CrossRef] [PubMed]

36. Park, C.W.; Ahn, J.H.; Lee, T.K.; Park, Y.E.; Kim, B.; Lee, J.C.; Kim, D.W.; Shin, M.C.; Park, Y.; Cho, J.H.; et al. Post-treatment with oxcarbazepine confers potent neuroprotection against transient global cerebral ischemic injury by activating nrf2 defense pathway. *Biomed. Pharmacother.* **2020**, *124*, 109850. [CrossRef]

37. Park, J.H.; Lee, T.K.; Kim, D.W.; Sim, H.; Lee, J.C.; Kim, J.D.; Ahn, J.H.; Lee, C.H.; Kim, Y.M.; Won, M.H.; et al. Neuroprotective effects of salicin in a gerbil model of transient forebrain ischemia by attenuating oxidative stress and activating pi3k/akt/gsk3beta pathway. *Antioxidants* **2021**, *10*, 629. [CrossRef]

38. Yousefi-Manesh, H.; Dehpour, A.R.; Nabavi, S.M.; Khayatkashani, M.; Asgardoon, M.H.; Derakhshan, M.H.; Moradi, S.A.; Sheibani, M.; Tavangar, S.M.; Shirooie, S.; et al. Therapeutic effects of hydroalcoholic extracts from the ancient apple mela rosa dei monti sibillini in transient global ischemia in rats. *Pharmaceuticals* **2021**, *14*, 1106. [CrossRef]

39. Jia, J.Y.; Tan, Z.G.; Liu, M.; Jiang, Y.G. Apurinic/apyrimidinic endonuclease 1 (ape1) contributes to resveratrolinduced neuroprotection against oxygenglucose deprivation and reoxygenation injury in ht22 cells: Involvement in reducing oxidative DNA damage. *Mol. Med. Rep.* **2017**, *16*, 9786–9794. [CrossRef]

40. Lee, J.C.; Won, M.H. Neuroprotection of antioxidant enzymes against transient global cerebral ischemia in gerbils. *Anat. Cell Biol.* **2014**, *47*, 149–156. [CrossRef]

41. Sugawara, T.; Noshita, N.; Lewen, A.; Gasche, Y.; Ferrand-Drake, M.; Fujimura, M.; Morita-Fujimura, Y.; Chan, P.H. Overexpression of copper/zinc superoxide dismutase in transgenic rats protects vulnerable neurons against ischemic damage by blocking the mitochondrial pathway of caspase activation. *J. Neurosci. Off. J. Soc. Neurosci.* **2002**, *22*, 209–217. [CrossRef]

42. Keller, J.N.; Kindy, M.S.; Holtsberg, F.W.; St Clair, D.K.; Yen, H.C.; Germeyer, A.; Steiner, S.M.; Bruce-Keller, A.J.; Hutchins, J.B.; Mattson, M.P. Mitochondrial manganese superoxide dismutase prevents neural apoptosis and reduces ischemic brain injury: Suppression of peroxynitrite production, lipid peroxidation, and mitochondrial dysfunction. *J. Neurosci. Off. J. Soc. Neurosci.* **1998**, *18*, 687–697. [CrossRef]

43. Chen, B.H.; Park, J.H.; Ahn, J.H.; Cho, J.H.; Kim, I.H.; Lee, J.C.; Won, M.H.; Lee, C.H.; Hwang, I.K.; Kim, J.D.; et al. Pretreated quercetin protects gerbil hippocampal ca1 pyramidal neurons from transient cerebral ischemic injury by increasing the expression of antioxidant enzymes. *Neural Regen. Res.* **2017**, *12*, 220–227. [PubMed]

44. Lee, T.K.; Kang, I.J.; Kim, B.; Sim, H.J.; Kim, D.W.; Ahn, J.H.; Lee, J.C.; Ryoo, S.; Shin, M.C.; Cho, J.H.; et al. Experimental pretreatment with chlorogenic acid prevents transient ischemia-induced cognitive decline and neuronal damage in the hippocampus through anti-oxidative and anti-inflammatory effects. *Molecules* **2020**, *25*, 3578. [CrossRef]

45. Yang, B.B.; Zou, M.; Zhao, L.; Zhang, Y.K. Astaxanthin attenuates acute cerebral infarction via nrf-2/ho-1 pathway in rats. *Curr. Res. Transl. Med.* **2021**, *69*, 103271. [CrossRef]

46. Radtke-Schuller, S.; Schuller, G.; Angenstein, F.; Grosser, O.S.; Goldschmidt, J.; Budinger, E. Brain atlas of the mongolian gerbil (*Meriones unguiculatus*) in ct/mri-aided stereotaxic coordinates. *Brain Struct. Funct.* **2016**, *221* (Suppl. 1), 1–272. [CrossRef]

47. Park, J.H.; Ahn, J.H.; Lee, T.K.; Park, C.W.; Kim, B.; Lee, J.C.; Kim, D.W.; Shin, M.C.; Cho, J.H.; Lee, C.H.; et al. Laminarin pretreatment provides neuroprotection against forebrain ischemia/reperfusion injury by reducing oxidative stress and neuroinflammation in aged gerbils. *Mar. Drugs* **2020**, *18*, 213. [CrossRef]

48. Ahn, J.H.; Shin, M.C.; Kim, D.W.; Kim, H.; Song, M.; Lee, T.K.; Lee, J.C.; Kim, H.; Cho, J.H.; Kim, Y.M.; et al. Antioxidant properties of fucoidan alleviate acceleration and exacerbation of hippocampal neuronal death following transient global cerebral ischemia in high-fat diet-induced obese gerbils. *Int. J. Mol. Sci.* **2019**, *20*, 554. [CrossRef]

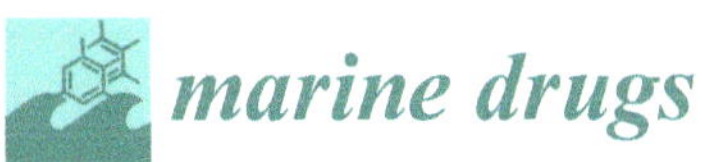

Article

Nitrogen-Containing Secondary Metabolites from a Deep-Sea Fungus *Aspergillus unguis* and Their Anti-Inflammatory Activity

Cao Van Anh [1,2], Yeo Dae Yoon [3], Jong Soon Kang [3], Hwa-Sun Lee [1], Chang-Su Heo [1,2] and Hee Jae Shin [1,2,*]

[1] Marine Natural Products Chemistry Laboratory, Korea Institute of Ocean Science and Technology, 385 Haeyang-ro, Yeongdo-gu, Busan 49111, Korea; caovananh@kiost.ac.kr (C.V.A.); hwasunlee@kiost.ac.kr (H.-S.L.); science30@kiost.ac.kr (C.-S.H.)

[2] Department of Marine Biotechnology, University of Science and Technology (UST), 217 Gajungro, Yuseong-gu, Daejeon 34113, Korea

[3] Laboratory Animal Resource Center, Korea Research Institute of Bioscience and Biotechnology, 30 Yeongudanjiro, Cheongju 28116, Korea; yunyd76@kribb.re.kr (Y.D.Y.); kanjon@kribb.re.kr (J.S.K.)

* Correspondence: shinhj@kiost.ac.kr; Tel.: +82-51-664-3341; Fax: +82-51-664-3340

Abstract: *Aspergillus* is well-known as the second-largest contributor of fungal natural products. Based on NMR guided isolation, three nitrogen-containing secondary metabolites, including two new compounds, variotin B (**1**) and coniosulfide E (**2**), together with a known compound, unguisin A (**3**), were isolated from the ethyl acetate (EtOAc) extract of the deep-sea fungus *Aspergillus unguis* IV17-109. The planar structures of **1** and **2** were elucidated by an extensive analysis of their spectroscopic data (HRESIMS, 1D and 2D NMR). The absolute configuration of **2** was determined by comparison of its optical rotation value with those of the synthesized analogs. Compound **2** is a rare, naturally occurring substance with an unusual cysteinol moiety. Furthermore, **1** showed moderate anti-inflammatory activity with an IC_{50} value of 20.0 µM. These results revealed that *Aspergillus unguis* could produce structurally diverse nitrogenous secondary metabolites, which can be used for further studies to find anti-inflammatory leads.

Keywords: deep-sea fungus; *A. unguis*; variotin; coniosulfide; anti-inflammatory

Citation: Anh, C.V.; Yoon, Y.D.; Kang, J.S.; Lee, H.-S.; Heo, C.-S.; Shin, H.J. Nitrogen-Containing Secondary Metabolites from a Deep-Sea Fungus *Aspergillus unguis* and Their Anti-Inflammatory Activity. *Mar. Drugs* **2022**, *20*, 217. https://doi.org/10.3390/md20030217

Academic Editors: Donatella Degl'Innocenti and Marzia Vasarri

Received: 2 March 2022
Accepted: 19 March 2022
Published: 20 March 2022

Publisher's Note: MDPI stays neutral with regard to jurisdictional claims in published maps and institutional affiliations.

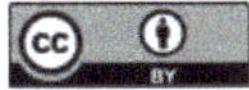

1. Introduction

Deep-sea hydrothermal vents are recognized as one of the most extreme and dynamic habitats on our planet [1]. These hotspot ecosystems are characterized by high temperature, high pressure, low oxygen supply, and the absence of sun light [2]. In addition, hydrothermal vent flows bring fluids with high concentrations of reduced sulfur-containing compounds and heavy metals [2]. Given this fact, microorganisms living in this specific environment are considered as a new frontier for discovery of natural products with unique structures and tremendous pharmacological activities [3].

Aspergillus is renowned as a prolific source of numerous fungal peptides, including lipo-, depsi-, linear-, and cyclic-peptides, which are structurally unique and demonstrated various bioactivities, such as anti-microbial, anti-fungal, anti-inflammatory, and cytotoxic activities [4,5]. Among the peptides derived from *Aspergillus* spp., unguisins are a unique cyclic heptapetide class commonly produced by *Aspergillus unguis*, and until now unguisins A–G have been reported [6,7].

Inflammation is a protective response of our body to a wide range of stimuli. This process plays a central role or is an important symptom in the pathogenesis of various chronic diseases for instance Alzheimer's disease, asthma, diabetes, and rheumatoid arthritis [8]. The inflammatory process is characterized by over secretion of nitric oxide (NO) and inflammatory cytokines such as interleukin 1 beta (IL-1β), tumor necrosis factor alpha

(TNF-α), and interleukin 6 (IL-6). Therefore, reducing the production of inflammatory mediators is a key indicator for the treatment of various diseases.

As part of our study on marine-derived microorganisms isolated near hydrothermal vents, we have reported some anti-inflammatory phenazine alkaloids from a yeast-like fungus *Cystobasidium laryngis*, and nidulin-related polyketides from *A. unguis* IV17-109, which showed anti-microbial and cytotoxic activities [9,10]. Based on NMR guided isolation, we found that the ^{1}H NMR spectra of non-polar fractions from *A. unguis* IV17-109 showed some minor interesting peaks in the olefinic region, which do not belong to unguisin peptides or nidulin-related polyketides. Further careful purification of these fractions led to the identification of two new compounds, variotin B (**1**) and coniosulfide E (**2**) (Figure 1). Anti-inflammatory activity of **1** and **2** was preliminarily evaluated and the result revealed that **1** has moderate activity. Here, we report the details of the isolation, structure identification, and anti-inflammatory nature of these compounds.

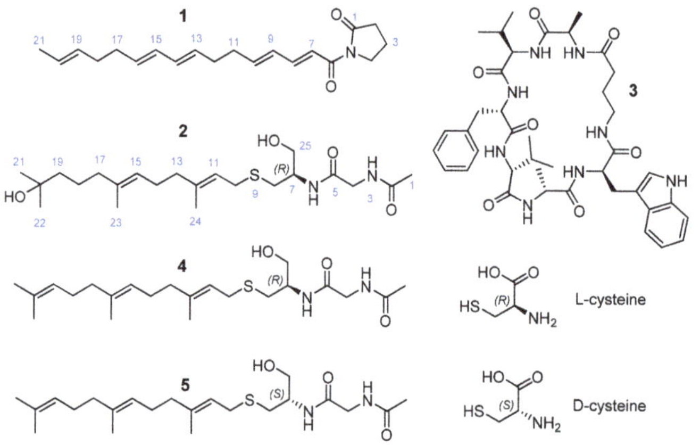

Figure 1. Structures of **1–3** isolated from *A. unguis* IV17-109, and the synthetic analogs (**4** and **5**).

2. Results and Discussion

Compound **1** was isolated as pale-yellow needles with the molecular formula of $C_{20}H_{27}NO_2$ based on its HRESIMS peak at *m/z* 336.1938, ([M+Na]$^+$, calculated for $C_{20}H_{27}NO_2Na$, 336.1939), requiring 8 indices of hydrogen deficiency. The ^{1}H NMR spectrum of **1** showed signals attributed to a methyl group at δ_H 1.62 (d, *J* = 4.5, H$_3$-21), seven methylene groups at δ_H 2.04–3.82, and ten olefinic protons at δ_H 5.42–7.37. The ^{13}C NMR spectrum in combination with HSQC data revealed signals of 20 resonances belonging to a methyl at δ_C 18.1, seven methylene carbons at δ_C 18.1–47.0, ten olefinic carbons at δ_C 121.7–146.9, and two carbonyl carbons at δ_C 168.2 and 177.8. Two carbonyl and ten sp^2 carbons, accounting for 7 out of 8 degrees of unsaturation, indicated **1** is a monocyclic compound. The structure of a five-membered lactam ring was determined by continuous ^{1}H-^{1}H COSY correlations from H$_2$-2 to H$_2$-4, and the HMBC correlation from H$_2$-4 to C-1. A substructure was identified as a C-16 polyunsaturated fatty acid by continuous ^{1}H-^{1}H COSY correlations from H-7 to H$_3$-21, and the HMBC correlations from H-7 and H-8 to C-6 (Figure 2). The connection of the fatty acid and the lactam ring was corroborated by the HMBC correlation from H$_2$-4 to C-6.

The geometries of $\Delta^{7,9,13,15}$ were deduced as *E*-form by their large coupling constants (Table 1) and the chemical shift of terminal methyl (C-21) was δ_C 18.1, revealing the geometry of Δ^{19} was *E*-form [11,12]. Therefore, **1** was determined as a new variotin derivative with a non-branched side chain and named variotin B [13].

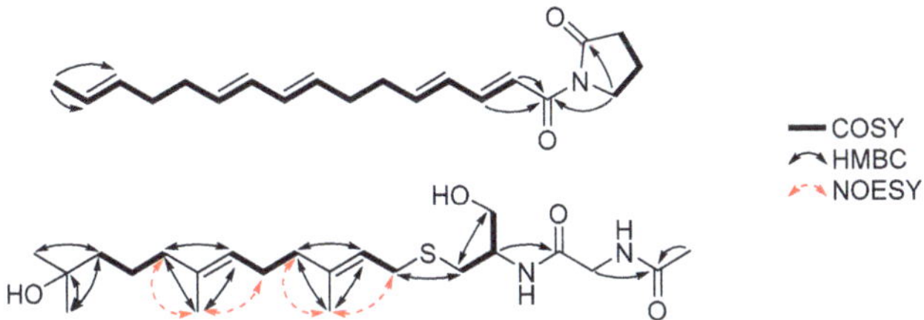

Figure 2. Key 2D NMR data of **1** and **2**.

Table 1. ^{1}H and ^{13}C NMR data of **1** and **2** in CD$_3$OD (600 MHz for ^{1}H and 150 MHz for ^{13}C).

Compound	1		2	
Position	δ_H, mult (*J* in Hz)	δ_C	δ_H, mult (*J* in Hz)	δ_C
1		177.8	2.01, s	22.5
2	2.61, t (8.1)	34.6		173.9
3	2.04, m	18.1		
4	3.82, m	47.0	3.86, m	43.6
5				171.5
6		168.2		
7	7.25, d (15.1)	121.7	4.03, m	52.3
8	7.37, dd (15.1, 10.8)	146.9	2.55–2.70	32.9
9	6.32, dd (15.1, 10.8)	130.7		
10	6.23, m	146.0	3.16–3.22	30.3
11	2.29, q (6.6)	34.0	5.23, td (7.8, 1.0)	121.8
12	2.21, m	32.8		140.1
13	5.56, td (13.6, 6.6)	131.6	2.06, m	40.7
14	6.01, m	132.6	2.13, m	27.4
15	6.01, m	131.8	5.13, td (6.8, 1.0)	125.2
16	5.56, td (13.6, 6.6)	133.1		136.3
17	2.10, dd (14.1, 6.8)	33.6	1.98, t (7.2)	41.3
18	2.04, m	33.8	1.46, m	23.7
19	5.44, m	131.9	1.40, m	44.3
20	5.44, m	126.1		71.4
21	1.62, d (4.5)	18.1	1.17, s	29.2
22			1.17, s	29.2
23			1.61, s	16.0
24			1.68, s	16.2
25			3.62, m	63.6

Compound **2** was isolated as a colorless solid and its molecular formula was determined as C$_{22}$H$_{40}$N$_2$O$_4$S, with four indices of hydrogen deficiency based on its HRESIMS peak at *m/z* 451.2607, ([M+Na]$^+$, calculated for C$_{22}$H$_{40}$N$_2$O$_4$SNa, 451.2606). The ^{1}H NMR spectrum of **2** showed signals attributed to five methyl groups at δ_H 1.17 (s, 6H, H$_3$-21 and H$_3$-22), 1.61 (s, H$_3$-23), 1.68 (s, H$_3$-24), and 2.01 (s, H$_3$-1); seven methylene groups at δ_H 1.40–3.22; an oxygenated methylene group at δ_H 3.60 and 3.64 (H-25$_{a,b}$); an amide methylene at δ_H 3.86 (m, H$_2$-4); an amide methine at δ_H 4.03 (m, H-7); and two olefinic protons at δ_H 5.13 and 5.23 (m, H-11 and H-15). The ^{13}C NMR spectrum in combination with HSQC data demonstrated signals of 22 resonances belonging to five methyls at δ_C 16.0 (C-23), 16.2 (C-24), 22.5 (C-1), and 29.2 (2C, C-21 and C-22); seven methylenes at δ_C 23.7–44.3; an oxygenated methylene at δ_C 63.6; an amide methylene at δ_C 43.6; an amide methine at δ_C 52.3; a tertiary alcohol at δ_C 71.4; four olefinic carbons at δ_C 121.8–140.1; and two carbonyl carbons at δ_C 171.5 and 173.9. Two carbonyl and four sp^2 carbons accounting for all 4 degrees of unsaturation indicated **2** is an acyclic compound.

The structure of a cysteinol unit was determined by sequential ^1H-^1H COSY correlations of H-8$_{a,b}$/H-7/H-25$_{a,b}$. A partial structure of *N*-acetylglycine, which was connected to the cysteinol moiety via a peptide bond, was determined by the HMBC correlations of H-7/C-5, H$_2$-4/C-2, and H$_3$-1/C-2. The remaining 15 carbons were assigned as a 10-hydro-11-hydroxyfarnesyl moiety based on a detailed analysis of ^1H-^1H COSY and HMBC data (Figure 2), and the connection of this moiety with the cysteinol residue via a thioether bond was determined by the HMBC correlations of H-8 $_{a,b}$/C-10 and H-10$_{a,b}$/C-8. The geometry of Δ^{11} was deduced as *E*-form by the strong NOESY correlations from H$_3$-24 to H-10$_{a,b}$ and H-13$_{a,b}$; and no-observed NOESY correlation from H$_3$-24 to H-11. Similarly, Δ^{15} was also determined as *E*-form (Figure 2). Consequently, the gross structure of **2** was determined as shown in Figure 1.

To determine the absolute configuration of **2**, we synthesized its analogs (**4** and **5**, a pair of enantiomers synthesized from *L*- and *D*-cysteine and farnesyl chloride, Scheme 1) from commercially available substances. By comparing the optical rotation sign of **2** $[\alpha]_D^{20} -$ 100 (*c* 0.3, MeOH) with that of **4** $[\alpha]_D^{20} - 110$ (*c* 0.3, MeOH) and **5** $[\alpha]_D^{20} + 120$ (*c* 0.3, MeOH), the absolute configuration of **2** was determined to be the same as that of **4** (7*R*). Thus, **2** was determined as a new derivative of sulfur-containing natural products, coniosulfides A-D [14], and named coniosulfide E.

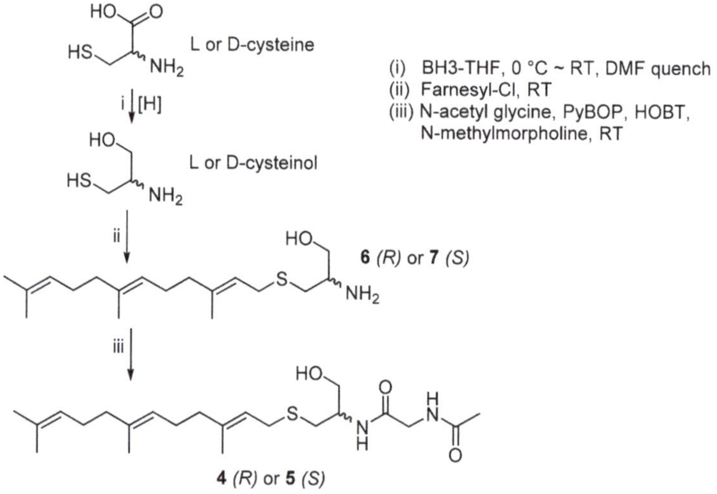

Scheme 1. Synthesis of **4** and **5**.

A co-isolated known compound was identified as unguisin A (**3**) by comparing its spectroscopic data with the corresponding literature values [6].

Since some fungal peptides were reported to show anti-inflammatory activity [4], **1** and **2** were evaluated for their anti-inflammatory activity. Subsequently, **1** showed moderate anti-inflammatory activity with an IC$_{50}$ value of 20.0 μM. Even though a literature review revealed many synthetic analogs of **2** demonstrated inhibitory effects on human isoprenylcysteine carboxyl methyltransferase (hIcmt) [15] or the inflammation process [16], unfortunately, **2** showed no anti-inflammatory activity at a concentration of 30.0 μM. Due to the limited amount of **2**, we were unable to check its effect on hIcmt. Therefore, further studies are needed to find the bioactivities of **2**.

To further investigate the anti-inflammatory activity of **1**, we examined the inhibitory effect of **1** on lipopolysaccharide (LPS)-induced production of inflammatory mediators, including NO, IL-6, and iNOS, in RAW 264.7 cells. The treatment of RAW 264.7 cells with LPS led to the accumulation of nitrite and IL-6, and **1** dose-proportionally inhibited LPS-induced production of nitrite and IL-6 in LPS-stimulated RAW 264.7 cells (Figure 3A,B). To further examine whether the effect of **1** were due to its effects on the mRNA expression of cognate genes, we investigated the effect of **1** on the mRNA expression of inducible nitric oxide synthase (iNOS) and IL-6 by quantitative polymerase chain reaction (qPCR). The mRNA levels of iNOS and IL-6 were induced by LPS treatment, and this induction was suppressed by **1** in a concentration-dependent manner (Figure 3C,D). Considering the above-mentioned data, it is noticeable that **1** showed anti-inflammatory activity by suppressing the production of NO and the expression of iNOS and IL-6 with no cytotoxicity at the treated concentrations. The results revealed that fungal natural products could be an important source of leads for the development of new anti-inflammatory drugs with minimal side effects.

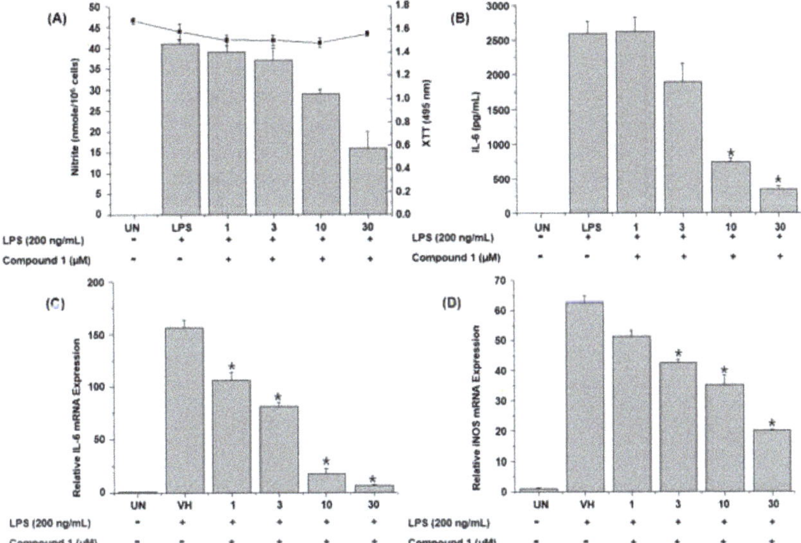

Figure 3. Inhibitory effects of **1** on LPS-induced nitrite production and IL-6 secretion in RAW 264.7 cells. RAW 264.7 cells were pretreated with **1** at the depicted concentrations (1~30 μM) for 1 h and stimulated with LPS (200 ng/mL) for 24 h. The levels of nitrite (**A**) and IL-6 (**B**) in culture supernatants were determined by Griess reaction and ELISA, respectively. The mRNA levels of IL-6 (**C**) and iNOS (**D**) were examined by qPCR. Data are represented as the mean ± SD of quadruplicate determinations. An asterisk (*) denotes that the response is significantly different from vehicle-treated group as determined by Dunnett's multiple comparison test at $p < 0.05$. The results shown are representatives of more than two independent experiments (UN: Untreated; VH: Vehicle (0.1% DMSO)).

3. Materials and Methods

3.1. General Experimental Procedures

HRESIMS data were obtained on a Waters Synapt G2 Q-TOF mass spectrometer (Waters Corporation, Milford, MA, USA). Optical rotations were measured on a Rudolph Research Analytical Autopol III polarimeter (Rudolph Research Analytical, Hackettstown, NJ, USA). 1D and 2D NMR spectra were acquired using a Bruker 600 MHz spectrometer (Bruker BioSpin GmbH, Rheinstetten, Germany). IR spectra were measured on a JASCO FT/IR-4100 spectrophotometer (JASCO Corporation, Tokyo, Japan). UV-visible spectra were measured by a Shimadzu UV-1650PC spectrophotometer. HPLC was carried out with a PrimeLine Binary pump (Analytical Scientific Instruments, Inc., El Sobrante, CA, USA) and a RI-101 detector (Shoko Scientific Co. Ltd., Yokohama, Japan). Semi-preparative HPLC was conducted using an ODS column (YMC-Pack-ODS-A, 250 × 10 mm i.d, 5 μM).

Analytical HPLC was performed with an ODS column (YMC-Pack-ODS-A, 250 × 4.6 mm i.d, 5 μM). All the used reagents were purchased from Sigma-Aldrich (Merck KGaA, Darmstadt, Germany).

3.2. Fungal Material, Fermentation, and Isolation of Secondary Metabolites

Fungal Material, Fermentation, and Isolation of **1–3** from *Aspergillus unguis* IV17-109

A. unguis IV17-109 (GenBank accession number OL700797) was isolated from a deep-sea shrimp sample as previously described [10]. The EtOAc extract was fractionated into 10 fractions (F1–F10), as described earlier [10]. The F7 fraction was purified by a semi-preparative reversed-phase HPLC (YMC-Pack-ODS-A, 250 × 10 mm i.d, 5 μm, flow rate 2.0 mL/min, 60% MeOH/H_2O, RI detector) to obtain **3** (2.0 mg, t_R = 32 min). The F8 fraction was subjected to a semi-preparative reversed-phase HPLC (YMC-Pack-ODS-A, 250 × 10 mm i.d, 5 μm, flow rate 2.0 mL/min, RI detector) using an isocratic elution with 70% MeOH/H_2O to yield a subfraction F8-1, and the subfraction was further purified by a semi-preparative HPLC (YMC-Pack-ODS-A, 250 × 10 mm i.d, 5 μm, flow rate 2.0 mL/min, RI detector) using an isocratic elution with 50% MeCN/H_2O to obtain **2** (1.0 mg, t_R = 15 min). Finally, the F9 fraction was purified by a semi-preparative reversed-phase HPLC (YMC-Pack-ODS-A, 250 × 10 mm i.d, 5 μm, flow rate 2.0 mL/min, RI detector) using an isocratic elution with 83% MeOH/H_2O to yield **1** (3.0 mg, t_R = 42 min).

Variotin B (**1**): pale-yellow needles; IR ν_{max} 3286, 2918, 1724, 1671, 1352, 1261, 989 cm^{-1}; UV(MeOH) λ_{max} (log ε) 283 (2.51), 229 (2.60) nm; HRESIMS m/z 336.1938 [M+Na]$^+$ (calcd for $C_{20}H_{27}NO_2Na$, 336.1939), ^{1}H NMR (CD$_3$OD, 600 MHz) and ^{13}C NMR (CD$_3$OD, 150 MHz) see Table 1.

Coniosulfide E (**2**): colorless solid, $[\alpha]_D^{20}$ − 100 (c 0.3, MeOH); IR ν_{max} 3303, 2929, 1653, 1547, 1374, 1038 cm^{-1}, HRESIMS m/z 451.2607 [M+Na]$^+$ (calcd for $C_{22}H_{40}N_2O_4SNa$, 451.2606), ^{1}H NMR (CD$_3$OD, 600 MHz) and ^{13}C NMR (CD$_3$OD, 150 MHz) see Table 1.

3.3. Synthesis of **4** and **5**

Compounds **4** and **5** were synthesized according to the reported procedures with minor modifications [17]. Borane-tetrahydrofuran (Borane-THF, 4 mL, 4 mmol) was added dropwise to *L*- or *D*-cysteine (0.121 g, 1 mmol) in dry THF (5 mL) at 0°C under a nitrogen atmosphere, and stirred at ambient temperature for 7 h. The reaction mixture was quenched with dry dimethylfomamide (DMF, 1 mL) and stirred for 1 h. Farnesyl chloride (0.5 mmol) was added to the reaction mixture and stirred at room temperature for 3 h. The volatiles were removed in vacuo. The residue was re-dissolved in EtOAC (20 mL) and washed with H_2O (20 mL) to remove the residue of cysteine. The EtOAc layer was evaporated under reduced pressure and the residue was purified by a semi-preparative HPLC using CH_3OH/H_2O (87:13) as an eluent to yield farnesyl-*L*-cysteinol (**6**) or farnesyl-*D*-cysteinol (**7**) (Figures S16 and S17).

To a dry DMF solution (500 μL) of **6** or **7** (5.0 mg) and *N*-acetylglycine (2.0 mg), benzotriazol-1-yloxytripyrrolidinophosphonium hexafluorophosphate (PyBOP, 12.0 mg), hydroxybenzotriazole (HOBT, 3.0 mg), and *N*-methylmorpholine (300 μL) were added [18]. The reaction mixture was stirred for 3 h at room temperature. Afterwards, 10 mL of water were added and the mixture was extracted twice with EtOAc (15 mL × 2). The EtOAC layer was dried, and the residue was purified by a semi-preparative HPLC (YMC-ODS column, 10 × 250 mm; MeCN-H_2O, 65:35) to give compounds **4** or **5** with an overall yield of 11%.

1-farnesyl-2-(*N*-aetylglycine)-*L*-cysteinol (**4**): white amorphous solid, $[\alpha]_D^{20}$ − 110 (c 0.3, MeOH), ^{1}H NMR (600 MHz, MeOD) δ_H 5.23 (t, *J* = 7.8 Hz, 1H), 5.14–5.07 (m, 2H), 4.05–4.00 (m, 1H), 3.90–3.82 (m, 2H), 3.64 (dd, *J* = 11.2, 5.2 Hz, 1H), 3.60 (dd, *J* = 11.1, 4.9 Hz, 1H), 3.22 (dd, *J* = 13.1, 8.0 Hz, 1H), 3.16 (dd, *J* = 13.1, 7.6 Hz, 1H), 2.70 (dd, *J* = 13.7, 6.5 Hz, 1H), 2.55 (dd, *J* = 13.7, 7.4 Hz, 1H), 2.11 (dt, *J* = 11.4, 5.8 Hz, 2H), 2.06 (dt, *J* = 14.2, 7.2 Hz, 4H), 2.01 (d, *J* = 1.0 Hz, 3H), 1.97 (t, *J* = 7.6 Hz, 2H), 1.68 (d, *J* = 7.2 Hz, 6H), 1.60 (s, 6H); ^{13}C NMR (150 MHz, MeOD) δ_C 173.8, 171.4, 140.1, 136.2, 132.1, 125.4, 125.2, 121.8, 63.6, 52.3,

43.6, 40.8, 40.7, 32.9, 30.4, 27.8, 27.5, 25.9, 22.5, 17.8, 16.2, 16.1; ESIMS *m/z* 433.2 [M + Na]$^+$ (Figures S18–S22).

1-farnesyl-2-(*N*-aetylglycine)-*D*-cysteinol (**5**): white amorphous solid, $[\alpha]_D^{20}$ + 120 (c 0.3, MeOH), ^{1}H and ^{13}C NMR, and ESIMS data of **5** were identical to those of **4** (Figures S23–S24).

3.4. Anti-Inflammatory Assay

Anti-inflammatory assay was conducted as described earlier [19]. Murine monocyte/macrophage RAW 264.7 (ATCC TIB-71) cell line was purchased from American Type Culture Collection (ATCC; Manassas, VA, USA).

4. Conclusions

In summary, based on NMR-guided isolation, two new (**1** and **2**) and one known (**3**) compounds were isolated from the culture broth of the deep-sea fungus *Aspergillus unguis* IV17-109. The planar structures of the new compounds were elucidated by a comprehensive analysis and comparison of their spectroscopic data with the values in the literature (HRESIMS, 1D, and 2D NMR). Compound **2** is a rare natural product with an unusual cysteinol moiety. The absolute configuration of **2** was determined by comparing its optical rotation sign with that of the synthesized analogs (**4** and **5**). Compounds **1** and **2** were preliminarily screened for their in vitro anti-inflammatory activity. Compound **1** showed moderate activity with an IC$_{50}$ value of 20.0 μM. To the best of our knowledge, this is the first report on linear nitrogenous secondary metabolites isolated from *Aspergillus unguis*. This research expanded the biological and chemical diversities of fungal natural products.

Supplementary Materials: The following are available online at https://www.mdpi.com/article/10.3390/md20030217/s1, Figures S1–S15, HRESIMS data, ^{1}H, ^{13}C, ^{1}H-^{1}H COSY, HSQC, HMBC, NOESY NMR experimental spectra of compounds **1** and **2**. Figures S16–S24, ESIMS, ^{1}H NMR, ^{13}C NMR experimental spectra of **4–7**.

Author Contributions: Conceptualization, H.J.S.; investigation, C.V.A. and Y.D.Y.; resources, H.-S.L. and C.-S.H.; writing—original draft preparation, C.V.A.; writing—review and editing, H.J.S.; visualization, J.S.K.; project administration, H.J.S.; funding acquisition, H.J.S. All authors have read and agreed to the published version of the manuscript.

Funding: This research was supported in part by the Korea Institute of Ocean Science and Technology (Grant PE99952) and the Ministry of Oceans and Fisheries, Republic of Korea (Grants PM62500 and no. 20170411).

Institutional Review Board Statement: Not applicable.

Informed Consent Statement: Not applicable.

Data Availability Statement: The data presented in the article are available in the Supplementary Materials.

Acknowledgments: The authors express gratitude to Jung Hoon Choi, Korea Basic Science Institute, Ochang, Korea, for providing mass data.

Conflicts of Interest: The authors declare no conflict of interest.

References

1. Skropeta, D.; Wei, L. Recent advances in deep-sea natural products. *Nat. Prod. Rep.* **2014**, *31*, 999–1025. [CrossRef] [PubMed]
2. Andrianasolo, E.; Lutz, R.; Falkowski, P. Chapter 3—Deep-Sea Hydrothermal Vents as a New Source of Drug Discovery. *Stud. Nat. Prod. Chem.* **2012**, *36*, 43–66.
3. Pan, C.; Shi, Y.; Chen, X.; Chen, C.-T.A.; Tao, X.; Wu, B. New compounds from a hydrothermal vent crab-associated fungus *Aspergillus versicolor* XZ-4. *Org. Biomol. Chem.* **2017**, *15*, 1155–1163. [CrossRef] [PubMed]
4. Youssef, F.S.; Ashour, M.L.; Singab, A.N.B.; Wink, M. A Comprehensive Review of Bioactive Peptides from Marine Fungi and Their Biological Significance. *Mar. Drugs* **2019**, *17*, 559. [CrossRef] [PubMed]

5. Henke, M.T.; Soukup, A.A.; Goering, A.W.; McClure, R.A.; Thomson, R.J.; Keller, N.P.; Kelleher, N.L. New Aspercryptins, Lipopeptide Natural Products, Revealed by HDAC Inhibition in *Aspergillus nidulans*. *ACS Chem. Biol.* **2016**, *11*, 2117–2123. [CrossRef] [PubMed]
6. Malmstrøm, J. Unguisins A and B: New Cyclic Peptides from the Marine-Derived Fungus *Emericella unguis*. *J. Nat. Prod.* **1999**, *62*, 787–789. [CrossRef] [PubMed]
7. Li, W.; Jiao, F.-W.; Wang, J.-Q.; Shi, J.; Wang, T.-T.; Khan, S.; Jiao, R.-H.; Tan, R.-X.; Ge, H.-M. Unguisin G, a new kynurenine-containing cyclic heptapeptide from the sponge-associated fungus *Aspergillus candidus* NF2412. *Tetrahedron Lett.* **2020**, *61*, 152322. [CrossRef]
8. Pahwa, R.; Goyal, A.; Jialal, I. *Chronic Inflammation*; StatPearls Publishing: Treasure Island, FL, USA, 2021. Available online: https://www.ncbi.nlm.nih.gov/books/NBK493173/ (accessed on 25 February 2022).
9. Lee, H.-S.; Kang, J.S.; Choi, B.-K.; Lee, H.-S.; Lee, Y.-J.; Lee, J.; Shin, H.J. Phenazine Derivatives with Anti-Inflammatory Activity from the Deep-Sea Sediment-Derived Yeast-Like Fungus *Cystobasidium laryngis* IV17-028. *Mar. Drugs* **2019**, *17*, 482. [CrossRef] [PubMed]
10. Anh, C.V.; Kwon, J.-H.; Kang, J.S.; Lee, H.-S.; Heo, C.-S.; Shin, H.J. Antibacterial and Cytotoxic Phenolic Polyketides from Two Marine-Derived Fungal Strains of *Aspergillus unguis*. *Pharmaceuticals* **2022**, *15*, 74. [CrossRef] [PubMed]
11. Yonehara, H.; Takeuchi, S.; Umezawa, H.; Sumiki, Y. Variotin, a new antifungal antibiotic, produced by *Paecilomyces varioti* Bainier var. antibioticus. *J. Antibiot.* **1959**, *12*, 109–110.
12. Podkorytov, I.S.; Lubnin, A.V. ^{13}C NMR spectra of the models for the end-group analysis of polybutadiene. *Magn. Reson. Chem.* **1991**, *29*, 561–565. [CrossRef]
13. Ishii, T.; Nonaka, K.; Sugawara, A.; Iwatsuki, M.; Masuma, R.; Hirose, T.; Sunazuka, T.; Ōmura, S.; Shiomi, K. Cinatrins D and E, and virgaricin B, three novel compounds produced by a fungus, *Virgaria boninensis* FKI-4958. *J. Antibiot.* **2015**, *68*, 633–637. [CrossRef] [PubMed]
14. Vertesy, L.; Ehrlich, K.; Segeth, P.; Toti, L. Coniosulfides and Their Derivatives, Processes for Preparing Them, and Their Use as Pharmaceuticals. U.S. Patent US 2005/0209308A1, 22 September 2005.
15. Majmudar, J.D.; Morrison-Logue, A.; Song, J.; Hrycyna, C.A.; Gibbs, R.A. Identification of a novel nanomolar inhibitor of hIcmt via a carboxylate replacement approach. *Med. Chem. Comm.* **2012**, *3*, 1125–1137. [CrossRef]
16. Voronkov, M.; Perez, E.; Healy, J.; Fernandez, J. Preparation of Amino Acids for Treating or Preventing Inflammation, Acne, and Bacterial Conditions. International Patent WO 2018/132759 Al, 19 July 2018.
17. Rodriguez, D.; Ramesh, C.; Henson, L.H.; Wilmeth, L.; Bryant, B.K.; Kadavakollu, S.; Hirsch, R.; Montoya, J.; Howell, P.R.; George, J.M.; et al. Synthesis and characterization of tritylthioethanamine derivatives with potent KSP inhibitory activity. *Bioorg. Med. Chem.* **2011**, *19*, 5446–5453. [CrossRef] [PubMed]
18. Hwang, J.-Y.; Park, S.C.; Byun, W.S.; Oh, D.-C.; Lee, S.K.; Oh, K.-B.; Shin, J. Bioactive Bianthraquinones and Meroterpenoids from a Marine-Derived *Stemphylium* sp. Fungus. *Mar. Drugs* **2020**, *18*, 436. [CrossRef] [PubMed]
19. Shin, H.J.; Heo, C.-S.; Anh, C.V.; Yoon, Y.D.; Kang, J.S. Streptoglycerides E–H, Unsaturated Polyketides from the Marine-Derived Bacterium *Streptomyces specialis* and Their Anti-Inflammatory Activity. *Mar. Drugs* **2022**, *20*, 44. [CrossRef]

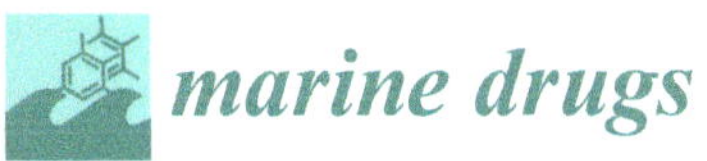 *marine drugs*

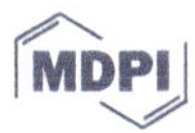

Article

Marginal Impact of Brown Seaweed *Ascophyllum nodosum* and *Fucus vesiculosus* Extract on Metabolic and Inflammatory Response in Overweight and Obese Prediabetic Subjects

Marlène Vodouhè [1], Julie Marois [2], Valérie Guay [2], Nadine Leblanc [2], Stanley John Weisnagel [3], Jean-François Bilodeau [3] and Hélène Jacques [1,*]

[1] School of Nutrition, Faculty of Agricultural and Food Sciences, Université Laval, Québec City, QC G1V 0A6, Canada; marlene.vodouhe.1@ulaval.ca
[2] Institute of Nutrition and Functional Foods, Université Laval, Québec City, QC G1V 0A6, Canada; julie.marois@fsaa.ulaval.ca (J.M.); valerie.guay@fsaa.ulaval.ca (V.G.); nadine.leblanc@fsaa.ulaval.ca (N.L.)
[3] Department of Medicine, Faculty of Medicine, Université Laval, CHU de Québec-Université Laval Research Centre, Québec City, QC G1V 4G2, Canada; john.weisnagel@crchudequebec.ulaval.ca (S.J.W.); jean-francois.bilodeau@crchudequebec.ulaval.ca (J.-F.B.)
* Correspondence: helene.jacques@fsaa.ulaval.ca; Tel.: +1-418-656-2131 (ext. 403864); Fax: +1-418-656-3353

Citation: Vodouhè, M.; Marois, J.; Guay, V.; Leblanc, N.; Weisnagel, S.J.; Bilodeau, J.-F.; Jacques, H. Marginal Impact of Brown Seaweed *Ascophyllum nodosum* and *Fucus vesiculosus* Extract on Metabolic and Inflammatory Response in Overweight and Obese Prediabetic Subjects. *Mar. Drugs* **2022**, *20*, 174. https://doi.org/10.3390/md20030174

Academic Editors: Donatella Degl'Innocenti and Marzia Vasarri

Received: 14 January 2022
Accepted: 24 February 2022
Published: 26 February 2022

Publisher's Note: MDPI stays neutral with regard to jurisdictional claims in published maps and institutional affiliations.

Abstract: The objective of the present study was to test whether a brown seaweed extract rich in polyphenols combined with a low-calorie diet would induce additional weight loss and improve blood glucose homeostasis in association with a metabolic and inflammatory response in overweight/obese prediabetic subjects. Fifty-six overweight/obese, dysglycemic, and insulin-resistant men and women completed a randomized, placebo-controlled, double-blind, and parallel clinical trial. Subjects were administrated 500 mg/d of either brown seaweed extract or placebo combined with individualized nutritional advice for moderate weight loss over a period of 12 weeks. Glycemic, anthropometric, blood pressure, heart rate, body composition, lipid profile, gut integrity, and oxidative and inflammatory markers were measured before and at the end of the trial. No effect was observed on blood glucose. We observed significant but small decreases in plasma C-peptide at 120 min during 2 h-OGTT (3218 ± 181 at pre-intervention vs. 2865 ± 186 pmol/L at post-intervention in the brown seaweed group; 3004 ± 199 at pre-intervention vs. 2954 ± 179 pmol/L at post-intervention in the placebo group; changes between the two groups, *p* = 0.002), heart rate (72 ± 10 at pre-intervention vs. 69 ± 9 (*n*/min) at post-intervention in the brown seaweed group; 68 ± 9 at pre-intervention vs. 68 ± 8 (*n*/min) at post-intervention in the placebo group; changes between the two groups, *p* = 0.01), and an inhibition in the increase of pro-inflammatory interleukin-6 (IL-6) (1.3 ± 0.7 at pre-intervention vs. 1.5 ± 0.7 pg/L at post-intervention in the brown seaweed group; 1.4 ± 1.1 at pre-intervention vs. 2.2 ± 1.6 pg/L at post-intervention in the placebo group; changes between the two groups, *p* = 0.02) following brown seaweed consumption compared with placebo in the context of moderate weight loss. Although consumption of brown seaweed extract had no effect on body weight or blood glucose, an early attenuation of the inflammatory response was observed in association with marginal changes in metabolic parameters related to the prevention of diabetes type 2.

Keywords: brown seaweed extract; metabolic and inflammatory markers; prediabetes

1. Introduction

The growing prevalence of type 2 diabetes worldwide is particularly alarming. Based on recent world statistics [1], 352 million adults aged from 20 to 79 years old were glucose intolerant (7.3%), and 425 million (8.8%) had type 2 diabetes in 2017 [1]. The association between the dramatic increase of the disease and the rising prevalence of obesity is often highlighted [2]. Obesity and overweight initiate several metabolic disorders [3] that include insulin resistance, which is considered to be the central feature leading to type 2 diabetes [4].

Prediabetes is an intermediate stage in the development of type 2 diabetes and is characterized by abnormal high fasting glucose, impaired glucose tolerance, and/or high-fasting insulin [5]. A number of other metabolic dysfunctions are linked to prediabetes and type 2 diabetes, such as chronic systemic low-grade inflammation [6,7], oxidative stress, endothelial dysfunction [8], and impaired gut integrity [9]. The extent to which these phenomena are observed differs with respect to diet composition, among other environmental factors. These disorders may be reversible at the prediabetes stage when nutritional interventions are implemented.

In a clinical setting, the implementation of a weight-loss approach is generally the first-line intervention in the prevention and management of type 2 diabetes among overweight or obese people. The main recommended nutritional treatment to lose weight and prevent type 2 diabetes is the reduction of energy intake [10]. Caloric restriction and weight loss have been shown to improve insulin sensitivity and reduce hyperglycemia [11,12]. A moderate caloric intake restriction of approximately 2093 KJ (500 kcal) per day is recommended [10,13] for a weight loss of 2 to 4 kg/month as suggested by the 2006 Canadian Obesity Guidelines [14].

Marine organisms are rich sources of compounds with diverse biological activities [15]. Among the most promising bioactive molecules in preventing type 2 diabetes are the phlorotannins, a class of polyphenols exclusively produced by brown seaweeds [16]. In vitro and in vivo studies [17,18] show that phlorotannin-rich extracts of brown seaweed *Ascophyllum nodosum* and *Fucus vesiculosus* reduce the α-amylase and α-glucosidase activities involved in the digestion of carbohydrates, resulting in a 90% reduction of glucose 30 min after a meal and a 40% decrease in peak insulin secretion in mice, as reported by Roy et al. [17]. In humans, it has been demonstrated that a single acute dose of 500 mg of a polyphenol-rich extract of *Ascophyllum nodosum* and *Fucus vesiculosus* had no significant effect on glycemia but induced a 12% reduction in the insulin incremental area under the curve (IAUC) following consumption of 50 g of bread compared with a placebo in healthy adults [19]. Fucoidan, a polysaccharide found in brown seaweeds, has also been recognized as a promising bioactive molecule with glucose-lowering potential [20,21], via a reduction of α-amylase and α-glucosidase activities, and therefore a diminution of intestinal absorption of glucose, and an enhancement of cellular glucose uptake via insulin through modulation of cellular glucose transporter GLUT-4 and AMP-activated protein kinase (AMPK). However, there are few studies addressing the chronic physiological effects of brown seaweed extract on metabolic and inflammatory markers in humans and particularly in people at high risk of type 2 diabetes.

Achieving normal blood glucose levels is one of the major goals in diabetes prevention, and it can be reached by different means, such as weight loss or an improvement of glucose homeostasis through a nutritional supplement [22]. From a biological perspective, the response to an energy-restricted diet varies between individuals [23], and this strategy alone is somewhat less effective in the long term [24]. Therefore, a nutritional supplement is often necessary in adjunction to energy restriction [25]. In this context, a brown seaweed extract, which has been shown to reduce waist circumference [26], could be administered in addition to a reduced-calorie diet to obtain additional effects.

The present study was thus undertaken to evaluate the effect of daily consumption of 500 mg of brown seaweed (*Ascophyllum nodosum* and *Fucus vesiculosus*) capsules rich in polyphenols associated with a reduced-energy diet on body weight and blood glucose homeostasis (glucose, insulin, and C-peptide in the fasting state and during a 2 h oral glucose tolerance test) for 12 weeks in overweight prediabetic subjects. Lipid profile, heart rate, markers of inflammation, oxidative stress, and integrity of the intestinal barrier were measured as secondary outcomes. We expect that brown seaweed extract lowers body weight and improves glucose homeostasis and metabolic and inflammatory markers in the context of moderate weight loss in this 12-week clinical trial.

2. Results

2.1. Demographic, Baseline Characteristics, and Compliance

In total, 56 subjects were enrolled in the study with 61% (n = 34) women and 39% (n = 22) men. Participants were comparable for age, body weight, BMI, waist and hip circumferences, systolic and diastolic blood pressures, heart rate, lipid profile, fasting glycemia, and OGTT 2 h glycemia (Supplementary Table S1). Forty-four subjects had impaired fasting glucose (5.6–6.9 mmol/L), 22 had high blood glucose levels after a 2 h test (7.7–11.0 mmol/L), and 24 had elevated glycated hemoglobin concentration (5.5–6.4%). Among those, 31 participants met one criterion, whereas 16 and 9 participants met two and three criteria, respectively.

2.2. Food Intake and Physical Activity

Food Frequency Questionnaire data show no difference in energy and macronutrient intake between groups at the baseline and after the 12-week intervention. The mean reduction in daily energy intake of the brown seaweed group was similar to that of the placebo group (p = 0.90). With regards to physical activity, no difference within and between groups was observed (Supplementary Table S2).

2.3. Anthropometric Measurement, Body Composition, Blood Pressure, and Heart Rate

There was no difference in anthropometric, body composition, and blood pressure parameters between the groups (Table 1). However, intragroup analysis revealed reductions in body weight, BMI, waist circumference, and total fat mass from the baseline in the two groups ($p \leq 0.01$) (Table 1). Results showed a 4% decrease in heart rate in the brown seaweed group and a 1.5% decrease in the placebo group. When we compared changes from the baseline (post vs. pre) between the two treatments, brown seaweed extract showed a reduction in the heart rate compared with control (p = 0.01) (Figure 1).

Table 1. Anthropometric, body composition, and blood pressure parameters over time within and between groups.

	Brown Seaweed Extract (n = 27)			Placebo (n = 29)			p_{IxG} [3]
	Pre [1]	Post [1]	p_I [2]	Pre [1]	Post [1]	p_I [2]	
Weight (kg)	91 ± 13	89 ± 13	<0.001	91 ± 14	89 ± 14	0.003	0.51
BMI (kg/m^2)	33 ± 4	32 ± 4	<0.001	33 ± 5	32 ± 4	0.003	0.55
Waist (cm)	109 ± 10	108 ± 10	0.003	108 ± 10	107 ± 10	0.007	0.76
Total fat mass (kg) †	38 ± 9	37 ± 9	0.001	39 ± 10	38 ± 10	0.001	0.93
Total lean mass (kg)	51 ± 8	50 ± 8	0.03	50 ± 10	50 ± 10	0.65	0.20
Visceral fat mass (kg)	1.9 ± 0.6	1.7 ± 0.6	0.04	1.6 ± 0.6	1.6 ± 0.5	0.23	0.52
SBP (mmHg)	119 ± 11	121 ± 12	0.27	118 ± 11	118 ± 12	0.93	0.39
DBP (mmHg)	75 ± 9	74 ± 9	0.51	76 ± 7	74 ± 8	0.14	0.58

BMI, body mass index; SBP, systolic blood pressure; DBP, diastolic blood pressure. † n = 56; n = 55 for total fat mass; n = 54 for visceral fat mass. [1] A repeated-measures ANOVA with two factors (treatment, post-pre phase) was performed to compare changes over time (post-pre) between groups. Mean ± SD pre-intervention (at the beginning of the 12-week trial) and post-intervention (at the end of the 12-week trial). [2] p-value to compare changes over time from the baseline to 12 weeks (pre vs. post) within each group (placebo or brown seaweed extract). [3] p-value to compare change over time (pre vs. post) between groups (placebo vs. brown seaweed extract).

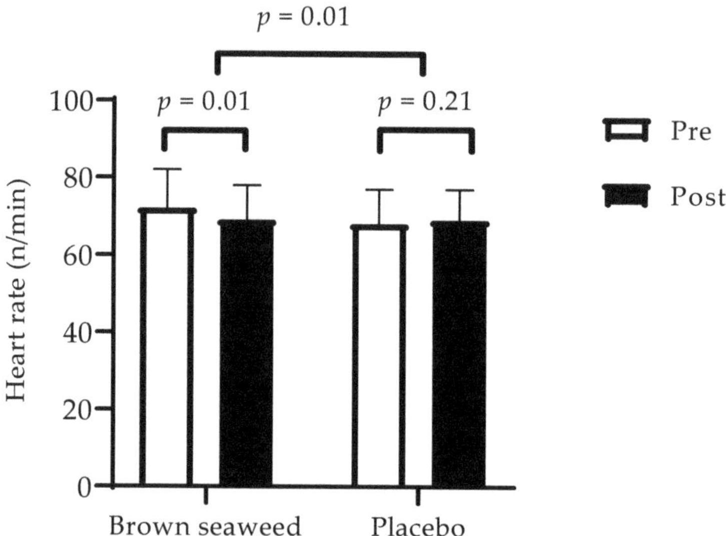

Figure 1. Variations of heart rate over time within and between groups. □ Pre-intervention (at the beginning of the 12-week trial). ■ Post-intervention (at the end of the 12-week trial). A repeated-measures ANOVA with two factors (treatment, post-pre phase) was performed to compare changes over time (post-pre) between groups. Values are means with standard deviations represented by vertical bars. $n = 56$.

2.4. Fasting Glycemic, Lipid, and Hepatic Biomarkers in the Fasting State

There were no significant differences in glycemic, lipid, and hepatic parameters in the fasting state between the two groups (Table 2).

Table 2. Glycemic, lipid, and hepatic markers over time within and between groups.

	Brown Seaweed Extract ($n = 27$)			Placebo ($n = 29$)			p_{IxG} [3]
	Pre [1]	Post [1]	p_I [2]	Pre [1]	Post [1]	p_I [2]	
Fasting glucose (mmol/L)	5.8 ± 0.5	5.7 ± 0.4	0.14	5.7 ± 0.6	5.6 ± 0.5	0.45	0.60
Fasting insulin (pmol/L) †	129 ± 49	123 ± 48	0.22	123 ± 63	114 ± 73	0.49	0.76
Fasting C-peptide (pmol/L)	1009 ± 298	957 ± 284	0.06	945 ± 307	916 ± 306	0.26	0.60
Hemoglobin A1c (%)	5.6 ± 0.3	5.6 ± 0.3	0.83	5.6 ± 0.2	5.6 ± 0.2	0.46	0.72
Total chol (mmol/L)	5.5 ± 0.8	5.2 ± 0.8	0.07	5.1 ± 0.8	5.1 ± 0.7	0.48	0.07
Triglycerides (mmol/L)	1.5 ± 0.7	1.7 ± 0.8	0.20	1.5 ± 0.5	1.5 ± 0.4	0.55	0.60
LDLc (mmol/L)	3.1 ± 0.7	2.9 ± 0.8	0.06	3.0 ± 0.7	3.0 ± 0.6	0.36	0.05
HDLc (mmol/L)	1.4 ± 0.3	1.3 ± 0.2	0.001	1.3 ± 0.3	1.3 ± 0.3	0.25	0.09
Chol/HDLc	4.4 ± 0.8	4.4 ± 0.9	0.12	4.4 ± 0.9	4.4 ± 0.8	0.17	0.86
HOMA-IR	4.8 ± 1.9	4.5 ± 1.8	0.18	4.5 ± 2.5	4.0 ± 2.8	0.65	0.57
AST (U/L)	23 ± 8	20 ± 5	0.02	25 ± 11	20 ± 8	0.004	0.69
ALT (U/L)	24 ± 8	24 ± 8	0.99	28 ± 20	31 ± 18	0.04	0.15
AST/ALT	1.1 ± 0.5	0.9 ± 0.2	0.07	1.1 ± 0.4	0.8 ± 0.3	0.001	0.23

Total Chol, total cholesterol; LDLc, low-density lipoprotein cholesterol; HDLc, high-density lipoprotein cholesterol; HOMA-IR, homeostasic model assessment of insulin resistance; AST, aspartate aminotransferase; ALT, alanine aminotransferase. † $n = 56$; $n = 53$ for fasting insulin; $n = 53$ for HOMA-IR. [1] A repeated-measures ANOVA with two factors (treatment, post-pre phase) was performed to compare changes over time (post-pre) between groups. Mean ± SD pre-intervention (at beginning of 12-week trial) and post-intervention (at end of 12-week trial). [2] p-value to compare changes over time from the baseline to 12 weeks (pre vs. post) within each group (placebo or brown seaweed extract). [3] p-value to compare change over time (pre vs. post) between groups (placebo vs. brown seaweed extract).

2.5. Glucose, Insulin, and C-Peptide during OGTT

We performed repeated-measures ANOVA for glucose (Figure 2A), C-peptide (Figure 2B), and insulin (Figure 2C) up to 120 min during OGTT. A reduction was observed in C-peptide concentrations at 120 min during OGTT in the brown seaweed group compared with the placebo group ($p = 0.002$) (Figure 2B). There were no differences between the two groups for fasting glucose, insulin, and C-peptide (Table 2) and their corresponding mean IAUC up to 120 min after OGTT (Figure 2D–F).

2.6. Inflammatory Status, Oxidative Stress Status, and Gut Integrity

High-sensitivity C-reactive protein (hsCRP) and F_2-isoprostane (8-iso-PGF$_{2\alpha}$) responses were similar between treatments (Table 3). However, there was a lower increase of plasma interleukin-6 (IL-6) concentration in the brown seaweed group (15%) compared with the placebo group (57%) ($p = 0.02$) (Figure 3). There was no difference in the gut integrity parameters between the groups.

2.7. Adverse Effects

No serious adverse event was reported in this study.

Table 3. Inflammatory, oxidative stress, and gut barrier integrity markers over time within and between groups.

	Brown Seaweed Extract ($n = 27$)			Placebo ($n = 29$)			p_{IxG} [3]
	Pre [1]	Post [1]	p_I [2]	Pre [1]	Post [1]	p_I [2]	
hsCRP (mg/L) †	3.0 ± 1.9	3.6 ± 2.7	0.67	2.7 ± 1.6	3.4 ± 2.6	0.88	0.84
F_2-isoprostane (8-iso PGF$_{2\alpha}$) $\times 10^{-1}$ ng/mL	2.2 ± 0.8	2.4 ± 0.8	0.65	2.5 ± 1.9	3.0 ± 2.3	0.53	0.76
LBP $\times 10^3$ (ng/mL)	6.4 ± 1.9	8.3 ± 1.8	0.002	6.8 ± 1.3	7.7 ± 1.9	0.17	0.20
Zonulin (ng/mL)	1.2 ± 0.6	1.2 ± 1.0	0.60	1.7 ± 1.0	1.9 ± 1.1	0.53	0.42

hsCRP, high-sensitivity C-reactive protein; LBP, lipopolysaccharide-binding protein. † $n = 53$ for hsCRP; $n = 54$ for LBP; $n = 55$ for zonulin. [1] A repeated-measures ANOVA with two factors (treatment, post-pre phase) was performed to compare changes over time (post-pre) between groups. Mean $\pm$ SD pre-intervention (at the beginning of the 12-week trial) and post-intervention (at the end of the 12-week trial). [2] p-value to compare changes over time from the baseline to 12 weeks (pre vs. post) within each group (placebo or brown seaweed extract). [3] p-value to compare change over time (pre vs. post) between groups (placebo vs. brown seaweed extract).

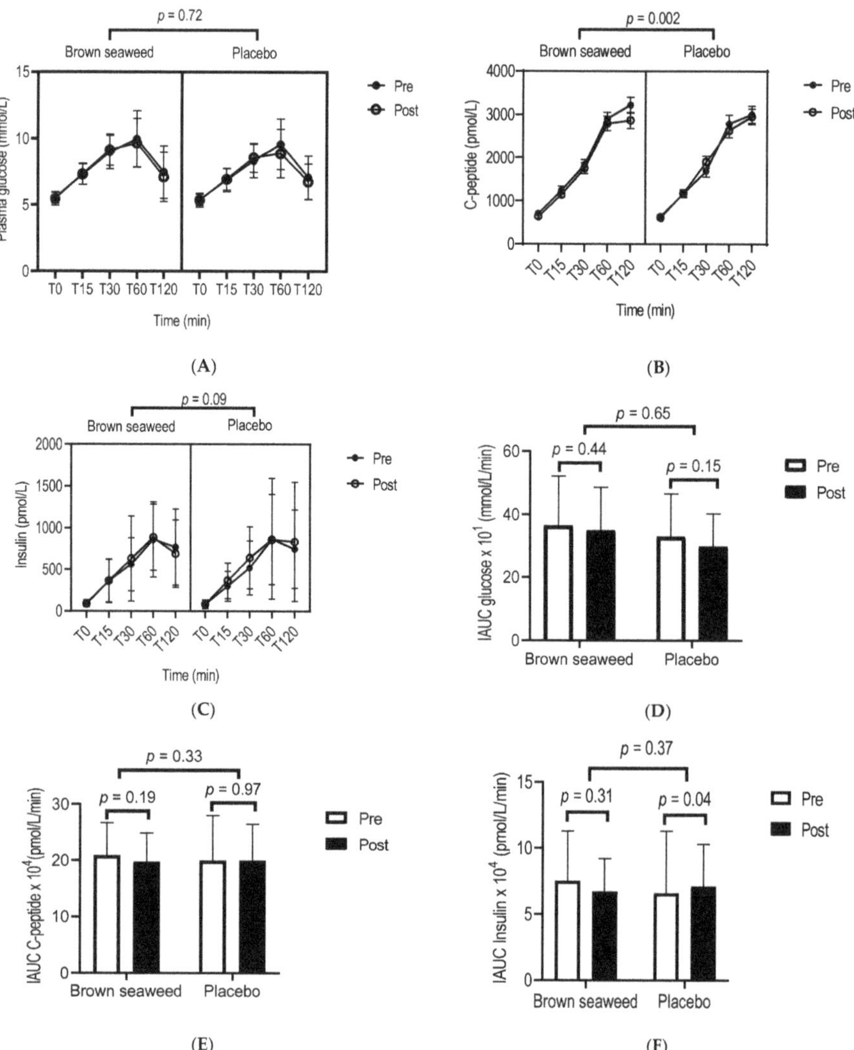

Figure 2. Glucose, insulin and C-peptide concentrations and IAUC during OGTT. □ Pre-intervention (at the beginning of the 12-week trial). ■ Post-intervention (at the end of the 12-week trial). Repeated measures ANOVA highlighting significant differences in the concentrations of glucose (**A**), C-peptide (**B**), and insulin (**C**), and in their respective IAUCs (**D–F**) over time between the brown seaweed and the placebo groups. A mixed model for repeated-measures ANOVA with three factors (treatment, OGTT time points, post-pre phase) (**A–C**) and with two factors (treatment, post-pre phase) (**D–F**) was performed. Incremental area under the curve (IAUC) for glucose, insulin, and C-peptide during the 2 h-OGTT was calculated from the trapezoidal rule and fasting baseline values. Values are means with standard deviations represented by vertical bars. $n = 56$ for glucose, $n = 44$ for insulin, and $n = 56$ for C-peptide.

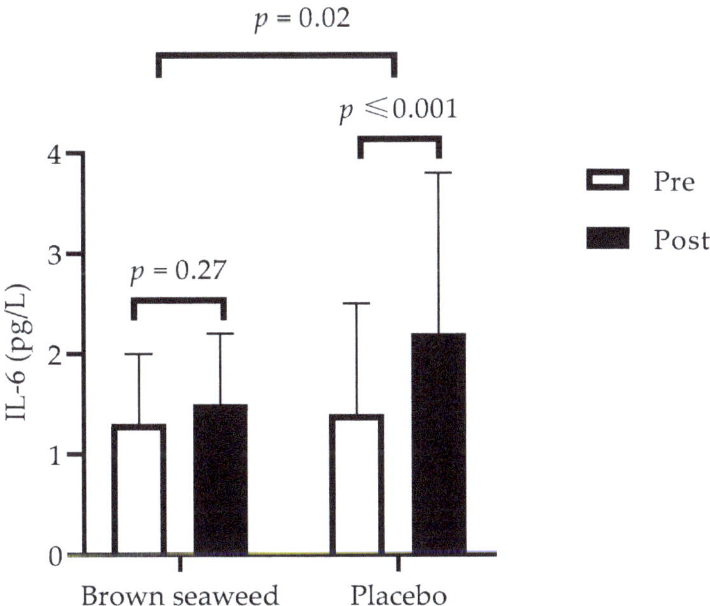

Figure 3. Variations of IL-6 concentrations over time within and between groups. ☐ Pre-intervention (at the beginning of the 12-week trial). ■ Post-intervention (at the end of the trial). A repeated-measures ANOVA with two factors (treatment, post-pre phase) was performed to compare changes over time (post-pre) between groups. Values are means with standard deviations represented by vertical bars. $n = 56$.

3. Discussion

The study investigated the effect of brown seaweed (*Ascophyllum nodosum* and *Fucus vesiculosus*) extract (InSea2®) rich in polyphenols combined with a moderate weight loss on glycemic and metabolic control among prediabetic overweight/obese subjects over 12 months. In this study, we advised both groups to follow a moderate energy-restricted balanced diet. Therefore, body weight, waist circumferences, and total fat mass decreased significantly in both groups. The main findings in this study indicate that daily consumption of 500 mg of brown seaweed extract had no effect on body weight and blood glucose, our primary outcomes, but had a modest beneficial impact on insulin secretion through the reduction of late C-peptide secretion during 2 h OGTT, heart rate and on the inhibition of the rise of IL-6 concentration in plasma compared with placebo in the context of moderate weight loss.

3.1. Weight Loss

With respect to anthropometric parameters, our results showed that the improvement in body weight and composition induced by consumption of 500 mg per day brown seaweed extract rich in polyphenols with dietary modifications aimed at moderate weight loss was not greater than that provoked by dietary modifications alone. The lack of additional weight loss is consistent with recent data from Derosa et al. [27], who reported no effect of 6-month administration of food supplement containing *Ascophyllum nodosum* and *Fucus vesiculosus* extract and chromium picolinate on body weight and BMI in dysglycemic subjects. On the other hand, De Martin and co-authors [26] reported a significant decrease in waist circumference in overweight and obese subjects after 6 months of treatment with the same nutraceutical combination that had been administered in the study by Derosa et al. [27]. In light of these studies, it is possible that a reducing effect of brown seaweed extract on body weight was masked by the effect of the low-calorie diet in the present study. It is also to be considered that the absence of additional weight loss could be attributed to the dysglycemic status of our subjects or to the absence of chromium picolinate in the supplement.

3.2. Glucose, Insulin, and C-Peptide

The lack of effect on blood glucose could be due, on the one hand, to the lack of effect on body weight [28] and, on the other hand, to taking the supplement once a day rather than three times a day (before breakfast, lunch, and dinner), as performed De Martin et al. [26]. There is a possibility that a single administration of the supplement intake during the day might have resulted in a less pronounced effect on the activities of intestinal α-amylase and α-glucosidase and, therefore, on the absorption of the glucose and blood levels.

It should also be considered that blood glucose is maintained primarily because of regulated pancreatic insulin secretion. In this respect, C-peptide is a byproduct of insulin synthesis from pro-insulin. It is secreted by pancreatic β-cells in equal amounts with insulin; however, unlike insulin, C-peptide is not extracted by the liver and has a constant peripheral clearance. It is considered a valuable and precise biomarker of insulin secretion due to its longer time life in circulation (20 to 30 min for C-peptide versus 5 min for insulin) [29]. Moreover, C-peptide hypersecretion occurred in prediabetic and diabetic patients in the fasting state and in the early and late phases of the OGTT [30]. In this context, a reduction in plasma C-peptide in these patients is desirable. In this study, we observed a modest decrease of C-peptide at the late phase of OGTT in participants consuming brown seaweed extract, suggesting a potential for reduced insulin secretion in the long term, thereby decreasing the risk for developing glucose intolerance and type 2 diabetes [31,32].

This effect may be associated with phlorotannins, polyphenolic compounds found in brown seaweeds only, and fucoidan, found as a sulfated polysaccharide in brown marine algae, known to decrease the α-amylase and α-glucosidase activities and, therefore, the digestion and assimilation of glucose [17,18,20,33]. This may result, in the long term, in an improvement of pancreatic function and, ultimately, in a reduction of glucose intolerance seen in prediabetic patients. Our results are in good agreement, but less pronounced than those of De Martin et al. [26] and Derosa et al. [27], who have recently reported a decrease in glycemia, insulin secretion, insulin resistance [26], and postprandial glycemia [27] following a 12-week consumption of 712.5 mg of *Ascophyllum nodosum* and *Fucus vesiculosus* extract with the addition of chromium picolinate. In light of these studies [26,27], it is important to consider that the presence of picolinate chromium, known as a hypoglycemic agent, could have accentuated the impact of the *Ascophyllum nodosum* and *Fucus vesiculosus* extract on glycemic response. Furthermore, in both previous studies [26,27], the effects were more pronounced after 6 months than after 3 months of treatment with an additional reduction of fasting plasma glucose, glycated hemoglobin, and insulin resistance. The differences in the impact of the extract on glucose homeostasis observed in the present study and the two former studies [26,27] could be explained by the frequency and doses, duration of the trial, and use of picolinate of chromium in the previous studies. However, our study is one of few to have explored the effects of brown seaweed extract alone and show that there is a beneficial impact, albeit modest, of the brown seaweed extract per se, without chromium picolinate, on insulin secretion.

3.3. Lipid Profile, Inflammation, and Heart Rate

Lipid-associated risk for cardiovascular disease events is gradual and continuous. LDL carries cholesterol from the liver throughout the body and leaves excess on the endothelium of the arteries, causing atherosclerotic plaques to develop. Consequently, a surplus of LDL cholesterol is associated with an increased risk of cardiovascular events in patients both with and without type 2 diabetes [34]. Therefore, as a primary goal of therapy, target LDL cholesterol levels for adults with diabetes are <2.60 mmol/L [35]. In the present study, no effect was observed on lipid parameters. Our results are not in accordance with those of Shin et al. [36], who observed a decrease in total and LDL cholesterol following daily consumption of 144 mg of *Ecklonia cava* brown seaweed during 12 weeks among hypercholesterolemic subjects, nor with those of Iacoviello et al. [37] who reported a decrease in triglycerides after the consumption of a high dose (900 mg) of *Ascophyllum nodosum* extract over 6 weeks. The difference could be explained by the nature of the seaweed, the dose, and the duration of the trial. Further studies with higher doses of *Ascophyllum nodosum* and *Fucus vesiculosus* extract are suggested to assess the impact of its consumption on lipid profile among people at risk of type 2 diabetes.

Inflammation and oxidative stress may play a pivotal role in the pathophysiology of type 2 diabetes. The elevated inflammatory and oxidative biomarkers observed at the post-intervention stage could be explained by the chronic inflammation process that is implicated in diabetes. Among several inflammatory biomarkers, Il-6 has been shown to predict the development of type 2 diabetes, promoting the development of inflammation, insulin resistance, and β-cell dysfunction [38]. In the present study, our results indicate that the extract inhibited the increase in IL-6 observed in overweight/obese placebo subjects, thereby attenuating early pro-inflammatory response, and suggesting that consumption of the extract might have potential anti-inflammatory properties. In line with this result, it has already been shown that *Ascophyllum nodosum* extract can inhibit pro-inflammatory IL-6 gene expression in the porcine colon ex vivo and in vitro [39,40]. Phlorotannins are proposed as the main compounds in marine brown seaweeds associated with this effect. Indeed, as reported by Catarino et al. [41], phlorotannins can inhibit the expression of pro-inflammatory cytokines and interfering with transcriptional regulation. Furthermore, in the present study, variations in Il-6 were strongly and positively correlated with glycemia in the fasting state ($r = 50$, $p = 0.001$). Furthermore, in post-intervention, we observed trends between Il-6 and insulin resistance measured by HOMA-IR ($r = 26$, $p = 0.07$), and Il-6 and plasma insulin values at 120 min during OGTT ($r = 0.24$, $p = 0.10$). These results suggest that the inhibition of IL-6 increase could be a mechanism responsible for the observed effects of the brown seaweed extract on parameters related to glucose homeostasis. However, in the present study, hs-CRP was not affected by treatment; therefore, indicating no effect of brown seaweed extract on the pro-inflammatory late regulation process. Interestingly, a late anti-inflammatory response, characterized by a decrease in inflammatory biomarkers TNF-α and hsCRP, was observed in an earlier 6-month study [27] investigating the metabolic and inflammatory effects of an extract of *Ascophyllum nodosum* and *Fucus vesiculosus* combined with chromium picolinate, therefore supporting the concept that the addition of chromium to brown seaweed extract might modulate inflammation differently [42].

Interestingly, heart rate is associated with inflammation [43] and plasma IL-6 concentrations [44]. We indeed observed a positive correlation between variations in heart rate and Il-6 ($r = 0.29$, $p = 0.04$). Therefore, the reduced heart rate seen in the brown seaweed group could be linked to the inhibition of increased pro-inflammatory marker Il-6. Interestingly, Jung et al. [45] previously observed that dieckol, a phlorotannin present in brown seaweed, can induce in vitro inhibition of cyclooxygenase 2 expression and prostaglandin E(2) production

3.4. Integrity of Gut Barrier

Dysregulation of intestinal mucosal barrier function and loss of integrity of the gut barrier can increase the passage to the intestinal pathogens and endotoxins, which cause infection or inflammation [46]. Animal models have provided evidence linking gut barrier dysfunction, activation of inflammation signaling pathways, and progression of insulin resistance to type 2 diabetes [47]. The potential of *Ecklonia radiata*, a brown seaweed from New Zealand, and its polysaccharides (fucoidan and alginate) were reported to improve gut health in a rat model by increasing stool bulk, short-chain fatty acids, and butyrate production [48]. However, Michiels et al. [49] showed no effect of a dried extract of *Ascophyllum nodosum* on gut microbiota in piglets. To our best knowledge, no studies have addressed the impact of brown seaweed on the health and integrity of the gut barrier in humans. In the context of our study, no effect of our brown seaweed extract was observed on LBP, an acute-phase protein secreted by the liver in the bloodstream in response to a bacterial infection, and zonulin, a protein associated with a loss of intestinal barrier function that modulates the permeability of tight junctions between cells of the wall of the digestive tract. Further studies measuring various parameters of gut integrity, such as occludin, claudins, or mucin, in addition to LBP and zonulin, are necessary to determine the impact of brown seaweed and their extracts on gut integrity among people at risk of type 2 diabetes.

The results of the present study showed a marginal beneficial impact of a polyphenol-rich extract obtained from two algae, *Ascophyllum nodosum* and *Fucus vesiculosus*, in the context of moderate weight loss over 12 weeks on metabolic risk factors of type 2 diabetes and cardiovascular disease, namely glucose homeostasis, heart rate, and Il-6 in prediabetic subjects. Moreover, our results should be interpreted with caution, given certain limitations. On the one hand, diet and physical activity were not strictly controlled, but on the other hand, our experimental approach was closer to the real context. Furthermore, we used 2 h OGTT instead of 3 h OGTT, which could have minimized the real effect of brown seaweed extract on glycemia, insulin, and C-peptide during OGTT. Finally, it might be worthwhile in subsequent studies to extend the duration of the trial to 6 months.

We acknowledge that this discussion has been focused on phlorotannins and fucoidans due to their known bioactive properties, but the extract contains other compounds such as small saccharides (mono- and disaccharide) as well as oligo- and polysaccharides, fatty acids, and phenolic compounds, as measured by Gabbia et al. [18]. For instance, the polysaccharide-rich composition of brown algae has shown the potential to act as prebiotics and to positively modulate the gut microbiota [50]. Moreover, in addition to phlorotannins, there are other polyphenolic compounds such as phenolic acids, flavonoids, phenolic terpenoids, and bromophenols in brown seaweeds, as reported by Cotas et al. [51]. On their own, each of these compounds can exhibit significant biological properties, including antidiabetic, anti-inflammatory, and antioxidant activities [51], and could potentially affect the parameters measured in this study. However, compared to phlorotannins, less is known about those polyphenols due to a lack of their characterization, isolation, and specific bioactivity analysis. Furthermore, it is possible that when combined, these compounds have interactions with each other, depending on the type and structure of these compounds, thereby modulating their effects.

In conclusion, the present results indicate that the consumption of a brown seaweed extract of *Ascophyllum nodosum* and *Fucus vesiculosus* for 12 weeks had no effect on body weight and blood glucose but induced a marginal beneficial impact on insulin secretion, heart rate, and Il-6 in overweight/obese prediabetic subjects. These results suggest that early attenuation of the inflammatory response by 500 mg of brown seaweed extract in the context of moderate weight loss could be associated with modest changes in metabolic parameters related to the prevention of type 2 diabetes. More studies with different doses and intervention durations are needed to determine the effects of this supplement on cardiovascular and type 2 diabetes risk factors.

4. Materials and Methods

4.1. Study Design

This study was a parallel, double-blind, randomized controlled 12-week clinical trial conducted from summer 2017 to winter 2018 at the Institute of Nutrition and Functional Foods in Quebec City (QC, Canada). The study was in accordance with the Declaration of Helsinki and was approved by the Université Laval's health-science research ethics committee. Participants were given a detailed written informed consent form to read and sign prior to their participation in the study. This trial was registered at clinicaltrials.gov as NCT03075943.

4.2. Population

Volunteers were recruited on a voluntary basis from the Institute of Nutrition and Functional Foods contacts database, Laval University network, and Diabète Québec Association website. Inclusion criteria included age between 18–70 years, body mass index (BMI) $\geq$ 27 cm, waist circumference $\geq$ 94 cm for men and $\geq$ 80 cm for women, fasting insulin $\geq$ 60 pmol/L, fasting glycemia between 5.6–6.9 mmol/L or/and 2 h glucose in oral glucose tolerance test (OGTT) between 7.8–11.0 mmol/L or/and glycated hemoglobin A1C (HbA1C) between 5.7–6.4% for prediabetes diagnostics [52], and stable weight during the last 3 months. Exclusion criteria included type 2 diabetes, uncontrolled hypertension, thyroid disorders, renal and hepatic dysfunction, gastro-intestinal disorders, or other chronic or acute diseases. People who intake medications, food supplements, or natural health products that affect glucose and lipid metabolisms or body weight were also excluded. Major surgery during the last 3 months, smoking, pregnancy or breastfeeding, and allergies to fish, seafood, or iodine were also considered as exclusion criteria. A total of 260 subjects, recruited in the Québec City metropolitan area through media advertising, were screened to examine their eligibility to participate in this study (Supplementary Figure S1). During the first screening visit, two self-administered online questionnaires were completed by all subjects to collect information on medical history, lifestyle, economic and socio-demographic characteristics. Of 260 subjects, 125 subjects were excluded, and 11 decided not to participate. During the second screening visit, blood was collected from 124 subjects, and 58 subjects were also excluded from the study because they did not meet the plasma inclusion criteria. Thus, of 66 eligible volunteers after the two screening visits, 56 completed the study (Supplementary Figure S1) because ten subjects among the eligible volunteers no longer met inclusion criteria, dropped out, or refused to pursue the study for personal reasons during the study. During a 2-week run-in phase, the participants were asked to maintain their dietary routine and refrain from vigorous activity. After the 2-week run-in phase, the participants were randomly assigned to either the placebo group or the brown seaweed extract group, based on weight, BMI, and gender, and received individualized nutritional counseling for a moderate weight loss.

4.3. Intervention

In the brown seaweed extract group, each participant received 500 mg of polyphenol-rich brown seaweed *Ascophyllum nodosum* and *Fucus vesiculosus* extract (2 capsules sold as a standardized extract under the registered trademark InSea2® of InnoVactiv Inc. (Rimouski, QC, Canada) to be taken daily 30 min before the main meal of the day for 12 weeks). The extract was prepared using an exclusive hot water extraction, followed by filtration and ultrafiltration processes and spray-drying. The extract used in the present study contained algae polyphenols (35%, as indicated in the certificate of analysis of the commercial product). The extraction process removed alginates and part of the salts, and the remaining constituents were mostly composed of algae polysaccharides, of which fucoidans were 11.5% fucose and minerals (iodine content = 67 mg/kg). The ability of InSea2® to inhibit α-amylase was 97.8% at a concentration of 0.1 g/L algae extract, as indicated in the certificate of analysis of the commercial product. Heavy metal analysis showed that inorganic arsenic (<0.41 mg/kg), cadmium (0.31 mg/kg), lead (0.77 mg/kg), and mercury (0.03 mg/kg) were less than the limit of quantification. The chemical characterization of InSea2® has previously been described in detail [18], confirming that the extract is mainly composed of saccharide derivatives and contains ~35% algae polyphenols, of which phloroglucinol derivatives, measured by NMR analysis and revealing the presence of fatty acids by GC-MS.

Participants of the control group received the same dose of placebo capsule to be taken in the same conditions as described above. Treatment and placebo capsules were similar in form, color, and taste and were supplied by innoVactiv Cie (Rimouski, Canada). The treatment capsule contained extract of brown seaweed (250 mg), dibasic calcium phosphate (150 mg), microcrystalline cellulose (100 mg), croscarmellose (3 mg), magnesium stearate (5 mg), titanium dioxide (1.8 mg), and hypromellose (94.3 mg). Placebo capsule contained microcrystalline cellulose (191 mg), dibasic calcium phosphate (287 mg), magnesium stearate (5 mg), caramel (25 mg), titanium dioxide (1.8 mg), hypromellose (94.3 mg).

The nutritional intervention aimed for moderate calorie restriction of about 500 kcal based on basal metabolism corrected for physical activity, using the traditional Harris Benedict–formula [53]. The individualized counseling intervention was given in the form of a dietary plan based on the "Food Guide for Diabetic Patients" [54] and "Health Plate Approach" [55]. Protein powders, fish oil, omega-3 or any marine supplements, as well as natural health products known to have effects on glucose or insulin levels, weight, satiety, or appetite, were forbidden. Moreover, it was not allowed to use weight loss products available on the market or to follow another weight loss program. In addition, slimming or anti-cellulite cosmetic creams were not permitted. A validated online Food Frequency Questionnaire [56] was completed by participants. Short International Physical Activity Questionnaire [57,58] and Side Effect Reporting Form were completed. Compliance was assessed by capsule counts [59]. Any change in medication, temporary medication, natural health product intake, or consumption of any other food supplements were monitored according to the exclusion criteria during the entire study period. To document compliance, subjects were asked to return unused capsules at the end of the study. Capsule counts indicated a minimum of 80% compliance in both groups.

4.4. Anthropometric and Body Composition Measurements

Bodyweight, height, and waist circumference were measured using conventional measurements. BMI was calculated as weight (kg)/height^2 (m^2). Body composition (total mass, fat mass, visceral mass) was determined using a dual-energy X-ray absorptiometry (DEXA) scanner (GE Lunar Prodigy Bone Densitometer, GE Lunar Healthcare, Madison, WI, USA), and data were analyzed using Lunar Prodigy Advance-enCORE 2010 software version 14.1.

4.5. Blood Pressure and Heart Rate Measurements

Blood pressure and heart rate were measured three times on the right arm using an automatic tensiometer (Digital Blood Pressure Monitor, model HEM-907XL; OMRON®, Kyoto, Japan) following a 10 min rest at the beginning and at the end of the experimental period using a Digital Blood Pressure Monitor (model HEM-907XL; OMRON® Blood pressure Monitor, Kyoto, Japan).

4.6. Oral Glucose Tolerance Test (OGTT)

At the beginning and end of the experimental periods, glucose tolerance was estimated by a two-hour, 75 g OGTT using a standard solution of glucose (Glucodex). Blood was collected before at T0 (0 min), T1 (15 min), T2 (30 min), T3 (60 min), and T4 (120 min). T0 (0 min) represented the fasting state.

4.7. Blood Collection and Storage

Blood samples were collected following a 12 h overnight fasting state before each OGTT. Venous blood samples were taken in tubes containing ethylenediaminetetraacetic acid (EDTA) and immediately centrifuged at $1100 \times g$ for 10 min. Plasma was stored at $-80\,^{\circ}C$ for further analysis of glycemic and lipid variables, inflammatory (hsCRP, IL-6), antioxidant (F$_2$-isoprostane as 8-iso PGF$_{2\alpha}$ isomer), and gut integrity markers (LBP and zonulin).

4.8. Glycemia, Insulin, C-Peptide, and Glycated Hemoglobin A1C Measurements

Glucose, insulin, and C-peptide concentrations were measured in fasting plasma and at different time points of the OGTT. Blood glucose was measured using The Dimension Vista® GLU method (REF K1039) (Siemens Healthcare Diagnostics Inc., Tarrytown, NY, USA), an adaptation of the hexokinase-glucose-6-phosphate dehydrogenase method [60]. Insulin and C-peptide, a marker of insulin secretion, were determined using ADVIA Centaur XPT

Immunoassay System test (Siemens Healthcare Diagnostics Inc., Tarrytown, NY, USA), a sandwich immunoassay using direct chemiluminescent technology, and specific insulin and C-peptide antibodies. HbA1c was determined using a 2.0 assay on a VARIANT II TURBO Hemoglobin Testing System (Bio-Rad Laboratories Inc., Hercules, CA, USA) using the principle of ion-exchange high-performance liquid chromatography. These analyses were performed at the Research Centre of Laval University Hospital (CHU of Québec) (QC, Canada).

The Homeostasis Model Assessment of Insulin Resistance (HOMA-IR) was used to estimate insulin sensitivity/resistance. HOMA-IR index was calculated according to the following formula: fasting insulin concentration (μL/mL) $\times$ fasting glucose concentration (mmol/L)/22.5 [61].

4.9. Lipid Profile Biomarkers Measurements

Plasma total triglycerides (TG), Low-Density Lipoprotein cholesterol (LDLc), High-Density Lipoprotein cholesterol (HDLc), Total cholesterol (Total chol), well-known markers of cardiovascular risk, were measured using enzymatic, colorimetric assay on a Cobas c701/702 instrument (Roche Diagnostics GmbH, Mannheim, Germany). Analyzes were performed at CHU of Québec (QC, Canada).

4.10. Hepatic Enzymes Measurements

Aspartate aminotransferase (AST) and alanine aminotransferase (ALT), plasma markers of hepatic function, were measured by Dimension Vista® AST and ALT methods, adapted from the recommended methods of International Federation of Clinical Chemistry [62] with the use of the coenzyme pyridoxal-5-phosphate (P5P). Laboratory analyzes were performed at CHU of Québec (QC, Canada).

4.11. Inflammatory, Oxidative Stress and Gut Integrity Biomarkers

Hs-CRP was determined at CHU of Québec (QC, Canada) using immunonephelometric technique (Siemens BN Prospec, Siemens Healthineers, Oakville, ON, Canada). Interleukin-6 was measured in plasma using Multiplex kits (EMD Millipore, Etobicoke, ON, Canada), and plates were read using Bio-Plex 200 system (Bio-Rad, Mississauga, ON, Canada). Total F2-isoprostane (as 8-iso-PGF$_{2\alpha}$ isomer) level from non-enzymatic peroxidation of arachidonic acid, a biomarker of oxidative stress, was measured in plasma, as previously described [63]. The latter analyses were conducted at the Québec Heart and Lung Institute (QC, Canada). LBP and zonulin were determined in plasma using commercially available enzyme-linked immunosorbent assay kits from Biomatik (Cambridge, ON, Canada). The analyses were conducted at the Institute of Nutrition and Functional Foods (QC, Canada).

4.12. Statistical Analysis

The sample size was determined based on insulin reduction after a single acute intake of 2 capsules of 250 mg of a polyphenol enriched brown seaweed extract from data published by Paradis et al. [19] with a statistical power of 80%, yielding a sample size of 27 for each group. Statistical analyses were performed using the statistical analysis software SPSS (version 22, 2007, IBM SPSS Statistics), except for data from OGTT, which were analyzed using SAS 9.4 (SAS Institute, Cary, NC, USA. Results are presented as means $\pm$ standard deviation. The primary analysis was to compare plasma glucose, insulin, and C-peptide obtained with OGTT before and after the intervention between the placebo and treatment. For that purpose, a mixed model for repeated-measures ANOVA with three factors (treatment, OGTT time points, post-pre phase) was performed. Incremental area under the curve (IAUC) for glucose, insulin, and C-peptide during the 2 h-OGTT was calculated from the trapezoidal rule and fasting baseline values. A repeated-measures ANOVA test with two factors (treatment, post-pre phase) was performed to compare changes over time (post-pre) between groups for the other parameters. Prior to performing repeated-measures ANOVA, normality was checked using a Shapiro–Wilk test, and distribution was normalized using logarithmic transformation when needed. Student's *t*-test (when data were normally distributed) and Mann–Whitney U test (when data were abnormally distributed) were performed to compare means at pre-intervention between groups, and F2-isoprostane changes from baseline between and within groups. Considering the small size of the experimental groups and the multiplicity of analysis, a Bonferroni correction was performed for the anthropometric ($p \leq 0.01$), blood pressure and heart rate ($p \leq 0.02$), glycemic ($p \leq 0.005$), lipid ($p \leq 0.01$), hepatic ($p \leq 0.02$), inflammatory and oxidative stress ($p \leq 0.02$), and gut integrity ($p \leq 0.03$) markers. To detect associations between variables, Pearson correlation coefficients were calculated using the Pearson correlation (CORR) procedure. Differences were considered significant at $p \leq 0.05$ (two-tailed) level.

Supplementary Materials: The following are available online at https://www.mdpi.com/article/10.3390/md20030174/s1, Table S1: Subjects' characteristics; Table S2: Nutritional intakes over time within and between groups; Figure S1: Flow chart.

Author Contributions: Conceptualization and design, J.M., S.J.W. and H.J.; data acquisition, analysis, interpretation, M.V., J.M., V.G., N.L., J.-F.B., S.J.W. and H.J.; critically revising the manuscript, M.V., J.M., V.G., N.L., J.-F.B., S.J.W. and H.J. All authors have read and agreed to the published version of the manuscript.

Funding: This research was funded by a grant from the Ministry of Agriculture, Fisheries, and Food of Québec (MAPAQ) and innoVactiv. InnoVactiv also provided the placebo and brown seaweed supplements. Marlène Vodouhè was supported by MITACS Acceleration Scholarship.

Institutional Review Board Statement: The study was in accordance with the Declaration of Helsinki and approved by the Health-Science Research Ethics Committee of Université Laval (protocol code 2016-227 and date of approval 11 January 2016).

Informed Consent Statement: Informed consent was obtained from all subjects involved in the study.

Data Availability Statement: Data available on request due to ethical restrictions.

Acknowledgments: The authors sincerely acknowledge volunteers who agreed to participate in this project. We are also grateful to Steeve Larouche and Danielle Aubin, nurses at the Institute of Nutrition and Functional Foods (INAF), Laval University, for performing blood collection and OGTTs, Amélie Charest and Iris Gigleux from INAF for their help in assessing body composition and Karine Greffard for F2-isoprostane assessment. We would like to also thank Hélène Crépeau, Anne-Sophie Julien, and Pierre Gagnon from Laval University for their help in statistical analyses.

Conflicts of Interest: Authors declare no potential conflict of interest.

References

1. International Diabetes Federation (IDF) (Ed.) *IDF Diabetes Atlas*, 8th ed.; International Diabetes Federation: Brussels, Belgium, 2017.
2. International Diabetes Federation (IDF) (Ed.) *IDF Diabetes Atlas*, 6th ed.; International Diabetes Federation: Brussels, Belgium, 2013.
3. Algoblan, A.; Alalfi, M.; Khan, M. Mechanism linking diabetes mellitus and obesity. *Diabetes Metab. Syndr. Obes.* **2014**, *7*, 587–591. [CrossRef]
4. Kahn, B.B.; Flier, J.S. Obesity and insulin resistance. *J. Clin. Investig.* **2000**, *106*, 473–481. [CrossRef]
5. Goldenberg, R.; Punthakee, Z. Definition, classification and diagnosis of diabetes, prediabetes and metabolic syndrome. *Can. J. Diabetes* **2013**, *37*, S8–S11. [CrossRef] [PubMed]
6. Tsalamandris, S.; Antonopoulos, A.S.; Oikonomou, E.; Papamikroulis, G.-A.; Vogiatzi, G.; Papaioannou, S.; Deftereos, S.; Tousoulis, D. The role of inflammation in diabetes: Current concepts and future perspectives. *Eur. Cardiol.* **2019**, *14*, 50–59. [CrossRef] [PubMed]
7. Huang, Z.; Chen, C.; Li, S.; Kong, F.; Shan, P.; Huang, W. Serum markers of endothelial dysfunction and inflammation increase in hypertension with prediabetes mellitus. *Genet. Test. Mol. Biomark.* **2016**, *20*, 322–327. [CrossRef] [PubMed]
8. Maschirow, L.; Khalaf, K.; Al-Aubaidy, H.; Jelinek, H. Inflammation, coagulation, endothelial dysfunction and oxidative stress in prediabetes—Biomarkers as a possible tool for early disease detection for rural screening. *Clin. Biochem.* **2015**, *48*, 581–585. [CrossRef] [PubMed]
9. Allin, K.H.; The IMI-DIRECT Consortium; Tremaroli, V.; Caesar, R.; Jensen, B.A.H.; Damgaard, M.T.F.; Bahl, M.I.; Licht, T.R.; Hansen, T.H.; Nielsen, T.; et al. Aberrant intestinal microbiota in individuals with prediabetes. *Diabetologia* **2018**, *61*, 810–820. [CrossRef]

10. American Diabetes Association. Obesity management for the treatment of type 2 diabetes. *Diabetes Care* **2017**, *40*, S57–S64. [CrossRef] [PubMed]

11. Markovic, T.P.; Jenkins, A.B.; Campbell, L.V.; Furler, S.M.; Kraegen, E.W.; Chisholm, D.J. The determinants of glycemic responses to diet restriction and weight loss in obesity and NIDDM. *Diabetes Care* **1998**, *21*, 687–694. [CrossRef]

12. Wing, R.R.; Blair, E.H.; Bononi, P.; Marcus, M.D.; Watanabe, R.; Bergman, R.N. Caloric restriction per se is a significant factor in improvements in glycemic control and insulin sensitivity during weight loss in obese NIDDM patients. *Diabetes Care* **1994**, *17*, 30–36. [CrossRef]

13. Sumithran, P.; Prendergast, L.A.; Delbridge, E.; Purcell, K.; Shulkes, A.; Kriketos, A.; Proietto, J. Long-term persistence of hormonal adaptations to weight loss. *N. Engl. J. Med.* **2011**, *365*, 1597–1604. [CrossRef]

14. Lau, D.C.W.; Douketis, J.D.; Morrison, K.M.; Hramiak, I.M.; Sharma, A.M.; for the Obesity Canada Clinical Practice Guidelines Steering Committee and Expert Panel. Synopsis of the 2006 Canadian clinical practice guidelines on the management and prevention of obesity in adults and children. *Can. Med. Assoc. J.* **2007**, *176*, 1103–1106. [CrossRef] [PubMed]

15. Blunt, J.W.; Copp, B.R.; Keyzers, R.A.; Munro, M.H.G.; Prinsep, M.R. Marine natural products. *Nat. Prod. Rep.* **2013**, *30*, 237–323. [CrossRef] [PubMed]

16. Lopes, G.; Andrade, P.B.; Valentão, P. Phlorotannins: Towards New pharmacological interventions for diabetes mellitus type 2. *Molecules* **2017**, *22*, 56. [CrossRef] [PubMed]

17. Roy, M.-C.; Anguenot, R.; Fillion, C.; Beaulieu, M.; Bérubé, J.; Richard, D. Effect of a commercially-available algal phlorotannins extract on digestive enzymes and carbohydrate absorption in vivo. *Food Res. Int.* **2011**, *44*, 3026–3029. [CrossRef]

18. Gabbia, D.; Dall'Acqua, S.; Di Gangi, I.M.; Bogialli, S.; Caputi, V.; Albertoni, L.; Marsilio, I.; Paccagnella, N.; Carrara, M.; Giron, M.C.; et al. The phytocomplex from *Fucus vesiculosus* and *Ascophyllum nodosum* controls postprandial plasma glucose levels: An in vitro and in vivo study in a mouse model of NASH. *Mar. Drugs* **2017**, *15*, 41. [CrossRef]

19. Paradis, M.-E.; Couture, P.; Lamarche, B. A randomised crossover placebo-controlled trial investigating the effect of brown seaweed (*Ascophyllum nodosum* and *Fucus vesiculosus*) on postchallenge plasma glucose and insulin levels in men and women. *Appl. Physiol. Nutr. Metab.* **2011**, *36*, 913–919. [CrossRef]

20. Kim, K.-T.; Rioux, L.-E.; Turgeon, S.L. Alpha-amylase and alpha-glucosidase inhibition is differentially modulated by fucoidan obtained from *Fucus vesiculosus* and *Ascophyllum nodosum*. *Phytochemistry* **2014**, *98*, 27–33. [CrossRef]

21. Shan, X.D.; Liu, X.; Hao, J.J.; Cai, C.; Fan, F.; Dun, Y.L.; Zhao, X.L.; Liu, X.X.; Li, C.X.; Yu, G.L. In vitro and in vivo hypoglycemic effects of brown algal fucoidans. *Int. J. Biol. Macromol.* **2016**, *82*, 249–255. [CrossRef]

22. Lee, T.; Dugoua, J.-J. Nutritional supplements and their effect on glucose control. *Curr. Diabetes Rep.* **2011**, *11*, 142–148. [CrossRef]

23. Khaodhiar, L.; Cummings, S.; Apovian, C.M. Treating diabetes and prediabetes by focusing on obesity management. *Curr. Diabetes Rep.* **2009**, *9*, 348–354. [CrossRef]

24. Padwal, R.S.; Sharma, A.M. Prevention of cardiovascular disease: Obesity, diabetes and the metabolic syndrome. *Can. J. Cardiol.* **2010**, *26*, 18C–20C. [CrossRef]

25. Lau, D.C. Current and emerging pharmacotherapies for type 2 diabetes. *Can. J. Diabetes* **2015**, *39*, S127–S128. [CrossRef]

26. De Martin, S.; Gabbia, D.; Carrara, M.; Ferri, N. The brown algae *Fucus vesiculosus* and *Ascophyllum nodosum* reduce metabolic syndrome risk factors: A clinical study. *Nat. Prod. Commun.* **2018**, *13*, 1934578X1801301228. [CrossRef]

27. DeRosa, G.; Cicero, A.F.; D'Angelo, A.; Maffioli, P. *Ascophyllum nodosum* and *Fucus vesiculosus* on glycemic status and on endothelial damage markers in dysglicemic patients. *Phytother. Res.* **2019**, *33*, 791–797. [CrossRef]

28. Kowall, B.; Rathmann, W.; Heier, M.; Holle, R.; Peters, A.; Thorand, B.; Herder, C.; Strassburger, K.; Giani, G.; Meisinger, C. Impact of weight and weight change on normalization of prediabetes and on persistence of normal glucose tolerance in an older population: The KORA S4/F4 study. *Int. J. Obes.* **2012**, *36*, 826–833. [CrossRef]

29. Gaillard, O. Le Peptide-C. *Immunoanal. Biol. Spec.* **2000**, *15*, 94–95. [CrossRef]

30. Zhang, H.; Bian, B.; Hu, F.; Su, Q. OGTT 1 h serum C-peptide to plasma glucose concentration ratio is more related to beta cell function and diabetes mellitus. *Oncotarget* **2017**, *8*, 51786–51791. [CrossRef]

31. Hayashi, T.; Boyko, E.J.; Sato, K.K.; McNeely, M.J.; Leonetti, D.L.; Kahn, S.E.; Fujimoto, W.Y. Patterns of insulin concentration during the OGTT predict the risk of type 2 diabetes in Japanese Americans. *Diabetes Care* **2013**, *36*, 1229–1235. [CrossRef]

32. Abdul-Ghani, M.A.; Jenkinson, C.P.; Richardson, D.K.; Tripathy, D.; DeFronzo, R.A. Insulin secretion and action in subjects with impaired fasting glucose and impaired glucose tolerance. Results from the veterans administration genetic epidemiology study. *Diabetes* **2006**, *55*, 1430–1435. [CrossRef]

33. Apostolidis, E.; Lee, C.M. In vitro potential of *Ascophyllum nodosum* phenolic antioxidant-mediated α-glucosidase and α-amylase inhibition. *J. Food Sci.* **2010**, *75*, H97–H102. [CrossRef]

34. Expert Panel on Detection, Evaluation, and Treatment of High Blood Cholesterol in Adults. Executive summary of the third report of the National Cholesterol Education Program (NCEP) expert panel on detection, evaluation and treatment of high blood cholesterol in adults (Adult treatment panel III). *JAMA* **2012**, *285*, 2486–2497.

35. American Diabetes Association. Dyslipidemia management in adults with diabetes. *Diabetes Care* **2004**, *27*, s68–s71. [CrossRef]

36. Shin, H.-C.; Kim, S.H.; Park, Y.; Lee, B.H.; Hwang, H.J. Effects of 12-week oral supplementation of *Ecklonia cava* polyphenols on anthropometric and blood lipid parameters in overweight Korean Individuals: A double-blind randomized clinical trial. *Phytother. Res.* **2012**, *26*, 363–368. [CrossRef]

37. Iacoviello, L.; Zito, F.; Rago, L.; Di Castelnuovo, A.; De Curtis, A.; Zappacosta, B.; de Gaetano, G.; Donati, M.B.; Cerletti, C. Prolonged administration of *Ascophyllum nodosum* to healthy human volunteers and cardiovascular risk. *Nutrafoods* **2013**, *12*, 137–144. [CrossRef]

38. Akbari, M.; Hassan-Zadeh, V. IL-6 signalling pathways and the development of type 2 diabetes. *Inflammopharmacology* **2018**, *26*, 685–698. [CrossRef]

39. Bahar, B.; O'Doherty, J.V.; Hayes, M.; Sweeney, T. Extracts of brown seaweeds can attenuate the bacterial lipopolysaccharide-induced pro-inflammatory response in the porcine colon ex vivo. *J. Anim. Sci.* **2012**, *90*, 46–48. [CrossRef]

40. Dutot, M.; Fagon, R.; Hemon, M.; Rat, P. Antioxidant, anti-inflammatory, and anti-senescence activities of a phlorotannin-rich natural extract from brown seaweed *Ascophyllum nodosum*. *Appl. Biochem. Biotechnol.* **2012**, *167*, 2234–2240. [CrossRef]

41. Catarino, M.D.; Amarante, S.J.; Mateus, N.; Silva, A.M.S.; Cardoso, S.M. Brown algae phlorotannins: A marine alternative to break the oxidative stress, inflammation and cancer network. *Foods* **2021**, *10*, 1478. [CrossRef]

42. Moradi, F.; Maleki, V.; Saleh-Ghadimi, S.; Kooshki, F.; Gargari, B.P. Potential roles of chromium on inflammatory biomarkers in diabetes: A systematic. *Clin. Exp. Pharmacol. Physiol.* **2019**, *46*, 975–983. [CrossRef]

43. Park, W.-C.; Seo, I.; Kim, S.-H.; Lee, Y.-J.; Ahn, S.V. Association between resting heart rate and inflammatory markers (white blood cell count and high-sensitivity C-reactive protein) in healthy Korean people. *Korean J. Fam. Med.* **2017**, *38*, 8–13. [CrossRef]

44. Whelton, S.P.; Narla, V.; Blaha, M.J.; Nasir, K.; Blumenthal, R.S.; Jenny, N.S.; Al-Mallah, M.; Michos, E. Association between resting heart rate and inflammatory biomarkers (high-sensitivity C-reactive protein, interleukin-6, and fibrinogen) (from the multi-ethnic study of atherosclerosis). *Am. J. Cardiol.* **2014**, *113*, 644–649. [CrossRef]

45. Jung, W.-K.; Heo, S.-J.; Jeon, Y.-J.; Lee, C.-M.; Park, Y.-M.; Byun, H.-G.; Choi, Y.H.; Park, S.-G.; Choi, I.-W. Inhibitory effects and molecular mechanism of dieckol isolated from marine brown alga on COX-2 and iNOS in microglial cells. *J. Agric. Food Chem.* **2009**, *57*, 4439–4446. [CrossRef]

46. König, J.; Wells, J.; Cani, P.D.; García-Ródenas, C.L.; Macdonald, T.; Mercenier, A.; Whyte, J.; Troost, F.; Brummer, R.-J. Human intestinal barrier function in health and disease. *Clin. Transl. Gastroenterol.* **2016**, *7*, e196. [CrossRef]

47. Cani, P.D.; Amar, J.; Iglesias, M.A.; Poggi, M.; Knauf, C.; Bastelica, D.; Neyrinck, A.M.; Fava, F.; Tuohy, K.M.; Chabo, C.W.; et al. Metabolic endotoxemia initiates obesity and insulin resistance. *Diabetes* **2007**, *56*, 1761–1772. [CrossRef]

48. Charoensiddhi, S.; Conlon, M.A.; Methacanon, P.; Franco, C.; Su, P.; Zhang, W. Gut health benefits of brown seaweed *Ecklonia radiata* and its polysaccharides demonstrated in vivo in a rat model. *J. Funct. Foods* **2017**, *37*, 676–684. [CrossRef]

49. Michiels, J.; Skrivanova, E.; Missotten, J.; Ovyn, A.; Mrazek, J.; De Smet, S.; Dierick, N. Intact brown seaweed (*Ascophyllum nodosum*) in diets of weaned piglets: Effects on performance, gut bacteria and morphology and plasma oxidative status. *J. Anim. Physiol. Anim. Nutr.* **2012**, *96*, 1101–1111. [CrossRef]

50. Shannon, E.; Conlon, M.; Hayes, M. Seaweed components as potential modulators of the gut microbiota. *Mar. Drugs* **2021**, *19*, 358. [CrossRef]

51. Cotas, J.; Leandro, A.; Monteiro, P.; Pacheco, D.; Figueirinha, A.; Gonçalves, A.M.M.; Da Silva, G.J.; Pereira, L. Seaweed phenolics: From extraction to applications. *Mar. Drugs* **2020**, *18*, 384. [CrossRef]

52. Diabetes Canada Clinical Practice Guidelines Expert Committee; Punthakee, Z.; Goldenberg, R.; Katz, P. Definition, classification and diagnosis of diabetes, prediabetes and metabolic syndrome. *Can. J. Diabetes* **2018**, *42*, S10–S15. [CrossRef]

53. Flack, K.D.; Siders, W.A.; Johnson, L.; Roemmich, J.N. Cross-validation of resting metabolic rate prediction equations. *J. Acad. Nutr. Diet.* **2016**, *116*, 1413–1422. [CrossRef]

54. Diabetes-Québec. Meal Planning for People with Diabetes. 2017. Available online: https://publications.msss.gouv.qc.ca/msss/fichiers/2016/16-215-01A.pdf (accessed on 20 February 2020).

55. Harvard Medical School. The Healthy Eating Plate. 2011. Available online: https://cdn1.sph.harvard.edu/wp-content/uploads/sites/30/2012/09/HEPJan2015.jpg (accessed on 6 September 2019).

56. Labonté, M.; Cyr, A.; Baril-Gravel, L.; Royer, M.-M.; Lamarche, B. Validity and reproducibility of a web-based, self-administered food frequency questionnaire. *Eur. J. Clin. Nutr.* **2012**, *66*, 166–173. [CrossRef]

57. IPAQ. Guidelines for Data Processing and Analysis of the International Physical Activity Questionnaire (IPAQ). Short and Long Forms. 2005. Available online: http://www.ipaq.ki.se/scoring.pdf (accessed on 15 March 2010).

58. Craig, C.L.; Marshall, A.L.; Sjöström, M.; Bauman, A.E.; Booth, M.L.; Ainsworth, B.E.; Pratt, M.; Ekelund, U.; Yngve, A.; Sallis, J.F.; et al. International physical activity questionnaire: 12-country reliability and validity. *Med. Sci. Sports Exerc.* **2003**, *35*, 1381–1395. [CrossRef]

59. Pullar, T.; Kumar, S.; Feely, M. Compliance in clinical trials. *Ann. Rheum. Dis.* **1989**, *48*, 871–875. [CrossRef]

60. Kunst, A.; Draeger, B.; Ziegenhorn, J. UV methods with hexokinase and glucose-6-phosphate dehydrogenase. In *Methods of Enzymatic Analysis*; Bergemeyer, H.Y., Ed.; Verlag Chemie: Deerfield, Germany, 1984; Volume VI, pp. 163–172.

61. Pacini, G.; Mari, A. Methods for clinical assessment of insulin sensitivity and β-cell function. *Best Pract. Res. Clin. Endocrinol. Metab.* **2003**, *17*, 305–322. [CrossRef]

62. Bergmeyer, H.U.; Scheibe, P.; Wahlefeld, A.W. Optimization of methods for aspartate aminotransferase and alanine aminotransferase. *Clin. Chem.* **1978**, *24*, 58–73. [CrossRef]

63. Bilodeau, J.F.; Bisson, M.; Larose, J.; Pronovost, E.; Brien, M.; Greffard, K.; Marc, I. Physical fitness is associated with prostaglandin F2alpha isomers during pregnancy. *Prostaglandins Leukot. Essent. Fat. Acids* **2019**, *145*, 7–14. [CrossRef]

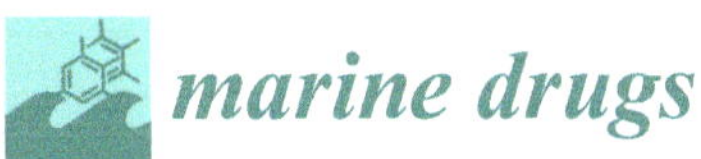

Article

Preparation and Characterization of Nano-Selenium Decorated by Chondroitin Sulfate Derived from Shark Cartilage and Investigation on Its Antioxidant Activity

Jianping Chen [1,2,*], Xuehua Chen [1], Jiarui Li [1], Baozhen Luo [1], Tugui Fan [1], Rui Li [1,2], Xiaofei Liu [1,2], Bingbing Song [1,2], Xuejing Jia [1,2] and Saiyi Zhong [1,2,*]

[1] Guangdong Provincial Key Laboratory of Aquatic Product Processing and Safety, Guangdong Provincial Engineering Technology Research Center of Seafood, Guangdong Province Engineering Laboratory for Marine Biological Products, Key Laboratory of Advanced Processing of Aquatic Product of Guangdong Higher Education Institution, Guangdong Provincial Science and Technology Innovation Center for Subtropical Fruit and Vegetable Processing, College of Food Science and Technology, Guangdong Ocean University, Zhanjiang 524088, China; 18977740415@163.com (X.C.); rain8413@163.com (J.L.); 13413650541@163.com (B.L.); ftg2693982106@163.com (T.F.); liruihn@163.com (R.L.); liuxf169@126.com (X.L.); 15891793858@163.com (B.S.); jiaxj@gdou.edu.cn (X.J.)
[2] Collaborative Innovation Center of Seafood Deep Processing, Dalian Polytechnic University, Dalian 116034, China
* Correspondence: cjp516555989@gdou.edu.cn (J.C.); zsylxc@126.com (S.Z.); Tel.: +86-187-1915-6629 (J.C.); +86-188-2669-9336 (S.Z.)

Abstract: In the present study, a selenium-chondroitin sulfate (SeCS) was synthesized by the sodium selenite (Na_2SeO_3) and ascorbic acid (Vc) redox reaction using chondroitin sulfate derived from shark cartilage as a template, and characterized by SEM, SEM-EDS, FTIR and XRD. Meanwhile, its stability was investigated at different conditions of pH and temperatures. Besides, its antioxidant activity was further determined by the DPPH and ABTS assays. The results showed the SeCS with the smallest particle size of 131.3 ± 4.4 nm and selenium content of 33.18% was obtained under the optimal condition (CS concentration of 0.1 mg/mL, mass ratio of Na_2SeO_3 to Vc of 1:8, the reaction time of 3 h, and the reaction temperature of 25 °C). SEM image showed the SeCS was an individual and spherical nanostructure and its structure was evidenced by FTIR and XRD. Meanwhile, SeCS remained stable at an alkaline pH and possessed good storage stability at 4 °C for 28 days. The results on scavenging free radical levels showed that SeCS exhibited significantly higher antioxidant activity than SeNPs and CS, indicating that SeCS had a potential antioxidant effect.

Keywords: nanoselenium; chondroitin sulfate derived from shark cartilage; structure characterization; antioxidant activity

Citation: Chen, J.; Chen, X.; Li, J.; Luo, B.; Fan, T.; Li, R.; Liu, X.; Song, B.; Jia, X.; Zhong, S. Preparation and Characterization of Nano-Selenium Decorated by Chondroitin Sulfate Derived from Shark Cartilage and Investigation on Its Antioxidant Activity. *Mar. Drugs* **2022**, *20*, 172. https://doi.org/10.3390/md20030172

Academic Editors: Donatella Degl'Innocenti and Marzia Vasarri

Received: 3 February 2022
Accepted: 24 February 2022
Published: 26 February 2022

Publisher's Note: MDPI stays neutral with regard to jurisdictional claims in published maps and institutional affiliations.

1. Introduction

Reactive oxygen species (ROS) are the result of the normal cell metabolism of living organisms. However, when the production of ROS exceeds the scavenging capacity of living organisms, oxidative stress occurs [1]. Excessive reactive oxygen species (ROS) not only affect normal metabolism, but also is closely related to the occurrence and development of various diseases, including cardiovascular diseases [2], Alzheimer's disease [3], nonalcoholic fatty liver disease [4], and so on. As an essential micronutrient for human health, selenium (Se) plays a vital role in protecting against oxidative stress [5]. Nevertheless, the beneficial and harmful doses of Se is an extremely narrow margin, which limits its practical applications in food and medicine [6]. Therefore, it is necessary to take effective measures to solve this problem.

Nanotechnology, as a technology developed in recent years, has been widely used in the field of biology. Selenium nanoparticles (SeNPs) have been widely used as drug carriers due to their advantages of small volume, large specific surface area, and unique physical and chemical properties. Previous studies have found that SeNPs can remove harmful peroxides from the body through glutathione peroxidase (GSH-PX) and protect the membrane structure of the body from damage [7]. Meanwhile, compared with organic and inorganic selenium compounds [8], SeNPs possesses higher bioactivity like antioxidant activity, better bioavailability and lower toxicity [9]. However, SeNPs are very unstable in the liquid phase and tend to aggregate and form gray or black selenium with a large particle size, thus losing the bioavailability and bioactivity of SeNPs [10]. Therefore, a suitable stabilizer is needed to improve its stability.

Natural bioactive polysaccharides have attracted more and more attention because they are rich in hydrophilic groups, such as hydroxyls, and are considered as ideal templates for SeNPs stabilization. A variety of polysaccharides have been reported to modify SeNPs and the modified SeNPs have been found to have strong antioxidant activity [6,11,12]. Chondroitin sulfate (CS), a natural anionic glycoaminoglycan, is extracted from various marine animal cartilages, such as shark, skate and so on [13,14]. Studies showed CS exhibited a variety of biological activities, such as antioxidant activity [15], anti-inflammatory activity [16] and anti-tumor activity [17]. Since it is rich in carboxyl and hydroxyl groups, it is often used to stabilize SeNPs. For example, Han et al. reported the preparation method of selenium–chondroitin sulfate (SeCS) using CS as a stabilizer to stable SeNPs, but the Se content in SeCS is only 10.1%, and the study on its stability has not been reported [18]. Since the Se content and stability of SeCS are related to its biological activity, it is necessary to further improve the Se content and investigate the stability of SeCS. Therefore, in this study, we screened the preparation conditions of SeCS, investigated its stability at a different pH and temperature, and evaluated its antioxidant activity using 2,2-diphenyl-1-picrylhydrazyl (DPPH) and 2,2′-azino-bis (3-ethylbenzo-thiazoline-6-sulfonic acid) diammonium salt (ABTS) assays. This study provides a theoretical basis for the application of SeCS as a fresh antioxidant agent in food and medicine.

2. Results and Discussion

2.1. Determination of Preparation Conditions of SeCS

2.1.1. Determination of CS Concentration

In order to evaluate the effect of CS concentration on the formation of SeCS, the particle sizes of SeCS prepared with different concentrations of CS were measured by nanoparticle size analyzer. As shown in Figure 1A, the particle sizes of SeNPs with 0.05 mg/mL CS surface decoration were 278.70 ± 9.47 nm. The average particle diameters of SeNPs were significantly decreased to 113.7 ± 2.89 nm in the presence of 0.1 mg/mL CS, indicating that CS between 0.05 mg/mL and 0.1 mg/mL could inhibit the aggregation of SeNPs with the increase of CS concentration. The result was in accordance with the previous study, which demonstrated that the particle diameters of SeNPs decorated with 1.0 mg/mL chitosan were smaller than that synthesized with 0.6 mg/mL chitosan [19]. However, when CS concentration is greater than 0.1 mg/mL, the particle size of SeCS in the system became larger. This might be because CS molecules aggregated to reduce its hydrophilic groups' function, resulting in the particle size become larger. Therefore, the optimal concentration of CS was selected as 0.1 mg/mL.

2.1.2. Determination of Molar Ratio of Na_2SeO_3 to Vc

According to the reaction equation, sodium selenite (Na_2SeO_3) reacts with ascorbic acid (Vc) at the coefficient of 1:2. However, in fact, an excess of V_C needs to be added to the system to prevent SeNPs from being oxidized. Therefore, in this study, fixing the CS concentration of 0.1 mg/mL, the reaction time of 3 h and the reaction temperature of 55 °C, the molar ratio of Na_2SeO_3 to Vc varied from 1:2 to 1:10. The particle sizes of SeCS prepared with different molar ratios of Na_2SeO_3 to Vc were shown in Figure 1B. The results showed that the average particle diameters of SeCS obtained with the molar ratio of Na_2SeO_3 to Vc of 1:2 were 187.3 ± 12.48 nm. As the molar ratio of Na_2SeO_3 to Vc increased to 1:8, the particle size reached the smallest. It was speculated that excessive Vc could improve the growth of the crystal nucleus to stabilize SeCS [20]. However, further increasing Vc concentration meant the particle size became larger due to the unstable reaction system. So, it might be the reason why the diameter of the SeCS prepared with a molar ratio of Na_2SeO_3 to Vc of 1:10 was larger than that obtained with a molar ratio of Na_2SeO_3 to Vc of 1:8. Therefore, the optimal molar ratio of Na_2SeO_3 to Vc was selected as 1:8.

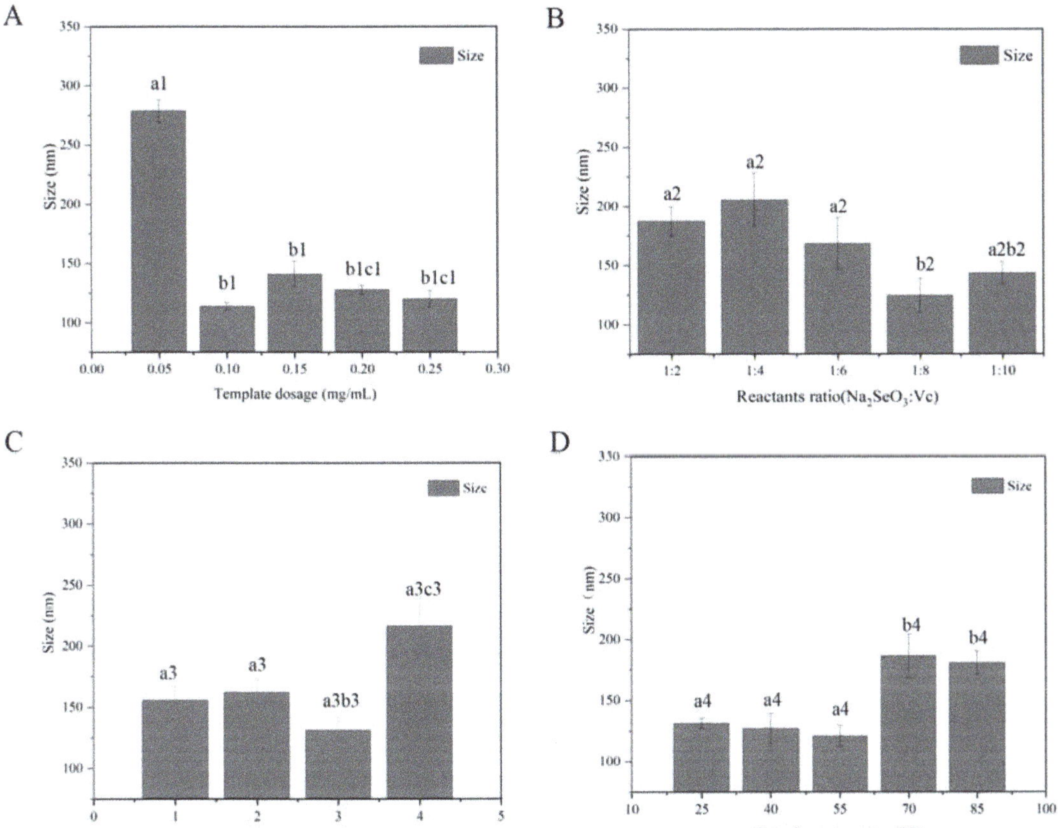

Figure 1. Effects of different template dosage (**A**), reactants ratio (**B**), reaction time (**C**), and reaction temperatures (**D**) on particle size of SeCS. Bars with a1, b1 and c1 represented a statistical difference ($p < 0.05$) among different template dosages. Bars with a2 and b2 represented a statistical difference ($p < 0.05$) among different reactants ratios. Bars with a3, b3 and c3 represented a statistical difference ($p < 0.05$) among different times. Bars with a4 and b4 represented a statistical difference ($p < 0.05$) among different reaction temperatures.

2.1.3. Determination of Reaction Time

Studies showed that reaction time had a vital role to regulate the SeNPs reaction system [21]. If the reaction time is too short, the reaction between Na_2SeO_3 and Vc is not sufficient. However, if the reaction time is too long, the SeNPs in the system will gather, leading to increasing the particle size. Therefore, we next further investigated the influence of reaction time on the particle size of system. Fixing the CS concentration of 0.1 mg/mL, the molar mass ratio of Na_2SeO_3 to Vc of 1:8 and the reaction temperature of 55 °C, the reaction time varied from 1 h to 4 h. The result was shown in Figure 1C. When the reaction time extended from 1 h to 2 h, no significant difference was observed in the particle size of the obtained SeCS. When the reaction time increased to 3 h, the particle size of the obtained SeCS reached to 131.2 ± 9.97 nm. When the reaction time exceeded 3 h, the particle size of the obtained SeCS remarkably increased. Therefore, we selected the reaction time of 3 h as the optimal reaction time to prepare SeCS.

2.1.4. Determination of Reaction Temperature

Fixing the CS concentration of 0.1 mg/mL, the molar mass ratio of Na_2SeO_3 to Vc of 1:8, reaction time of 3 h, the reaction temperature varied from 25 to 85 °C. The particle size of the obtained SeCS is shown in Figure 1D. It could be seen that although the particle size of the obtained SeCS slightly decreased at 55 °C, there was no significant difference between 25 °C and 55 °C. When the reaction temperature was further separately increased to 70 °C and 85 °C, the particle size of the obtained SeCS both significantly increased. The reason might be that heating easily led to the violent movement of nanoparticles, thus increasing the chance and intensity of collisions and intensifying aggregation [22]. Therefore, in terms of saving energy, the optimal reaction temperature was selected as 25 °C.

In summary, these above results demonstrated that we optimized conditions for preparing SeCS as a CS concentration of 0.1 mg/mL, the molar mass ratio of Na_2SeO_3 to Vc of 1:8, reaction time of 3 h and reaction temperature of 25 °C, so SeCS used in subsequent experiments were obtained in optimal reaction conditions. Under the optimal reaction conditions, the SeCS was successfully prepared and inductively coupled plasma mass spectrometry (ICP-MS) was used to measure the Se content of the SeCS obtained. It was found that the Se content in SeCS was 33.18%, which is higher than that reported in previous studies [18,23].

2.2. Characterization of SeCS

2.2.1. Scanning Electron Microscopy (SEM)

In order to verify the above results, SEM was used to analyze the morphology of SeNPs and SeCS. As shown in Figure 2, the SEM results of SeNPs clearly revealed that SeNPs without CS surface decoration showed serious aggregation and formed large particles chunks (Figure 2A,C). Nevertheless, the addition of CS accelerated the production of homogeneous spherical SeCS with high dispersibility (Figure 2B,D), which further confirmed the formation of SeCS.

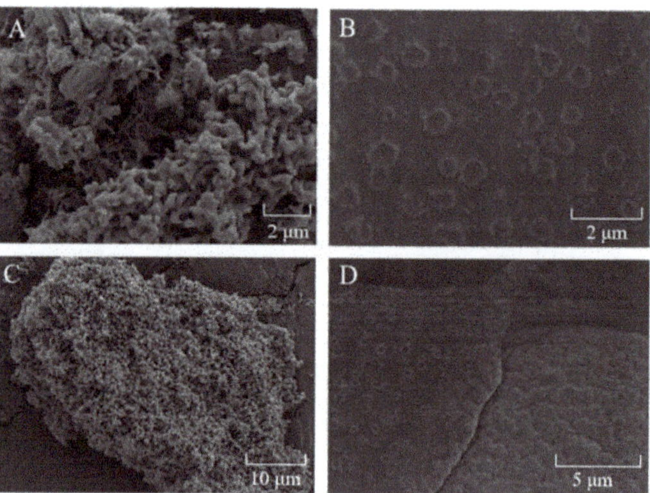

Figure 2. SEM images of SeNPs (**A,C**) and SeCS (**B,D**) powders. The SeNPs were obtained in the same procedure of SeCS without CS.

2.2.2. Element Analysis of SeCS

To determine chemical compositions of SeCS samples, scanning electron microscopy equipped with an energy dispersion spectrum detector (SEM-EDS) was employed. The results were shown in Figure 3. It was found that C (44.16%), O (37.74%), and Na (18.1%) were the chemical compositions of CS (Figure 3A). Furthermore, an SEM-EDS investigation of SeNPs showed the percentages of Se, C and O atoms were 92.27%, 7.43% and 0.30% (Figure 3B), which were similar to previous findings of Ye et al. [21]. An EDS investigation of SeCS (Figure 3C) showed that the presence of a strong Se atoms signal (65.73%). The existence of the Na atom (1.27%), C atom (25.55%) and O atom (7.44%) in SeCS suggested that CS successfully combined to the surface of the SeNPs.

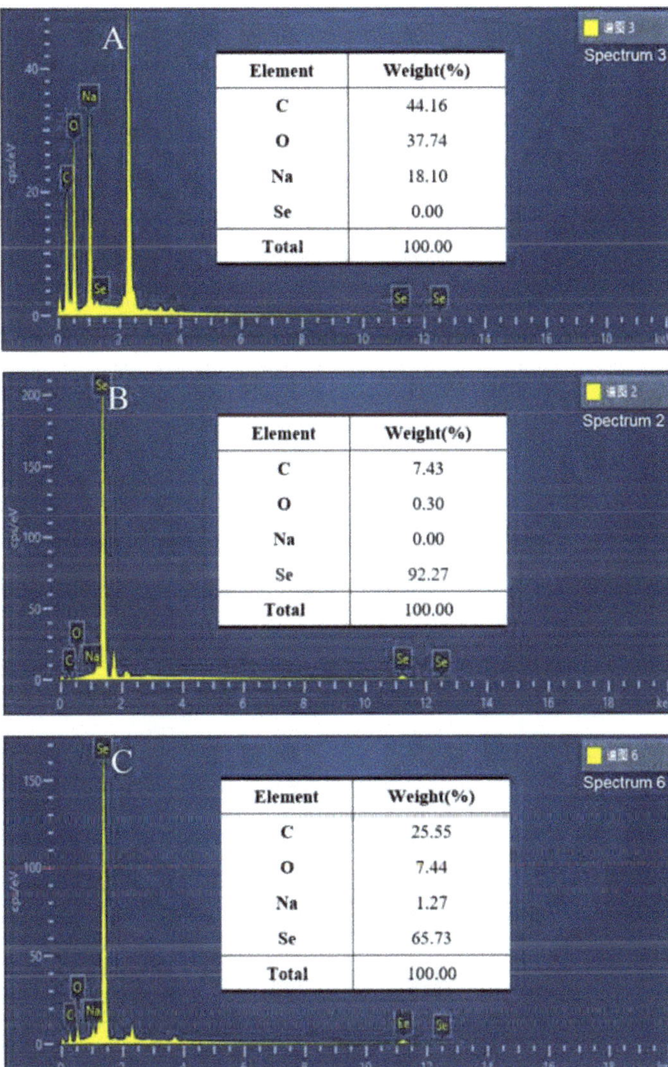

Figure 3. SEM-EDS element analysis of CS (**A**), SeNPs (**B**) and SeCS (**C**). The SeNPs were obtained in the same procedure of SeCS without CS.

2.2.3. Fourier Transform Infrared Spectroscopy (FT-IR) Analysis

To confirm the chemical binding of CS to the surface of the SeNPs, FTIR spectroscopy is used to ascertain the formation of SeCS. The FTIR spectra of CS and SeCS were shown in Figure 4. The typical IR spectrum of CS was presented in Figure 4 which was in good agreement with the literature [23]. The FTIR spectrum of CS exhibited an absorption band at 3402 cm^{-1}, indicating the overlapping of –OH and –NH stretching vibrations. Additionally, the absorption peaks of CS were 1070 cm^{-1} and 1128 cm^{-1}, 1224 cm^{-1}, 1419 cm^{-1}, and 1635 cm^{-1}, which corresponded to the characteristic asymmetric stretching vibrations of the C–O–C bridge (β-1,4 glycosidic bonds), asymmetric stretching vibrations of –S=O, stretching vibrations of the -COOH and stretching vibrations of the –C=O of –NHCO–. By comparing the FTIR spectra of CS, SeCS resembled that of CS and there were no new absorption peaks in the FTIR spectrum of SeCS, indicating that the reaction between CS and SeNPs did not generate any new covalent bonds. However, an obvious change occurred in the peak locations of SeCS, indicating that the main interaction between CS and SeNPs was physical adsorption.

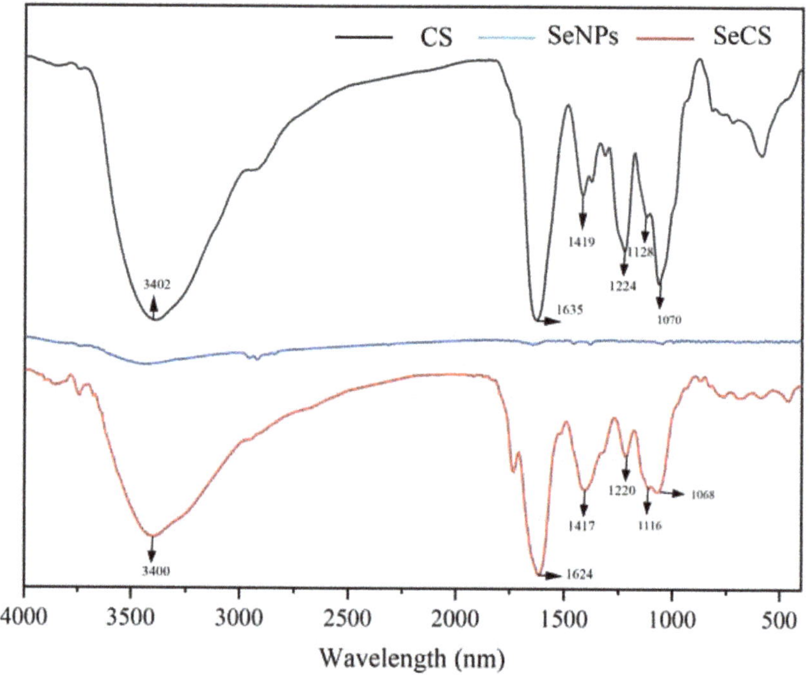

Figure 4. FT-IR spectra of CS, SeNPs and SeCS. The SeNPs were obtained in the same procedure of SeCS without CS.

2.2.4. Powder X-ray Diffractometry (XRD) Analysis

On this basis of FT-IR analysis, XRD was used to characterize the formation of SeCS. XRD analysis could detect phase identification of crystalline materials. The intensity and sharpness of XRD peaks reflected the crystalline nature of the sample. The XRD spectra of CS, SeNPs and SeCS were shown in Figure 5. As shown in Figure 5, the X-ray diffractogram of SeNPs showed two broad peaks in the ranges of 20–40° and 40–60° (2θ), indicating that SeNPs existed in an amorphous form. This result was in good agreement with the literature [21]. No sharp peaks were found in the XRD pattern of CS and SeCS, confirming their amorphous characteristic in nature. Compared with the XRD diffraction patterns of

CS and SeNPs, both the peak positions and intensity of SeCS shifted, suggesting that the formation of SeCS.

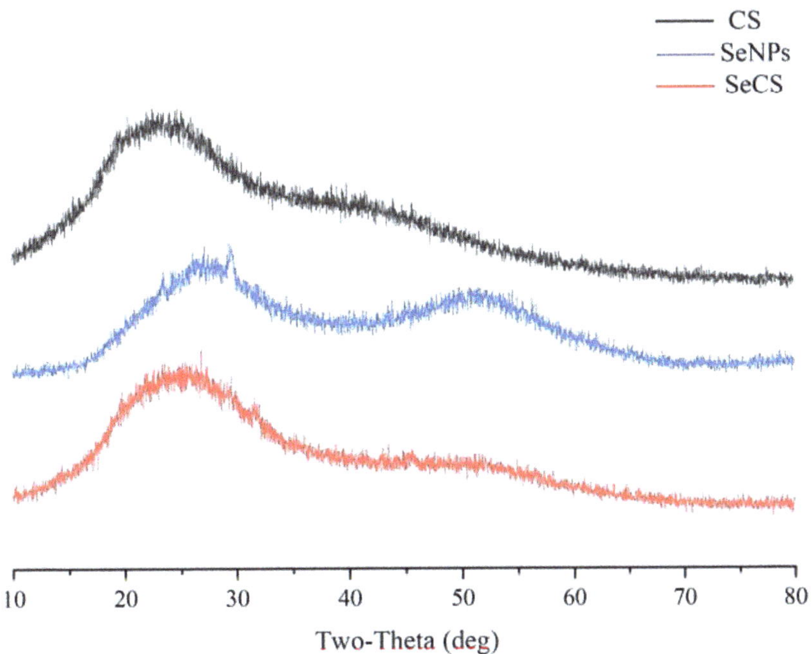

Figure 5. XRD patterns of CS, SeNPs and SeCS. The SeNPs were obtained in the same procedure of SeCS without CS.

2.2.5. Stability of SeCS

The stability of nanoparticles is one of the key factors for their biological function. Studies have shown that the stability of nanoparticles is closely related to pH, storage temperature and storage time in the application medium [24,25]. Therefore, we next investigated the influence of different pHs and storage temperatures on the stability of SeCS. The influence of pH on the stability of SeCS was shown in Figure 6A. The particle diameters of SeCS notably decreased to approximately 98.9 ± 5.9 nm at the 2–8 pH range. Then, no significant shift occurred at the 8–12 pH range. This was probably attributed to the strongest electrostatic interaction between anionic CS and SeNPs at pH 8.0 due to the sensitivity of CS at a low pH [26]. The effect of storage temperature on the stability of SeCS was shown in Figure 6B. When the SeCS solution was stored at 4 °C for 28 days, the particle size showed no obvious change. Yet, the particle diameter of the SeCS solution stored at 25 °C for 28 days significantly increased to 262.7 ± 13.6 nm. It was speculated that an increase in particle diameter might be related with the changes of the internal structure of the SeCS because the increasing temperature resulted in a change in the amorphous state of SeCS to the crystalline state. Moreover, our results were consistent with previous studies that high temperature was not conducive to the stability of selenium nanoparticles [10,26]. These results indicated that SeCS exerted excellent stability under a refrigerating temperature and alkaline environment.

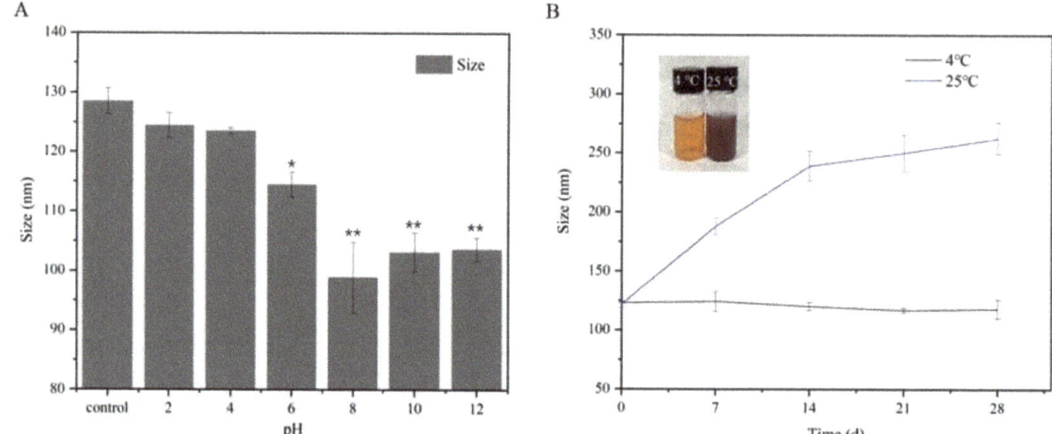

Figure 6. Effects of different pHs (**A**) and storage temperatures (**B**) on the size of SeCS. The initial pH value of the control group was 6.8. $p < 0.05$ (*) or $p < 0.01$ (**) means that columns between control group and other groups are significantly different.

2.3. The Antioxidant Property of SeCS

The antioxidant potential of SeCS was analyzed using the DPPH assay and ABTS assay in which ascorbic acid was used as a standard. As shown in Figure 7, the DPPH and ABTS radical scavenging rates of CS and SeNPs were extremely low. However, comparing with CS and SeNPs, the DPPH and ABTS radical scavenging rates of SeCS significantly increased. With the concentration of SeCS increased, the DPPH and ABTS radical scavenging rates of SeCS increased from $29.13 \pm 3.28\%$ (0.1 mg/mL) and $13.92 \pm 2.57\%$ (20 µg/mL) to $66.69 \pm 2.71\%$ (0.5 mg/mL) and $52.44 \pm 2.29\%$ (100 µg/mL), respectively. Our results indicated that SeCS could effectively scavenge the DPPH and ABTS free radical in a dose-dependent manner. However, the DPPH and ABTS scavenging activities of SeCS were lower than the V_C, particularly in the ABTS scavenging assay.

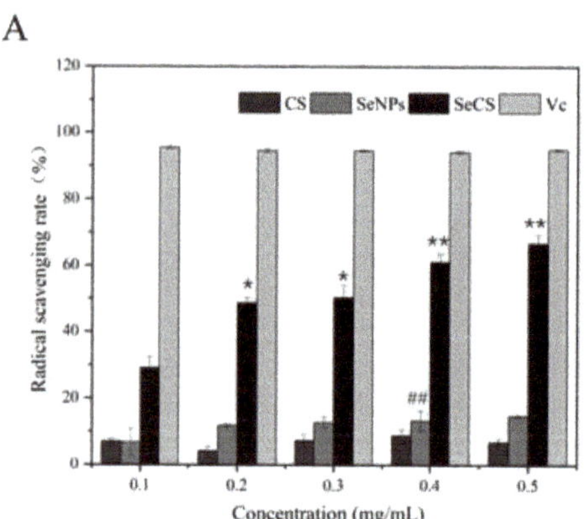
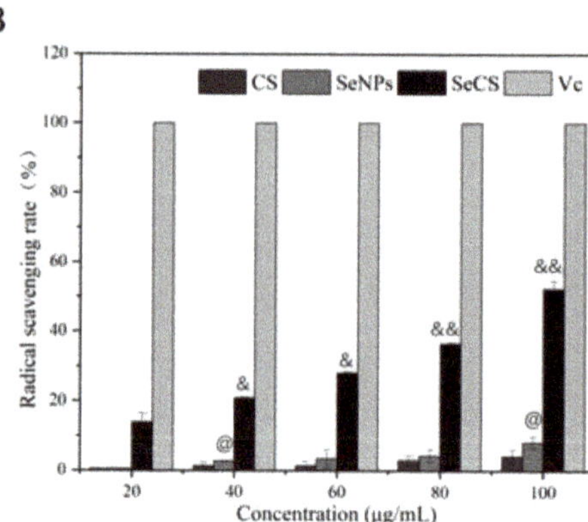

Figure 7. DPPH radical scavenging rate (**A**) and ABTS radical scavenging rate (**B**) of SeCS. $p < 0.05$ (*) or $p < 0.01$ (**) means that columns between SeCS at 0.1 mg/mL and SeCS at other concentrations are significantly different. $p < 0.01$ (##) means that columns between SeNPs at 0.1 mg/mL and SeNPs at 0.4 mg/mL are significantly different. $p < 0.05$ (&) or $p < 0.01$ (&&) means that columns between SeCS at 20 µg/mL and SeCS at other concentrations are significantly different. $p < 0.05$ (@) means that columns between SeNPs at 20 µg/mL and SeNPs at other concentrations are significantly different.

3. Materials and Methods

3.1. Materials

Chondroitin sulfate (CS) derived from shark cartilage (95% purity, Mw = 499.37, C107703) was purchased from Aladdin. CS is composed of chondroitin 6-sulfate and chondroitin 4-sulfate, and the proportion of chondroitin 6-sulfate and chondroitin 4-sulfate detected by high performance liquid chromatography is equal to or greater than 0.33:1. Na_2SeO_3, ascorbic acid (Vc), DPPH and ABTS were supplied by Shanghai Yuanye Biotechnology Co., Ltd. (Shanghai, China). The other chemicals and reagents were of analytical purity grade.

3.2. Determination of Preparation Conditions of SeCS Nanoparticles

SeCS nanoparticles were prepared according to the method as described in previous study with some modifications [23]. CS was dissolved in 30 mL of deionized water and the concentration of CS was 0.05, 0.1, 0.15, 0.2, and 0.25 mg/mL. Different molar ratios of Na_2SeO_3 to Vc (Na_2SeO_3: Vc = 1:2, 1:4, 1:6, 1:8, 1: 10) were added to CS solution and stirred at different temperatures (25 °C, 40 °C, 55 °C, 70 °C, 85 °C) for different times (1 h, 2 h, 3 h, 4 h). Then, the solution was dialyzed against double-distilled water for 48 h with a dialysis bag (M_W = 3500). The optimum preparation process of SeCS was determined by particle size analysis. The final solution was freeze-dried to preserve the bioactivity of SeCS.

3.3. Measurement of Se Content in SeCS

The selenium content of SeCS was measured using 7500 CX ICP-MS (Agilent, Palo Alto, CA, USA). The following measurement conditions of the instrument: incident power of 1550 W; plasma gas flow rate at 15 L/min; carrier gas flow rate at 1.0 L/min; auxiliary gas flow rate at 1.0 L/min; helium flow rate at 4.0 mL/min; atomization chamber temperature of 2 °C; sampling depth of 10.0 mm; sampling rate at 1.0 L/min.

3.4. Characterization of SeCS

The surface morphologies of the samples were detected using MIRA4 SEM (Tescan, Brno, Czech). The elemental compositions of the samples were measured using a MIRAL SEM-EDS (Tescan, Brno, Czech). The FT–IR spectrums of the samples were measured using a Tensor 27 spectrometer (Bruker, Karlsruhe, Germany) from 4000 to 400 cm^{-1} with a 4 cm^{-1} resolution, i.e., 2 mg of the sample was completely ground with the spectroscopic grade potassium bromide (KBr) powder and a transparent tablet was used for measurement. The X-ray diffractometer of the samples was obtained using an Ultima VI diffractometer (Rigaku, Tokyo, Japan) operated at 40 kV and 40 mA. Moreover, the samples were investigated in the range of 10–80 degree (2θ angle).

3.5. Stability of SeCS in Different Environments

3.5.1. Effects of Different pH on the Size of SeCS Nanoparticles

After dialysis, the system solution pH (6.8) was adjusted to 2, 4, 6, 8, 10 and 12 using 0.1 M sodium hydroxide (NaOH) or 0.1 M hydrochloric acid (HCl). After 10 min, the particle size of SeCS was determined by Malvern Zeizer Nano ZS particle analyzer (Malvern, Worcestershire, UK).

3.5.2. Effects of Different Storage Temperatures on the Size of SeCS Nanoparticles

The SeCS solutions were stored in 4 °C and 25 °C, respectively. After 0, 7, 14 and 28 days, the size of SeCS was measured by Malvern Zetasizer Nano ZS particle analyzer (Malvern, Worcestershire, UK).

3.6. Antioxidant Activity Evaluation of SeCS

3.6.1. DPPH Radical Scavenging Assay

The antioxidant activity of SeCS was evaluated using 2,2-diphenyl-1-picrylhydrazyl (DPPH) reagent according to a previously described method with some modifications [27].

Different concentrations (0.1–0.5 mg/mL) of CS, SeNPs and SeCS solutions were respectively added into 0.2 mM DPPH solution in methanol. After 30 min incubation in a dark place, the color change of the reaction mixture was read at 517 nm using a TU-1901 double beam UV-visible spectrophotometry (Persee, Beijing, China). Positive control in this assay was ascorbic acid. The formula of the DPPH scavenging rate was listed below:

$$\text{DPPH scavenging rate (\%)} = [A_0 - (A_1 - A_2)]/A_0 \times 100\%$$

In the equation, A_0, A_1 and A_2 separately represented the absorbance values of control, the samples with DPPH solution and the samples without DPPH solution.

3.6.2. ABTS Radical Scavenging Assay

ABTS radical scavenging activity was detected as reported in previous research with some modifications [28]. Potassium persulfate (2.6 mM) was added into ABTS (7.4 mM) to obtain the ABTS stock solution. Then, the solution was incubated at room temperature in dark for 12 h. Deionized water was used to dilute the solution to prepare the ABTS working solution (0.70 ± 0.02 absorbance at 734 nm). After that, 4 mL ABTS working solution with 1 mL sample were mixed for 6 min in the dark. Subsequently, the absorbance of mixture was recorded at a wavelength of 734 nm using a TU-1901 double beam UV-Visible spectrophotometer (Persee, Beijing, China). Ascorbic acid was selected as a positive control. The formula of the ABTS scavenging rate was listed below:

$$\text{ABTS scavenging rate (\%)} = (1 - A_i/A_0) \times 100$$

In the equation, A_0 and A_i separately indicated the absorbance values of the blank control and the sample.

3.7. Statistical Analysis

All assays were repeated three times and the values were indicated as mean $\pm$ standard deviation (SD). Statistical analysis was done using SPSS 23.0 software and Origin 2020. The comparison between two groups was analyzed by Two-tailed Student's *t*-test. *p* value less than 0.05 or 0.01 was considered significantly shift.

4. Conclusions

This study provided an effective strategy to prepare SeCS using CS as a stabilizing agent. Using the reaction system at reaction conditions of a Na_2SeO_3:Vc ratio of 1:8, 0.1 mg/mL CS, a 3 h reaction time and a 25 °C reaction temperature could generate spherical SeCS nanoparticles of 131.3 ± 4.4 nm in diameter with a high selenium entrapment efficiency (33.18%). These amorphous SeNPs were suggested to interact with CS via physical adsorption, and exhibited pH stability (pH > 8) and storage stability at 4 °C for 28 days. Moreover, SeCS exerted a stronger in vitro antioxidant capacity than SeNPs and CS. These results confirmed the higher stability and the improved antioxidant properties of SeNPs capped with CS compared to SeNPs. Taken together, SeCSs have the potential to further develop a dietary supplement to apply in the prevention and alleviation of oxidative stress-related diseases.

Author Contributions: J.C. and X.C. designed the experiment and wrote the paper. X.C., J.L., B.L. and T.F. performed the experiments. J.C. and X.C. analyzed the data. R.L., X.L., B.S., X.J. and S.Z. participated in experimental design and contributed regents and materials. J.C. and S.Z. coordinated the studies. All authors have read and agreed to the published version of the manuscript.

Funding: This research was funded by Key-Area Research and Development Program of Guangdong Province (grant number: 2020B1111030004), Guangdong Basic and the Applied Basic Research Foundation (grant number: 2020A1515010860 and 2021A1515012455), the Guangdong Ocean University Innovation Program (grant number: 230419100), the Nanhai Youth Scholar Project of Guangdong Ocean University (grant number: QNXZ201909), the Project of Science and Technology of Zhanjiang

City (grant number: 2020A01034), the Scientific Research Foundation of Guangdong Ocean University (grant number: R17034), the Guangdong Province ordinary universities characteristic innovation project (grant number: 2020KTSCX051), and the Guangdong Provincial Department of Education and the Innovative Team Program of High Education of the Guangdong Province (grant number: 2021KCXTD021).

Institutional Review Board Statement: Not applicable.

Data Availability Statement: Not applicable.

Conflicts of Interest: The authors declare no conflict of interest.

References

1. Birben, E.; Sahiner, U.M.; Sackesen, C.; Erzurum, S.; Kalayci, O. Oxidative stress and antioxidant Defense. *World Allergy Organ.* **2012**, *5*, 9–19. [CrossRef] [PubMed]
2. Taleb, A.; Ahmad, K.A.; Ihsan, A.U.; Qu, J.; Lin, N.; Hezam, K.; Koju, N.; Hui, L.; Ding, Q.L. Antioxidant effects and mechanism of silymarin in oxidative stress induced cardiovascular diseases. *Biomed. Pharmacother.* **2018**, *102*, 689–698. [CrossRef] [PubMed]
3. Ionescu-Tucker, A.; Cotmana, C.W. Emerging roles of oxidative stress in brain aging and Alzheimer's disease. *Neurobiol. Aging* **2021**, *107*, 86–95. [CrossRef] [PubMed]
4. Chen, Z.; Tian, R.F.; She, Z.G.; Cai, J.J.; Li, H.L. Role of oxidative stress in the pathogenesis of nonalcoholic fatty liver disease. *Free. Radic. Bio. Med.* **2020**, *152*, 116–141. [CrossRef] [PubMed]
5. Wang, Y.Y.; Qiu, Y.; Sun, L.; Ding, Z.C.; Yan, J.K. Preparation, characterization, and antioxidant capacities of selenium nanoparticles stabilized using polysaccharide–protein complexes from Corbicula fluminea. *Food Biosci.* **2018**, *26*, 177–184. [CrossRef]
6. Liu, G.Y.; Yang, X.; Zhang, J.X.; Liang, L.; Miao, F.; Ji, T.; Ye, Z.Q.; Chu, M.; Ren, J.Y.; Xu, X. Synthesis, stability and anti-fatigue activity of selenium nanoparticles stabilized by Lycium barbarum polysaccharides. *Int. J. Biol. Macromol.* **2021**, *179*, 418–428. [CrossRef]
7. Forootanfar, H.; Adeli-Sardou, M.; Nikkhoo, M.; Mehrabani, M.; Amir-Heidari, B.; Shahverdi, A.R.; Shakibaie, M. Antioxidant and cytotoxic effect of biologically synthesized selenium nanoparticles in comparison to selenium dioxide. *J. Trace Elem. Med. Bio.* **2014**, *28*, 75–79. [CrossRef]
8. Zhang, S.Y.; Zhang, J.; Wang, H.Y.; Chen, H.Y. Synthesis of selenium nanoparticles in the presence of polysaccharides. *Mater. Lett.* **2004**, *58*, 2590–2594. [CrossRef]
9. Soumaya, M.; Shrudhi, D.K.S.; Santhiya, R.; Rajeshkumar, S.; Venkat, K.S. Selenium nanoparticles: A potent chemotherapeutic agent and an elucidation of its mechanism. *Colloid. Surface. B* **2018**, *170*, 280–292.
10. Zhang, J.L.; Teng, Z.; Yuan, Y.; Zeng, Q.Z.; Lou, Z.Y.; Lee, S.H.; Wang, Q. Development, physicochemical characterization and cytotoxicity of selenium nanoparticles stabilized by beta-lactoglobulin. *Int. J. Biol. Macromol.* **2018**, *107*, 1406–1413. [CrossRef]
11. Tang, L.; Luo, X.; Wang, M.; Wang, Z.; Guo, J.; Kong, F.; Bi, Y. Synthesis, characterization, in vitro antioxidant and hypoglycemic activities of selenium nanoparticles decorated with polysaccharides of Gracilaria lemaneiformis. *Int. J. Biol. Macromol.* **2021**, *193*, 923–932. [CrossRef] [PubMed]
12. Xiao, Y.; Huang, Q.; Zheng, Z.; Guan, H.; Liu, S. Construction of a cordyceps sinensis exopolysaccharide-conjugated selenium nanoparticles and enhancement of their antioxidant activities. *Int. J. Biol. Macromol.* **2017**, *99*, 483–491. [CrossRef]
13. Martel-Pelletier, J.; Farran, A.; Montell, E.; Vergés, J.; Pelletier, J.P. Discrepancies in composition and biological effects of different formulations of chondroitin sulfate. *Molecules* **2015**, *20*, 4277–4289. [CrossRef] [PubMed]
14. Cunha, A.L.; Oliveira, L.G.; Maia, L.F.; Oliveira, L.F.C.; Michelacci, Y.M.; Aguiar, J.A.K. Pharmaceutical grade chondroitin sulfate: Structural analysis and identification of contaminants in different commercial preparations. *Carbohyd. Polym.* **2015**, *134*, 300–308. [CrossRef]
15. Müller, A.J.; Letelier, M.E.; Galleguillos, M.A.; Molina-Berríos, A.E.; Adarmes, H.H. Comparison of the antioxidant effects of synovial fluid from equine metacarpophalangeal joints with those of hyaluronic acid and chondroitin sulfate. *Am. J. Vet. Res.* **2010**, *71*, 399–404. [CrossRef] [PubMed]
16. Krylov, V.B.; Grachev, A.A.; Ustyuzhanina, N.E.; Ushakova, N.A.; Preobrazhenskaya, M.E.; Kozlova, N.I.; Portsel, M.N.; Konovalova, I.N.; Novikov, V.Y.; Siebert, H.C.; et al. Preliminary structural characterization, anti inflammatory and anticoagulant activities of chondroitin sulfates from marine fish cartilage. *Russ. Chem. Bull.* **2011**, *60*, 746–753. [CrossRef]
17. Palhares, L.; Barbosa, J.S.; Scortecci, K.C.; Rocha, H.A.O.; Brito, A.S.; Chavante, S.F. In vitro antitumor and anti-angiogenic activities of a shrimp chondroitin sulfate. *Int. J. Biol. Macromol.* **2020**, *162*, 1153–1165. [CrossRef]
18. Han, J.; Guo, X.; Lei, Y.X.; Dennis, B.S.; Wu, S.X.; Wu, C.Y. Synthesis and characterization of selenium–chondroitin sulfate nanoparticles. *Carbohyd. Polym.* **2012**, *90*, 122–126. [CrossRef] [PubMed]
19. Zeng, S.Q.; Ke, Y.; Liu, Y.X.; Shen, Y.B.; Zhang, L.; Li, C.; Liu, A.P.; Shen, L.; Hua, X.J.; Wu, H.J.; et al. Synthesis and antidiabetic properties of chitosan-stabilized selenium nanoparticles. *Colloid. Surface. B* **2018**, *170*, 115–121. [CrossRef]
20. Liu, Y.T.; Zeng, S.Q.; Liu, Y.X.; Wu, W.J.; Shen, Y.B.; Zhang, L.; Li, C.; Liu, A.P.; Shen, L.; Hu, B.; et al. Synthesis and antidiabetic activity of selenium nanoparticles in the presence of polysaccharides from Catathelasma ventricosum. *Int. J. Biol. Macromol.* **2018**, *114*, 632–639. [CrossRef]

21. TableYe, X.G.; Chen, Z.Z.; Zhang, Y.Y.; Mu, J.J.; Chen, L.Y.; Li, B.; Lin, X.R. Construction, characterization, and bioactive evaluation of nano-selenium stabilized by green tea nano-aggregates. *LWT-Food Sci. Technol.* **2020**, *129*, 109475.
22. Song, X.; Chen, Y.; Sun, H.; Liu, X.; Leng, X. Physicochemical stability and functional properties of selenium nanoparticles stabilized by chitosan, carrageenan, and gum Arabic. *Carbohyd. Polym.* **2021**, *255*, 117379. [CrossRef] [PubMed]
23. Gao, F.; Zhao, J.; Liu, P.; Ji, D.S.; Zhang, L.T.; Zhang, M.X.; Li, Y.Q.; Xiao, Y.L. Preparation and in vitro evaluation of multi-target-directed selenium chondroitin sulfate nanoparticles in protecting against the Alzheimer's disease. *Int. J. Biol. Macromol.* **2020**, *142*, 265–276. [CrossRef]
24. Ding, L.; Huang, Y.; Cai, X.X.; Wang, S.Y. Impact of pH, Ionic Strength and Chitosan Charge Density on Chitosan/Casein Complexation and Phase Behavior. *Carbohyd. Polym.* **2019**, *208*, 133–141. [CrossRef]
25. Jiang, W.T.; Fu, Y.T.; Yang, F.; Yang, Y.F.; Liu, T.; Zheng, W.J.; Zeng, L.L.; Chen, T.F. Gracilaria lemaneiformis polysaccharide as integrin-targeting surface decorator of selenium nanoparticles to achieve enhanced anticancer efficacy. *ACS Appl. Mater. Inter.* **2014**, *6*, 13738–13748. [CrossRef]
26. Gao, X.; Li, X.F.; Mu, J.J.; Ho, C.T.; Su, J.Y.; Zhang, Y.T.; Lin, X.R.; Chen, Z.Z.; Li, B.; Xie, Y.Z. Preparation, Physicochemical Characterization, and Anti-Proliferation of Selenium Nanoparticles Stabilized by Polyporus Umbellatus Polysaccharide. *Int. J. Biol. Macromol.* **2020**, *152*, 605–615. [CrossRef] [PubMed]
27. Chen, W.; Yue, L.; Jiang, Q.; Liu, X.; Xia, W. Synthesis of varisized chitosan-selenium nanocomposites through heating treatment and evaluation of their antioxidant properties. *Int. J. Biol. Macromol.* **2018**, *114*, 751–758. [CrossRef] [PubMed]
28. Catarina Guedes, A.; Amaro, H.M.; Gião, M.S.; Xavier Malcata, F. Optimization of ABTS radical cation assay specifically for determination of antioxidant capacity of intracellular extracts of microalgae and cyanobacteria. *Food Chem.* **2013**, *13*, 638–643. [CrossRef]

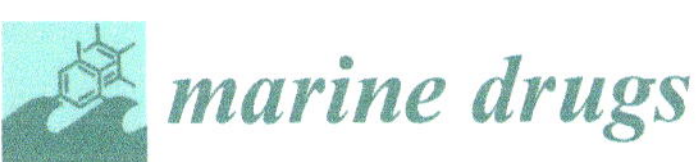

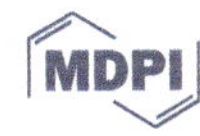

Review

Anti-Inflammatory Effects of Compounds from Echinoderms

Hardik Ghelani, Md Khursheed, Thomas Edward Adrian and Reem Kais Jan *

College of Medicine, Mohammed Bin Rashid University of Medicine and Health Sciences,
Dubai P.O. Box 505055, United Arab Emirates
* Correspondence: reem.jan@mbru.ac.ae; Tel.: +971-4-383-8733

Abstract: Chronic inflammation can extensively burden a healthcare system. Several synthetic anti-inflammatory drugs are currently available in clinical practice, but each has its own side effect profile. The planet is gifted with vast and diverse oceans, which provide a treasure of bioactive compounds, the chemical structures of which may provide valuable pharmaceutical agents. Marine organisms contain a variety of bioactive compounds, some of which have anti-inflammatory activity and have received considerable attention from the scientific community for the development of anti-inflammatory drugs. This review describes such bioactive compounds, as well as crude extracts (published during 2010–2022) from echinoderms: namely, sea cucumbers, sea urchins, and starfish. Moreover, we also include their chemical structures, evaluation models, and anti-inflammatory activities, including the molecular mechanism(s) of these compounds. This paper also highlights the potential applications of those marine-derived compounds in the pharmaceutical industry to develop leads for the clinical pipeline. In conclusion, this review can serve as a well-documented reference for the research progress on the development of potential anti-inflammatory drugs from echinoderms against various chronic inflammatory conditions.

Keywords: anti-inflammatory activity; inflammatory pathways; marine drugs; echinoderm; sea cucumber; sea urchin; starfish

Citation: Ghelani, H.; Khursheed, M.; Adrian, T.E.; Jan, R.K. Anti-Inflammatory Effects of Compounds from Echinoderms. *Mar. Drugs* **2022**, *20*, 693. https://doi.org/10.3390/md20110693

Academic Editors: Donatella Degl'Innocenti and Marzia Vasarri

Received: 27 September 2022
Accepted: 31 October 2022
Published: 3 November 2022

Publisher's Note: MDPI stays neutral with regard to jurisdictional claims in published maps and institutional affiliations.

1. Introduction

Inflammation is an innate immune response to a variety of stimuli, such as infections and tissue injury. The onset of inflammation is characterized by the secretion of several types of chemokines, including cytokines and chemoattractants, which draw leukocytes to the site of injury or infection through the process of extravasation. The immune function of inflammation is mediated by several classes of soluble antimicrobial peptides, including defensins, cathelicidins, marginins, and C-reactive proteins (CRP), and immune cells, including neutrophils, macrophages, natural killer cells, and dendritic cells. All these components of inflammation combine and stimulate opsonization and phagocytosis to clear infections. Phagocytosis and opsonization are induced by several classes of reactive oxygen species (ROS) or reactive nitrogen species induced in neutrophils by the activation of specific signaling pathways [1–3]. The process of acute inflammation is necessary to fight infection and tissue injury. However, there are several physiological conditions in which the process of inflammation is persistently stimulated, leading to chronic disease [4,5]. Immune-mediated inflammatory diseases are diverse and manifest in several conditions, such as asthma, rheumatoid arthritis, ulcerative colitis, and Crohn's disease [6,7].

1.1. Inflammatory Pathways and Models

Multiple inflammatory pathways play a role in innate immunity and activate adaptive immunity to combat the cause of inflammation. These pathways are initiated by several classes of receptors present on leukocytes known as pattern recognition receptors. Common examples of such receptors are (1) the toll-like receptor family (TLR), (2) C-type lectin receptors, (3) retinoic acid-inducible gene-I-like receptors, and (4) nucleotide-binding and oligomerization domain (NOD)-like receptors (NLR) [8,9]. The activation of immune cells such as macrophages, neutrophils, and other immune cells leads to the secretion of cytokines, which sustain the inflammatory response. These cytokines bind to the immune cells and activate their function. The common cytokine receptor families are the: (1) immunoglobulin superfamily, (2) class I cytokine receptor family, (3) class II cytokine receptor family, (4) tissue necrosis factor (TNF) receptor superfamily, and (5) chemokine receptor family. Ligand binding on the pattern recognition receptors or cytokine receptors activates several signaling pathways, which ultimately induces the transcription of several inflammation regulatory genes. There are four broad categories of signaling pathways activated during the inflammation process: (1) the mitogen-activated protein kinase (MAPK) pathway, (2) phosphoinositide 3-kinase signaling pathway, (3) Janus kinase (JAK) signal transducer and activator of transcription (STAT), and (4) I kappa B kinase (IκB)/nuclear factor kappa B (NF-κB) signaling pathways [10,11].

The sustained activation of these signaling pathways underlies the cause of several inflammatory diseases. For instance, the NF-kB signaling pathway is a classic pathway in the regulation of inflammation. The activation of NF-kB via IκBα increases the expression of various downstream inflammatory mediators, such as proinflammatory cytokines (interleukin 1β (IL-1β), IL-6, and TNFα); key proinflammatory enzymes, including inducible nitric oxide synthase (iNOS) and cyclooxygenase-2 (COX-2); and their derivatives nitric oxide (NO) and prostaglandin E2 (PGE2) [12,13]. Multiple experimental models are available to study the activation of inflammatory signaling and transcription for various inflammatory diseases. These experimental models are also widely used to evaluate potential anti-inflammatory compounds and to understand the mechanism(s) of their therapeutic effects. Various experimental models have been designed and implemented to study the preliminary efficacy of anti-inflammatory compounds. For example, carrageenan-induced paw edema in mouse [14] and 12-O-tetradecanoylphorbol-13-acetate (TPA) mouse ear inflammation models [15]. Other specific experimental models are also available and have been used for the assessment of chronic inflammatory diseases, including the dextran sodium sulfate (DSS)-induced colitis model [16], which has been widely used to screen the anti-inflammatory effects of marine drugs. For example, this model was recently used to study the anti-inflammatory effects of polysaccharides isolated from the mussel *Mytilus couscous* [17]. Another well-known model to study cytokine-mediated inflammatory signaling pathways is TNFα-induced intestinal inflammation in colon cancer cell lines [18]. For example, krill oil was screened for its anti-inflammatory effects by using this model in HT-29 and Caco-2 cells [19]. The free fatty acid (FFA)-mediated activation of inflammatory signaling in hepatocytes is a well-known model for nonalcoholic steatohepatitis [20]. Jiena et al. [21] demonstrated that fucoxanthin, a popular marine-derived compound, attenuated FFA-induced inflammation via the AMP-activated protein kinase/nuclear factor erythroid 2–related factor 2/TLR4 signaling pathway in normal human Chang liver cells.

1.2. Marine-Derived Anti-Inflammatory Drugs

Chronic inflammatory conditions pose a major burden on our healthcare system, despite the availability of several synthetic compounds used for the management of these conditions. Over the past decade, the research and development of model systems and evaluation of the efficacy of various compounds have led to the identification of several anti-inflammatory compounds from natural origins [22–24]. Marine sources produce a vastly diverse range of bioactive compounds, several of which possess anti-inflammatory potential. Indeed, anti-inflammatory compounds have been derived from marine microorganisms such as seaweeds, corals, and algae [25]. These fall into several classes of bioactive compounds with therapeutic potential for several chronic inflammatory conditions. For example, marine alkaloids from a diverse range of marine organisms have been evaluated for their potential anti-inflammatory activity [26]. Another class of marine compounds act as inhibitors of NF-κB, a mediator that is activated in the inflammation process [27]. Pigments from various marine organisms have been shown to have anti-inflammatory activity and can be used in the management of chronic inflammation [28,29]. For instance, Echinochrome A (EchA, a pigment isolated from sea urchin), briaviodiol A (a cembranoid from a soft coral), and cucumarioside A2 (a triterpene glycoside from sea cucumbers) have been shown to suppress inflammation via the reprogramming of macrophages from M1 to M2 [30]. Seaweeds are classically used as food supplements and have great potential as a source of anti-inflammatory compounds [31,32]. Overall, because of the diversity of classes of bioactive compounds from marine sources with potential applications as anti-inflammatory agents, there is a need to comprehensively catalogue these resources.

Over the past few decades, attempts have been made to isolate and purify biologically active compounds with potent anti-inflammatory activity from different marine sources. However, very few compounds have been selected for clinical trials and even fewer have reached the market. Despite this low success rate, the hunt for new anti-inflammatory compounds from the diverse marine environment continues. Recently, Li et al. reviewed the anti-inflammatory metabolites from marine organisms such as sponges and corals but did not include larger organisms such as sea cucumbers, sea urchins, and starfish [25]. In this review article, we describe promising anti-inflammatory compounds and crude extracts isolated from echinoderms such as sea cucumbers, sea urchins, and starfish and review their potential molecular mechanisms of action in an effort to shed light on the current state of the research on anti-inflammatory compounds from echinoderms.

2. Methods

During the period between December 2021 and June 2022, separate database searches were conducted on PubMed, Scopus, Web of Science, American Chemical Society (ACS), MDPI, Elsevier, and SpringerLink using various relevant keywords and combinations of keywords, such as "Sea cucumber" + "Anti inflammatory", "Sea urchin" + "Anti inflammatory", and "Starfish" + "Anti inflammatory". The inclusion criteria encompassed only original research articles published in the English language between 2010 and 2022. Editorials, review articles, and any duplicated publications were excluded. As a final step in the screening process, we included only studies thoroughly aligned with the theme of this review. For easier readership and referencing, the review is divided into sections according to the three types of echinoderms and subsections describing the anti-inflammatory activities of the various compounds that originate from them.

3. Anti-Inflammatory Compounds from Sea Cucumbers

Sea cucumbers belong to the class of Holothuroidea and the phylum of Echinodermata. They are globally found in deep seas in benthic areas. Sea cucumbers are harvested for food and are widely consumed in China, Korea, Japan, Malaysia, Indonesia, and Russia. There are approximately 1500 species of sea cucumbers, of which approximately 100 are known for human consumption [33]. Sea cucumbers have received particular attention for their potential therapeutic benefits owing to the availability of a variety of active compounds originating from them that possess medicinal properties [33]. Sea cucumbers are a rich source of bioactive polysaccharides, terpenoids, peptides, lipids, and fatty acids. As a result, sea cucumbers are used as a tonic food and folk medicine in Eastern Asia to cure numerous ailments. East Asian consumers consider sea cucumbers as one of the most luxurious and nutritious foods and use them as a traditional remedy for hypertension, rheumatism, asthma, cuts and burns, joint pain, back pain, wound injuries, kidney problems, reproductive disorders, constipation, and cancer [34,35]. The bioactive substances derived from various species of sea cucumbers and their proposed mechanisms of anti-inflammatory activity are described in the below sections and are summarized in Table 1.

3.1. Anti-Inflammatory Activity of Polysaccharides from Sea Cucumbers

Several studies have emphasized the valuable anti-inflammatory effects of polysaccharides obtained from sea cucumbers. Sulphated fucan, fucoidan, and fucosylated chondroitin sulfate (FCS) are major polysaccharides isolated from several species of sea cucumbers, such as *Thelenota ananas, Stichopus variegatus, Holothuria nobilis, Ypsilothuria bitentaculata, Cucumaria frondosa, Stichopus (Apostichopus) japonicus, Stichopus choloronotus,* and *Isostichopus badionotus*. These polysaccharides have shown potent anti-inflammatory activity in various cellular, as well as animal, models of chronic inflammation. The chronic administration of fucoidan (Figure 1: (**1**)) derived from *Isostichopus badionotus* reduced the hepatic expression and serum concentrations of inflammatory cytokines and other inflammatory markers (TNFα, IL-1β, IL-6, IL-10, macrophage inflammatory protein 1 (MIP-1), and CRP) in diet-induced obese mice. The anti-inflammatory response of fucoidan was achieved by the inactivation of JNK and IκB/NF-κB pathways in hepatocytes [36]. Moreover, fucoidan isolated from *Apostichopus japonicus* reduced the expression of TNFα, IL-1β, and IL-6 by inactivating the MAPK/ NF-κB pathway in the lipopolysaccharide (LPS)-challenged liver injury mouse model [37]. Fucoidan, isolated from *Acaudina molpadioides*, alleviated renal fibrosis and inflammation by decreasing the expression of transforming growth factor β1 (TGFβ1), plasminogen activator inhibitor 1, and phosphorylated Smad3 in diabetic mice [38]. Fucoidans derived from *Thelenota ananas* prevented ethanol-induced gastric ulceration by downregulating the expression of proinflammatory cytokines and related transcription factors (TNFα, IL-6, and NF-κB) [39]. Fucoidan oligosaccharides isolated from *Pearsonothuria graeffei* and *Isostichopus Badionotus* alleviated high-fat diet (HFD)-induced low-grade inflammation by lowering the serum TNFα and LPS levels in mice [40]. The primary glycosaminoglycan FCS was purified from *Isostichopus badionotus* and screened in vivo and in vitro for anti-inflammatory activity. FCS downregulated the NF-kB gene expression and thereby suppressed the expression of downstream genes such as COX-2, iNOS, and TNFα and attenuated the inflammation and tissue damage caused by TPA in a mouse ear inflammation model [15]. Furthermore, FCS (Figure 1: (**2**)) isolated from edible sea cucumbers *Apostichopus japonicus, Stichopus chloronotus, Cucumaria djakonovi,* and *Acaudina molpadioidea* reduced carrageenan-induced paw edema in a mouse model [14,41]. More recently, Zhu et al. [42] demonstrated that the sulfated fucan/FCS-dominated polysaccharide fraction from low-edible-value sea cucumber species reduced the levels of proinflammatory cytokines (such as TNFα and IL-6) of HFD and streptozotocin (STZ)-induced type 2 diabetic rats, indicating a decreased inflammatory response. FCS, isolated from *Lymantria grisea*, inhibited neutrophil recruitment and TNFα production in thioglycollate-induced peritonitis and LPS-induced lung inflammation mouse models [43]. Interestingly, the heteroglycan (sulphated polysaccharide) fractions derived from the cartilage of *Curcumaria frondosa* (at concentrations of 0.1–100 µg/mL) increased the oxidative stress and decreased cell viability, as evidenced by the induced levels of TNFα, IL-6, and IL-10 in THP-1 macrophages [44].

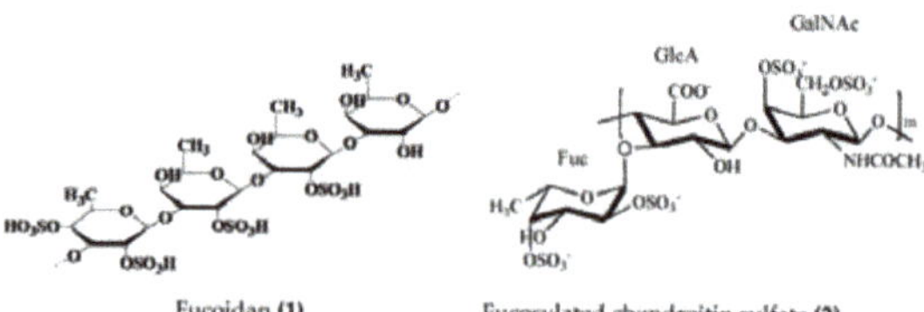

Figure 1. Structures of anti-inflammatory polysaccharides derived from sea cucumbers (structure (**1**) re-used with permission from reference [36], Elsevier, 2016; structure (**2**) re-used with permission from reference [14], Elsevier, 2018).

3.2. Anti-Inflammatory Activity of Triterpenoid Glycosides from Sea Cucumbers

Triterpenoid glycosides are broadly distributed in plants, animals, and marine organisms such as holothurians and sponges. Triterpenoid glycosides play a crucial role in chemical defenses and possess a variety of pharmacological activities. Approximately 300 triterpenoid glycosides have been identified and categorized from sea cucumbers. Relatively few anti-inflammatory triterpenoid glycosides from sea cucumbers are documented in the literature. Triterpenoid glycosides isolated from the Egyptian sea cucumber *Holothuria thomasi* significantly decreased the serum levels of TNFα and IL-6, as well as glucose, adiponectin, liver malondialdehyde, and α-amylase activity, in STZ-induced diabetic rats [45]. Similarly, a liposomal preparation of triterpenoid glycoside (Holothurin A (Figure 2: (3)) and Echinoside A (Figure 2: (4)) isolated from *Pearsonothuria graeffei* reduced the inflammation by inhibiting the release of proinflammatory cytokines and infiltration of macrophages in the adipose tissue of HFD-fed obese mice. Moreover, this liposomal triterpenoid glycoside preparation significantly reduced the PGE2 levels in adipose tissue by modulating the p-ERK/cPLA2/COX-1 pathway [46]. Moreover, holothurin A and echinoside A also attenuated inflammation by downregulating the expression of proinflammatory cytokines in vascular and peritoneal macrophages of ApoE$^{-/-}$ mice [47].

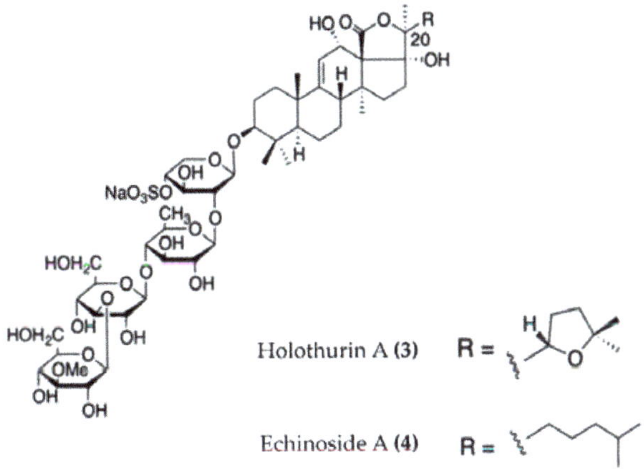

Figure 2. Structures of anti-inflammatory triterpenoid glycosides derived from sea cucumbers (structures (3) and (4) re-used from reference [47]).

3.3. Anti-Inflammatory Activity of Peptides from Sea Cucumbers

Marine bioactive peptides are short amino acid sequences, generally 2–20 amino acids in length, that are biologically inactive within their respective precursor proteins until released by enzymic hydrolysis. Hydrolysates derived from marine sources have attracted considerable interest within the scientific community due to their diverse biological activities and applications in clinical treatment [48]. Protein constitutes more than 70% of the sea cucumber body and is an effective source of food-borne bioactive peptides. The enzymatic hydrolysates extracted from *Apostichopus japonicus* and *Acaudina leucoprocta* exhibited potent anti-inflammatory activity in a diet-induced hyperuricemic renal inflammation mouse model. The hydrolysates downregulated the proinflammatory cytokines (TNFα, IL-1β, and IL-6) and upregulated the anti-inflammatory cytokines TGFβ and IL-10 by modification of the TLR4/myeloid differentiation primary response 88(MyD88)/NF-κB signaling pathway. The amino acid sequences of peptides found in hydrolysates of *Apostichopus japonicus* and *Acaudina leucoprocta* have been characterized by MALDI-TOF/TOF-MS. GPS-GRP (Gly-Pro-Ser-Gly-Arg-Pro) and GPAGPR (Gly-Pro-Ala-Gly-Pro-Arg) were identified as the two major anti-inflammatory peptides from *Apostichopus japonicus*, while PQGETGA (Pro-Gln-Gly-Glu-Thr-Gly-Ala) and GFDGPEGPR (Gly-Phe-Asp-Gly-Pro-Glu-Gly-Pro-Arg) were detected with the highest abundance in *Acaudina leucoprocta* [49]. Zhang et al. [50] also reported two peptides (Gly-Lys (Figure 3: (5)) and Ala-Pro-Arg (Figure 3: (6))) from *Apostichopus japonicus* that showed marked anti-inflammatory activity in a CuSO4-induced zebrafish inflammation model. Moreover, a molecular docking analysis revealed that both peptides have a high affinity to bind and inhibit angiotensin-I converting enzyme (ACE-1), a therapeutic target in the treatment of inflammatory conditions [50]. Low molecular weight sea cucumber peptides (SCP, rich in aspartic acid, glycine, proline, and glutamic acid) isolated from *Stichopus japonicus*, a sea cucumber widely distributed along the coasts of China and Japan, displayed potent anti-inflammatory activity in LPS-stimulated RAW264.7 murine macrophages by the inhibition of NF-κB and activation of MAPK in macrophages [51]. Moreover, the anti-inflammatory activity of another SCP (rich in glycine, glutamic acid, and proline) isolated from *Stichopus japonicus* was also demonstrated in vivo, where it significantly inhibited serum proinflammatory cytokines and downregulated the overexpression of TLR4 and NF-κB in gastrocnemius muscles of rats [52]. The hydrolysate bioactive fraction, isolated from the sea cucumber species *Holothuria forskali*, reduced the vascular cell adhesion molecule (VCAM)-1 and IL-6 expression levels in endothelial cells and intercellular adhesion molecule (ICAM)-1 expression in subcutaneous adipose tissue and was shown to inhibit ACE-1 enzyme activity in an in vitro assay [53]. Recently, Jo et al. [54] isolated sea cucumber extracellular matrices (body wall collagen) from *Stichopus japonicus*, which possessed potent anti-inflammatory activity in a TNFα and IL-1β-induced osteoarthritis in vitro model. Moreover, the major yolk protein isolated from *Stichopus japonicus* attenuated experimental DSS-induced colitis by preventing tissue damage, promoting the expression of anti-inflammatory cytokines, and increasing the levels of short-chain fatty acids [55]. Similarly, sea cucumber (*Stichopus japonicus*) enzymatic hydrolysates have been shown to alleviate the inflammatory response via the downregulation of RANKL (receptor activator of NF-kB) and thereby inhibiting the NF-kB pathway in ovariectomized rats [56].

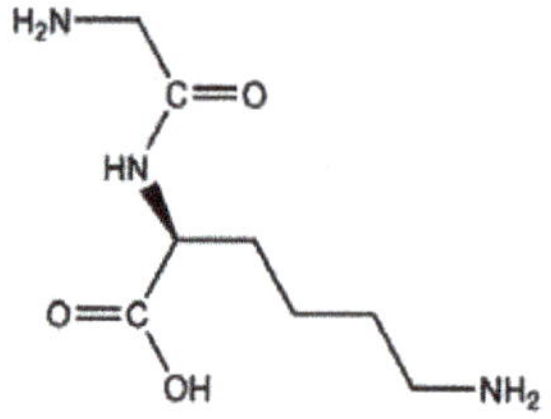

Gly-Lys (**5**) 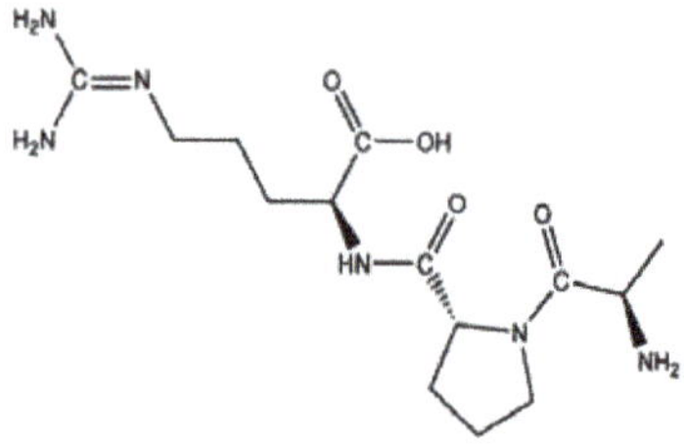   Ala-Pro-Arg (**6**)

Figure 3. Structures of anti-inflammatory peptides derived from sea cucumbers (structures (**5**) and (**6**) re-used with permission from reference [50], John Wiley and Sons, 2021).

3.4. Anti-Inflammatory Activity of Lipids and Fatty Acids from Sea Cucumbers

Lipids are best known for their integral role in biological membranes and as signaling molecules in the cytoplasm. Sea cucumbers are rich sources of lipids, phospholipids, and various fatty acids that exert a wide variety of biological activities. Eicosapentaenoic acid (EPA), isolated from *Cucumaria frondosa*, has a potent anti-obesity effect and modulates the peroxisome proliferator activated receptor γ (PPARγ) signaling in the inflammatory condition of insulin resistance, as well as type 2 diabetes [57,58]. Phosphatidylcholine (EPA-PC) (Figure 4: (**7**)) and phosphatidylethanolamine (EPA-PE) (Figure 4: (**8**)) from *Cucumaria frondosa* improve chronic inflammation and alter the interaction between macrophages and adipocytes [59,60]. Moreover, EPA-PC and EPA-PE diminish chronic inflammation by promoting the M2-dominant polarization of macrophages in white adipose tissue, as observed in 3T3L1 and RAW264.7 transwell coculture. EPA-PC and EPA-PE also inhibit the transactivation of NF-κB in RAW264.7 macrophages and upregulate PPARγ expression in 3T3-L1 adipocytes in the coculture, indicating that they may alleviate adipose tissue inflammation [59,60]. Both EPA-PC and EPA-PE reduced the serum TNFα, IL-6, and monocyte chemoattractant protein (MCP), increased the serum heme oxygenase-1 (HO-1) levels (one of the most abundant enzymes involved in oxidative stress and with anti-inflammatory properties), and attenuated macrophage infiltration in the liver and adipose tissue of high-fat high-sucrose diet-induced inflammation in mice [61]. Moreover, EPA-PC inhibited amyloid β-protein-induced neurotoxicity by alleviating the NLR family pyrin domain-containing 3 (NLRP3) inflammasome in an Alzheimer's disease rat model [62]. EPA phospholipids derived from *Cucumaria frondosa* mitigated obesity-induced inflammation by reducing TNFα and IL-6 in the serum of diet-induced obese mice [63]. A fatty acid-rich fraction (n-hexane phase) of *Apostichopus japonicus* has shown several immunomodulatory activities in an ovalbumin-induced allergic airway inflammation mouse model and in splenocytes [64]. This fraction reduced eosinophil infiltration and goblet cell hyperplasia and attenuated IL-4, IL-5, IL-13, and IL-17 in the spleen and bronchoalveolar lavage fluid of mice. It also increased the expression of anti-inflammatory cytokines (TGFβ and IL-10) in bronchoalveolar lavage fluid and a splenocyte culture medium [64]. Frondanol™ is a nutraceutical lipid extract (rich in 12-methyltetradecanoic acid (Figure 4: (**9**)) and myristoleic acid (Figure 4: (**10**))) of the intestines of the edible Atlantic sea cucumber *Cucumaria frondosa*. Frondanol has potent anti-inflammatory activity and has been shown to attenuate inflammation in an adjuvant arthritis rat model, as well as an ear edema mouse model [65]. It also potently inhibits lipoxygenase (LOX) pathways, reducing leukotriene production in human polymorphonuclear cells [65]. More recently, Subramanya et al. [16] demonstrated that chronic treatment with Frondanol decreased inflammation in a DSS-induced colitis mouse model. Frondanol markedly reduced proinflammatory cytokine mRNA expression in colon tissue and cytokine levels in the circulation, while inhibiting production of the proinflammatory mediator leukotriene B4 (LTB4) [16]. Sphingolipids isolated from *Cucumaria frondosa* decrease the serum proinflammatory cytokines, as well as mRNA expression in the adipose tissue of obese mice by the inhibition of phosphorylated JNK, IκB, and NF-κB nuclear translocation [66]. Furthermore, these sphingolipids attenuated renal fibrosis and inflammation via the inactivation of TGFβ/Smad signaling pathway in STZ-HFD-fed type 2 diabetic mice [67]. The cerebrosides and glucosylceramides extracted from *Cucumaria frondosa* reduced the expression of proinflammatory cytokines and thereby improved the insulin sensitivity in adipose tissues of high-fructose diet-fed rats [68].

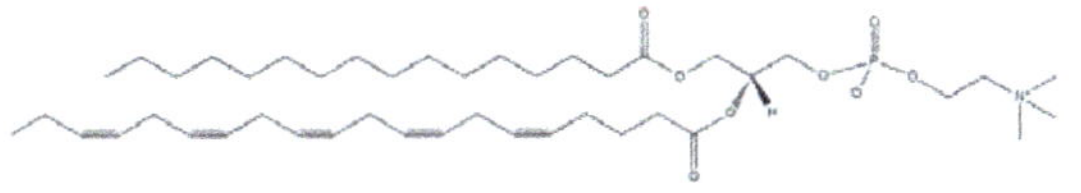

Eicosapentaenoic acid-phosphatidylcholine (**7**)

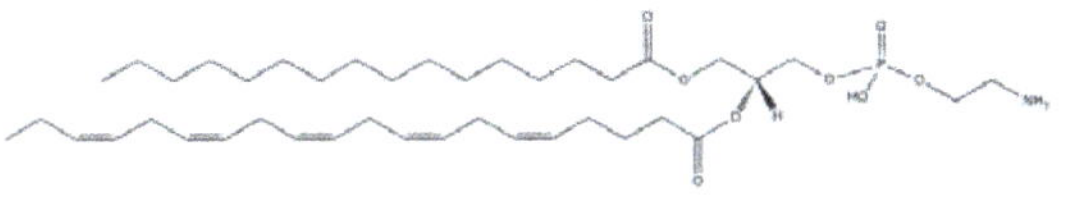

Eicosapentaenoic acid-phosphatidylethanolamine (**8**)

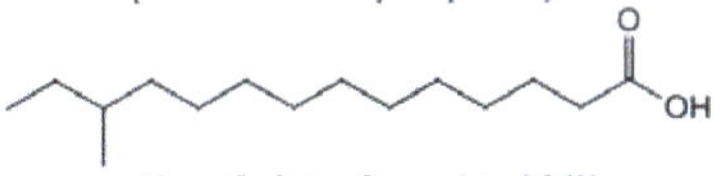

12-methyltetradecanoic acid (**9**)

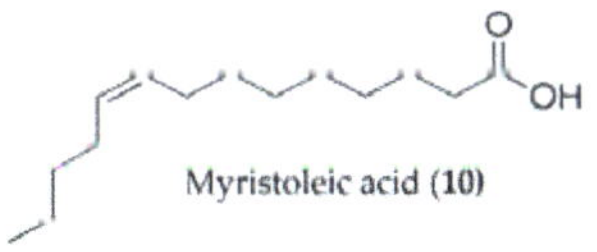

Myristoleic acid (**10**)

Figure 4. Structures of anti-inflammatory fatty acid derivatives derived from sea cucumbers (structures (**7**) and (**8**) re-used from reference [59]).

3.5. Anti-Inflammatory Activity of Miscellaneous Crude Extracts of Sea Cucumbers

Several aqueous and organic solvent-extracted fractions of various sea cucumber species have shown marked anti-inflammatory activity in various in vivo and in vitro models. Frondanol A5 (isopropyl alcohol/water extract of epithelium from the sea cucumber *Cucumaria frondosa*) decreased the production of inflammatory cytokines, such as IL-1α, IL-1β, IL-2, IL-4, IL-6, IL-10, IL-12, IL-17A, interferon gamma (IFNγ), and TNFα, in an

APC$^{\text{Min}/+}$ mouse model [69]. Additionally, Frondanol A5 also suppressed the mRNA expression of inflammatory markers (5-LOX and 5-lipoxygenase activating protein (FLAP)) and an angiogenesis marker in intestinal tumors [69]. An ethyl-acetate fraction (which contains mostly phenolic compounds) of the sea cucumber *Holothuria scabra* attenuates inflammation in vitro by inhibiting the production of NO and proinflammatory cytokines via the NF-κB and JNK pathways [70]. The ethyl-acetate fraction from another sea cucumber species, *Stichopus japonicus*, markedly reduced inflammation by inhibiting the production of NO and PGE2 (via downregulating the iNOS and COX-2 gene expression). Moreover, the fraction was shown to suppress the transcription of proinflammatory cytokines in LPS-stimulated murine macrophages through suppression of the phosphorylation of MAPK [71]. An aqueous fraction of *Stichopus japonicus* reduced production of the proinflammatory cytokines IL-6, and TNFα in LPS-stimulated macrophages and inhibited antigen-induced mast cell degranulation and IL-4 mRNA expression in antigen-stimulated RBL-2H3 rat basophil [72]. An aqueous extract of the sea cucumber *Stichopus chloronotus* demonstrated both anti-inflammatory and antioxidative activities by upregulating cartilage-specific markers such as collagen type II, aggrecan core protein, and SRY-Box transcription factor 9 (sox-9) expression and downregulating collagen type 1, IL-1, IL-6, IL-8, matrix metalloproteinases (MMP)-1, MMP-3, MMP-13, COX-2, iNOS, and protease-activated receptor 2 (PAR-2) expression [73]. An aqueous extract of *Holothuria polii* attenuated the levels of the inflammatory markers IL-6, NO, and MMP-9 in mouse mammary epithelial SCp2 cells and the levels of IL-1β produced in THP-1 human monocytes [74]. A methanol body wall extract of the sea cucumber *Holothuria atra* downregulated the proinflammatory cytokines TNFα, and IL-1β in a cecal ligation and puncture rat model [75]. The body wall preparation of *Isostichopus badionotus* suppressed the expression of proinflammatory genes, including TNFα, iNOS, COX-2, NF-κB, and IL-6, in a mouse ear inflammation model [76]. Ethanol extracts obtained from four species of sea cucumbers belonging to the family Holothuriidae (namely, Holothuriidae ni1, Holothuriidae ni2, Holothuriidae ni3, and Holothuriidae ni4) showed potent antioxidant and COX-2 inhibitory activities in vitro [77].

Table 1. Anti-inflammatory bioactive compounds and extracts derived from sea cucumbers.

Species	Bioactive Compounds/Extracts	Model	Mechanism of Anti-Inflammatory Activity	Ref.
Apostichopus japonicus and *Stichopus chloronotus*	Fucosylated chondroitin sulfate	Carrageenan-induced paw edema in rats	Reduces neutrophil migration, decreases paw edema	[14]
Isostichopus badionotus	Fucosylated chondroitin sulfate	TPA-induced ear inflammation in mice	Suppresses TPA-mediated up-regulation of TNFα, IL-6, NF-kB, iNOS, IL-10, IL-11, COX-2 and STAT3 genes in mouse ear tissue	[15]
Isostichopus badionotus	Fucoidan	High-fat high-sucrose diet induced obese mouse model	Regulates serum inflammatory cytokines (TNFα, CRP, MIP-1, IL-1β, IL-6, and IL-10) and their mRNA expression, inactivates JNK and IκB/NF-κB pathways	[36]
Holothuria albiventer and *Cucumaria frondosa*	Sulfated fucan /FCS	HFD and STZ-induced type 2 diabetes mellitus model	Suppresses production of proinflammatory cytokines (TNFα and IL-6)	[42]
Holothuria thomasi	Triterpenoid Glycoside	STZ-induced diabetic rats	Decreases serum IL-6, TNFα levels	[45]
Pearsonothuria graeffei	Triterpenoid glycoside liposomes	HFD-fed obese mice	Reduces TNFα, IL-1β, and IL-6 and infiltration of macrophages in obese mice via p-ERK/cPLA2/COX-1 pathway and reduces the PGE2 levels	[46]

Table 1. *Cont.*

Species	Bioactive Compounds/Extracts	Model	Mechanism of Anti-Inflammatory Activity	Ref.
Apostichopus japonicus and *Acaudina leucoprocta*	Small peptides (GPSGRP, GPAGPR, PQGETGA, GFDGPEGPR)	Diet-induced renal inflammation in mice	Downregulates the transcription of proinflammatory cytokines, upregulates anti-inflammatory cytokines, and inhibits TLR4/MyD88/NF-κB signaling pathway	[49]
Apostichopus japonicus	Peptide (GL, APA)	CuSO4-induced neuromast damage in zebrafish model	Suppresses leukocyte migration, ACE enzyme inhibition	[50]
Stichopus japonicus	Peptides	LPS-stimulated RAW264.7 macrophages	Suppresses NO production and mRNA expression of inflammatory mediators (iNOS, TNFα, IL-1β and IL-6) through inhibition of NF-κB and MAPK signaling pathways	[51]
Stichopus japonicus	Peptides	Endurance swimming rat model	Reduces inflammation by suppression of TLR4 expression and NF-κB activation in gastrocnemius muscle tissue of rat	[52]
Holothuria forskali and *Parastichopus tremulus*	Hydrolysate	In vitro assay of ACE-1, human umbilical endothelial and Caco-2 cells co-culture	Reduces VCAM-1, ICAM-1 and IL-6 expression in endothelial cells, inhibits ACE-1	[53]
Stichopus japonicus	Collagen	Synoviocytes osteoarthritis model	Suppresses mRNA expression of inflammatory cytokines in synoviocytes	[54]
Stichopus japonicus	Major yolk protein from body wall	DSS-induced colitis in mice	Prevents tissue damage, promotes IL-4 and IL-10, increases short-chain fatty acids	[55]
Apostichopus japonicus	Body wall hydrolysate	Ovariectomized-induced osteoporosis in rat	Blocks NF-kB activation by downregulating RANKL, suppresses proinflammatory cytokines	[56]
Cucumaria frondosa	Eicosapentaenoic acids	LPS-stimulated RAW264.7 macrophages and 3T3-L1 adipocytes, high-fat high-sucrose diet-induced inflammatory mouse model	Reduces elevated levels of serum TNFα, IL-6 and MCP-1, attenuates macrophage infiltration in the liver in mice, attenuates the phosphorylation of NF-κB in Raw264.7 macrophages and increased PPARγ expression in 3T3-L1 adipocytes	[60]
Cucumaria frondosa	Frondanol	DSS-induced colitis in mice	Reduces inflammation-associated changes in colon in mice, reduces proinflammatory cytokine content at the protein and mRNA level, reduces proinflammatory LTB4 levels	[16]
Apostichopus japonicus	Fatty acids	Allergic airway inflammation mouse model and in splenocytes	Reduces eosinophil infiltration and goblet cell hyperplasia, attenuates IL-4, IL-5, IL-13, IL-17 and increases level of anti-inflammatory cytokines TGFβ and IL-10	[64]
Cucumaria frondosa,	Sphingolipids	High-fat high-fructose diet-induced obese mice	Decreases serum proinflammatory cytokines IL-1β, IL-6 and TNFα, increases anti-inflammatory IL 10, via inhibition of phosphorylation of JNK and translocation of NF-κB	[66]
Cucumaria frondosa	Frondanol A5	APC$^{Min/+}$ mouse model	Attenuates circulating inflammatory cytokines and suppresses mRNA expression of inflammatory markers such as 5-LOX and FLAP	[69]
Holothuria scabra	Ethyl acetate Extract	LPS stimulated RAW264.7 macrophages	Inhibits proinflammatory cytokines mRNA and protein, suppresses NO production via inhibition of iNOS, down-regulates IκB/NF-κB and JNK expression in macrophages	[70]

Table 1. *Cont.*

Species	Bioactive Compounds/Extracts	Model	Mechanism of Anti-Inflammatory Activity	Ref.
Stichopus japonicus	Ethyl acetate fraction	LPS-stimulated RAW264.7 macrophages	Inhibits proinflammatory cytokines via suppression of the phosphorylation of MAPK, ERK and p38 MAPK signaling pathway	[71]
Stichopus japonicus	Aqueous Fraction	LPS-stimulated RAW264.7 macrophages and antigen-stimulated RBL-2H3 rat basophil.	Reduces proinflammatory cytokines IL-6 and TNFα, inhibits antigen-induced mast cell degranulation and IL-4 mRNA expression	[72]
Stichopus chloronotus	Aqueous Extract	Osteoarthritis-articular cartilage model	Upregulates cartilage specific markers, downregulates IL-1β, IL-6, IL-8, MMP-1, MMP-3, MMP-13, COX-2, iNOS and PAR-2 expression, increases glycosaminoglycans and reduces NO and PGE2 production	[73]
Holothuria polii	Aqueous Extract	TPA-activated THP-1 cells and endotoxin-induced mammary epithelial SCp2 cells	Decreases levels of inflammatory markers IL-6, NO and MMP-9 in the mouse mammary SCp2 cells, decreases the level of IL-1β in THP1 cells	[74]

4. Anti-Inflammatory Compounds from Sea Urchins

Sea urchins are seafloor-dwelling invertebrates belonging to the phylum Echinodermata that have high nutritional and medicinal properties. They are rich in vitamins, minerals, proteins, fatty acids, and polysaccharides and possess anticancer, anticoagulant/antithrombotic, antimicrobial, anti-inflammatory, and antioxidant properties. The extracts and hydrolysates of sea urchins contain various bioactive compounds, especially glycosides, pigments, sphingolipids, glycolipids, sulphate, and phospholipids [78]. The anti-inflammatory properties of various active components isolated from sea urchins are summarized in Table 2.

4.1. Anti-Inflammatory Activity of Pigments from Sea Urchins

Pigments isolated from the shells and spines of sea urchins are currently being widely studied for biological activity. EchA (Figure 5: (**11**)) is widely distributed in various species of sea urchins and has been screened for its biological activity [28]. The anti-inflammatory activity of EchA, isolated from different species, has been evaluated using various in vivo and in vitro models. EchA from *Scaphchinus mirabilis* attenuated macrophage activation and neutrophil infiltration in a bleomycin (BLM)-induced scleroderma mouse model. In the same study, EchA cotreatment markedly attenuated the BLM-induced increase in the TNFα and IFNγ levels [79]. The intravenous injection of EchA in DSS-induced colitis mice significantly reduced the disease activity index (DIA), improved the colon length, and reduced the accumulation of excessive immune cells (neutrophils and macrophages) within the epithelia and mesenchymal layers of damaged colons [80]. Furthermore, EchA treatment suppressed the in vitro activation of proinflammatory M1-type macrophages and increased the production of M2-type macrophages, which abate the inflammation and initiate tissue repair [80]. EchA also reduced the level of the inflammatory cells in the aqueous humor and reduced the levels of TNFα, NF-κB, and ROS in the aqueous humor in an endotoxin-induced uveitis rat model [81]. EchA attenuated the phosphorylation of p38, ERK1/2, and JNK and thereby effectively modulated the MPAK pathway in cardiac myoblast H9c2(2-1) cells and isolated rat cardiomyocytes [82]. Histochrome®(containing 1% EchA) is a commercially available antioxidant product permitted for subconjunctival and intravenous use in Russia. Histochrome®reduced the expression of MMPs, collagen degradation, and dermal mast cell recruitment in an ultraviolet B-exposed hairless mouse model [83]. EchA treatment also reduced the inflammatory response-induced mast cell infiltration, as well as the expression of proinflammatory cytokines such as IFNγ, IL-4, and IL-13, in an acute dermatitis mouse model [84]. Spinochromes A (Figure 5: (**12**)) and B (Figure 5: (**13**)) isolated from the shells and spine of *Evechinus chloroticus* have anti-inflammatory activity in the cotton pellet granuloma rat model of chronic inflammation [85,86]. Seven major spinochromes (including EchA and Spinochromes A–D) isolated from different sea urchin species reduced TNFα production in LPS-stimulated J774A.1 macrophages [87]. In addition, the pigment isolated from the spines and shells of sea urchin *Strongylocentrotus nudus* inhibited the production of NO, IL-6, TNFα, PGE2, and 6-keto-prostaglandin F (PGF)1α in LPS-stimulated RAW264.7 macrophages [88].

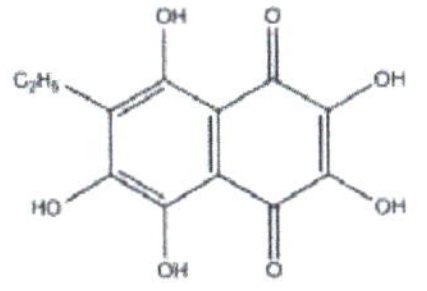

Echinochrome A (**11**) 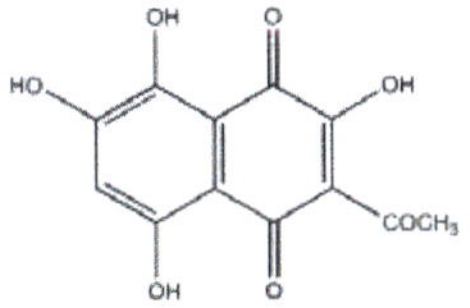   Spinochrome A (**12**)

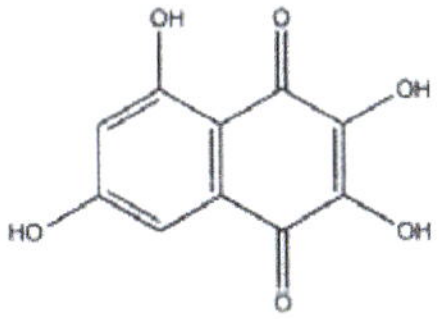

Spinochrome B (**13**)

Figure 5. Structures of anti-inflammatory pigments derived from sea urchins (structures (**11–13**) re-used with permission from reference [85], Elsevier, 2020).

4.2. Anti-Inflammatory Activity of Polysaccharides from Sea Urchins

Like other echinoderms, sea urchins are a rich source of bioactive polysaccharides, though few of them have been evaluated for anti-inflammatory activity. A high molecular weight sulphated polysaccharide from the eggs of the sea urchin *Paracentrotus lividus*, attenuated carrageenan-induced rat paw edema by inhibiting the production or antagonizing action of various chemical mediators such as serotonin, histamine, prostanoids, and leukotrienes [89]. In another study, gonadal polysaccharides isolated from a sea chestnut (*Anthocidaris crassispina*) reduced NO production in LPS-stimulated RAW264.7 macrophages [90].

4.3. Anti-Inflammatory Activity of Peptides from Sea Urchins

Centrocin 1, a peptide isolated from the green sea urchin *Strongylocentrotus droebachiensis* has shown potent anti-inflammatory activity. Centrocin 1 significantly reduced the expression of various inflammatory cytokines such as IL-12p40, IL-6, IL-1β, TNFα, and TLR 2 in *Propionibacterium acnes*-challenged monocytes [91], as well as in LPS-induced THP-1 monocytes [92]. Furthermore, Centrocin 1 attenuated proinflammatory cytokines IL-8, TNFα, and MMP-2 in the ear tissue of *Propionibacterium acnes* induced ear swelling inflammation rat model [91]. The anti-inflammatory effect of centrocin 1 could be due to the downregulation of TLR2, which further triggers an innate immune response and the inhibition of proinflammatory cytokines [91]. Interestingly, vanadium binding protein, isolated from the blood of fresh sea urchin *Halocynthia roretzi*, reduced NO production and cytokines (COX 2, IL 1β, IL 6, and TNFα) secretion by inactivating the NF-kB and MAPK pathways in LPS-stimulated RAW264.7 macrophages [93].

4.4. Anti-Inflammatory Activity of Miscellaneous Compounds from Sea Urchins

Several bioactive compounds such as lactones, polyketides, terpenes, and sulphonic acid derivatives have been isolated from various species of sea urchins and tested for anti-inflammatory activity. Salmachroman (Figure 6: (**14**)), a polyketide isolated from *Salmacis bicolor*, possesses dual-inhibition potential against proinflammatory enzymes COX-2 and 5-LOX [94]. The polyoxygenated furanocembranoids salmacembranes A (Figure 6: (**15**)) and B (Figure 6: (**16**)) from this species also exhibited significant COX-1, COX-2, and 5-LOX inhibitory activity [95]. Several compounds have been isolated from the long-spined sea urchin *Stomopneustes variolaris* and tested for their potential to inhibit the proinflammatory eicosanoid pathway enzymes COX-2 and 5-LOX [96].

A cembrane diterpenoid, characterized as 4-hydroxy-1-(16-methoxyprop-16-en-15-yl)-8-methyl-21,22 dioxatricyclo [11.3.1.15,8], and octadecane-3,19-dione (Figure 6: (**17**)) exhibited greater inhibitory potential against inflammatory agent 5-LOX than ibuprofen. The selectivity ratio of COX-1 to COX-2 inhibition was also higher for this compound in comparison to ibuprofen [96]. The macrocyclic lactone stomopneulactone D (Figure 7: (**18**)) inhibited the generation of iNOS and inhibited COX-2 and 5-LOX in LPS-stimulated macrophages [97]. Fourteen-membered macrocyclic pyrone derivatives named stomopnolides A (Figure 7: (**19**)) and B (Figure 7: (**20**)) also showed marked 5-LOX inhibitory activity [98]. A crude lipid extract from the body wall of the sea urchin *Strongylocentrotus droebachiensis* exhibited MAPK p38, COX-1, and COX-2 inhibitory activity in LPS-stimulated human mononuclear U-937 monocytes [99]. A sulfonic acid derivative, (Z)-4-methylundeca-1,9-diene-6-sulfonic acid (Figure 8: (**21**)), isolated from the cold-water sea urchin *Brisaster latifrons* suppressed the production of proinflammatory cytokines and inflammatory responses by inactivation of the JNK/p38 MAPK and NF-κB pathways in LPS-stimulated RAW264.7 macrophages [100]. Hp-S1 ganglioside (Figure 8: (**22**)), isolated from the sperm of sea urchin *Hemicentrotus pulcherrimus* or the ovary of *Diadema setosum*, decreased the expression of iNOS and COX-2, as well as the proinflammatory cytokines TNFα, IL-1β, and IL-6. These effects of Hp-S1 were mediated through downregulating the MyD88-mediated NF-κB and JNK/p38 MAPK signaling pathways in LPS-stimulated microglial cells [101]. Ovithiol A, isolated from sea urchin *Paracentrotus lividus* eggs, decreased the expression of adhesion molecules ICAM-1 and VCAM-1 and decreased the monocyte–human umbilical vein endothelial cells interaction [102]. Phenolics, flavonoids, and proteins extracted from viscera, spines, shells, and gonads from the sea urchin *Stomopneustes variolaris* exhibit antioxidant and anti-inflammatory activities in vitro [103].

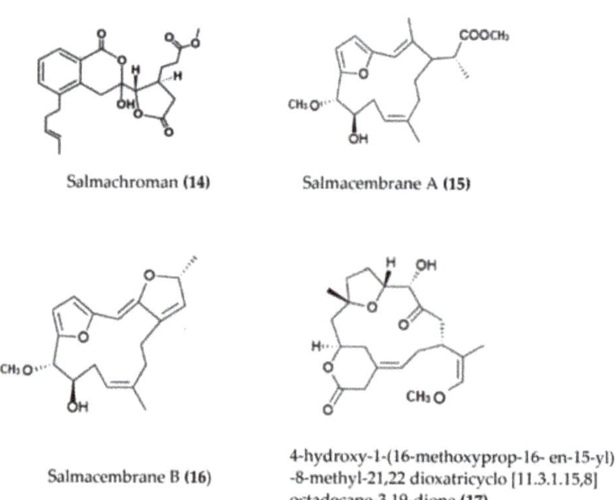

Figure 6. Structures of anti-inflammatory polyketides, furanocembranoids, and cembrane diterpenoids derived from sea urchins (structure (**14**) re-used with permission from [94], Taylor & Francis, 2021; structures (**15**) and (**16**) re-used with permission from reference [95], Springer Nature, 2020; structure (**17**) re-used with permission from reference [96], Springer Nature, 2020).

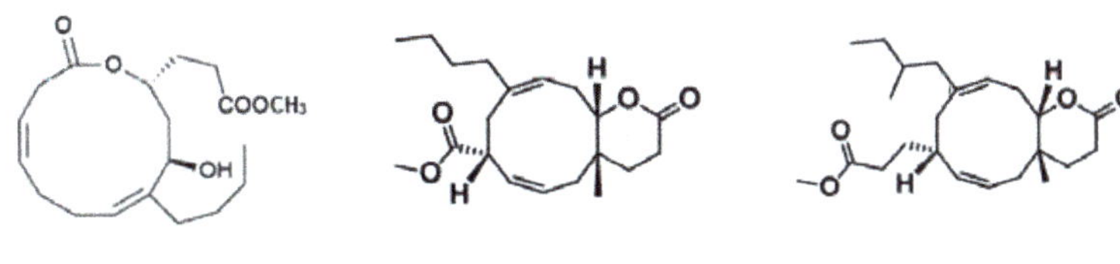

Stomopneulactone D (**18**)   Stomopnolide A (**19**)   Stomopnolide B (**20**)

Figure 7. Structures of anti-inflammatory macrocyclic compounds derived from sea urchins (structure (**18**) re-used with permission from reference [97], Elsevier, 2020; structures (**19**) and (**20**) re-used with permission from reference [98], Taylor & Francis, 2021).

(Z)-4-methylundeca-1,9-diene-6-sulfonic acid (**21**)   Hp-S1 ganglioside (**22**)

Figure 8. Structures of anti-inflammatory miscellaneous compounds from sea urchins (structure (**21**) re-used with permission from reference [100], Springer Nature, 2013; structure (**22**) re-used from reference [101]).

Table 2. Anti-inflammatory bioactive compounds derived from sea urchins.

Species	Bioactive Compounds/Extracts	Model	Mechanism of Anti-Inflammatory Activity	Ref.
Scaphechinus mirabilis	EchA	Bleomycin-induced scleroderma mouse model	Attenuates macrophage activation and infiltration (neutrophils), inhibits production of TNFα and IFNγ	[79]
-	EchA	DSS-induced colitis mice	Decreases DIA, improves colon length and suppresses tissue damage, suppresses macrophage activation.	[80]
-	EchA	Endotoxin-induced uveitis rat model	Reduces levels of TNFα, NF-κB antibody positive cells and ROS in aqueous humor	[81]
-	Histochrome® (1% EchA)	UV-B exposed hairless mouse model	Reduces MMPs expression, collagen degradation and dermal inflammatory cell recruitment	[83]
Paracentrotus lividus	EchA	Stabilization of the RBCs membrane, cecal ligation and puncture model for sepsis	Potent stabilizing effect on the human RBCs, suppresses the production of IL-6 and TNFα	[104]
Scaphechinus mirabilis	Spinochromes A and B	Cotton-pellet granuloma rat model	Reduces chronic inflammation	[86]
Echinometra mathaei, Diadema savignyi, Tripneustes gratilla and *Toxopneustes pileolus*	Spinochromes and EchA	LPS stimulated J774A.1 macrophages	Reduces TNFα production	[87]
Strongylocentrotus nudus	Spines and shells pigments	LPS-stimulated RAW264.7 macrophages	Decreases production of NO, IL-6, TNFα, PGE2 and 6-keto-PGF 1α	[88]
Paracentrotus lividus	Sulfated polysaccharide	Carrageenan-induced rat paw edema	Reduces the paw-edema	[89]
Anthocidaris crassispina	Gonad polysaccharide	LPS-stimulated RAW264.7 macrophages	Reduces NO production	[90]

Table 2. *Cont.*

Species	Bioactive Compounds/Extracts	Model	Mechanism of Anti-Inflammatory Activity	Ref.
Strongylocentrotus droebachiensis	Centrocin 1 (CEN1HC-Br)	LPS-induced THP-1 cells, Ear swelling inflammation rat model	Reduces expression of various inflammatory cytokines such as IL-12p40, IL-6, IL-1β, TNFα	[91,92]
Salmacis bicolor	Salmachroman	In vitro COX and 5-LOX inhibitory assays	Inhibits COX-2 and 5-LOX	[94]
Salmacis bicolor	Salmacembranes A and B	In vitro COX and 5-LOX inhibitory assays	Inhibits COX-1, COX-2, and 5-LOX	[95]
Stomopneustes variolaris	Cembrane type of diterpenoid	In vitro COX and LOX assay	Inhibits 5-LOX, high COX-1/COX-2 ratio than ibuprofen	[96]
Stomopneustes variolaris	Stomopneulactones D	LPS-stimulated RAW264.7 macrophages	Inhibits COX-2 and 5-LOX, reduces generation of iNOS and intracellular ROS	[97]
Stomopneustes variolaris	Stomopnolides A and B	In vitro 5-LOX inhibitory assays	Inhibits 5-LOX	[98]
Strongylocentrotus droebachiensis	Fatty acid derivatives	LPS-stimulated human mononuclear U-937 monocyte	Inhibits p38 MAPK, COX-1 and COX-2	[99]
Brisaster latifrons	(Z)-4-methylundeca-1,9-diene-6-sulfonic acid	LPS-stimulated RAW264.7 macrophages	Inhibits production of proinflammatory cytokines by inactivation of JNK/p38 MAPK and NF-κB pathways	[100]
Hemicentrotus pulcherrimus and *Diadema setosum*	Hp-s1 ganglioside	LPS-stimulated microglial cells	Decreases iNOS and COX-2 expression. Suppresses cytokine production. Downregulates the NF-κB and JNK/p38 MAPK signaling pathway	[101]

5. Anti-Inflammatory Compounds from Starfish

Starfish (sea stars) are invertebrates that belong to the class Asteroidea, phylum Echinodermata. There are over 1500 species around the world, mostly inhabiting oceans, while a few occur in brackish water [105,106]. Several starfish species have been used in traditional Chinese medicine to treat various ailments such as goiters, body aches, and rheumatism [105]. In this section, we summarized the findings on the anti-inflammatory potential of various bioactive components isolated from starfish, such as glycosides, triterpenoid glycosides, steroids, and fatty acid derivatives. Several glycosides have been isolated from different species of starfish that exhibited promising preliminary anti-inflammatory activity, such as the inhibition of ROS and NO production in macrophages. Table 3 summarizes the anti-inflammatory effects displayed on LPS-stimulated RAW264.7 macrophages and bone marrow-derived dendritic cells (BMDCs) by bioactive compounds isolated from different species of starfish. Astrosterioside A (Figure 9: (**23**)) and D (Figure 9: (**24**)) and sulphated steroidal hexasaccharides isolated from starfish *Astropecten monacanthus* showed potent anti-inflammatory activity, inhibiting the secretion of proinflammatory cytokines (TNFα, IL-6, and IL-1) in LPS-stimulated BMDCs [107]. The fatty acid-rich fraction of the skin and gonads of starfish *Asterias amurensis* significantly downregulated the expression of the inflammatory mediators IL-1 β, IL-6, TNFα, iNOS, and COX-2 in LPS-stimulated RAW264.7 macrophages. This anti-inflammatory effect of fatty acids is driven through activation of the NF-κB and MAPK pathways [108]. The lipidomic profiling of spiny starfish *Marthasterias glacialis* led to the discovery of cis-11-eicosenoic and cis-11,14 eicosadienoic acids (fatty acids), as well as the unsaturated sterol ergosta-7,22-dien-3-ol. These lipids were thought to have potent anti-inflammatory activity through the reduction of ROS, NO, and proinflammatory cytokines in LPS-stimulated macrophages. Furthermore, these compounds downregulate the expression of various inflammatory genes, including iNOS, COX-2, IkBα, C/EBP homologous protein (CHOP), and NF-κB, in stimulated macrophages [109]. Oxygenated steroid derivatives (Figure 10: (**25–28**)) isolated from a methanol extract of the

Vietnamese starfish *Protoreaster nodosus* exhibit potent anti-inflammatory activity in LPS-stimulated BMDCs, inhibiting the secretion of proinflammatory cytokines, including IL-12 p40, IL-6, and TNFα [110]. Steroids (Figure 11: (**29–35**)) from another Vietnamese starfish *Astropecten polyacanthus*, used as a tonic in Vietnamese ancient medicine, also exhibited potent anti-inflammatory activity when tested against LPS-stimulated BMDCs [111].

Astrosterioside A **(23)**   Astrosterioside D **(24)**

Figure 9. Structures of anti-inflammatory steroidal hexasaccharides derived from starfish *Astropecten monacanthus* (structures (**23**) and (**24**) re-used with permission from reference [107], ACS Publications, 2013).

(25S) 5α-cholestane-
3β,6α,8β,15α,16β,26-hexol **(25)**   (25S) 5α-cholestane-
3β,6α,7α,8β,15α,16β,26-heptol **(26)**

(25S) 5α-cholestane-
3β,6α,7α,8β,15α,16β,26-octol **(27)**   Nodososide **(28)**

Figure 10. Structures of anti-inflammatory steroid derivatives derived from starfish *Protoreaster nodosus* (structures (**25–28**) re-used with permission from reference [110], Springer Nature, 2015).

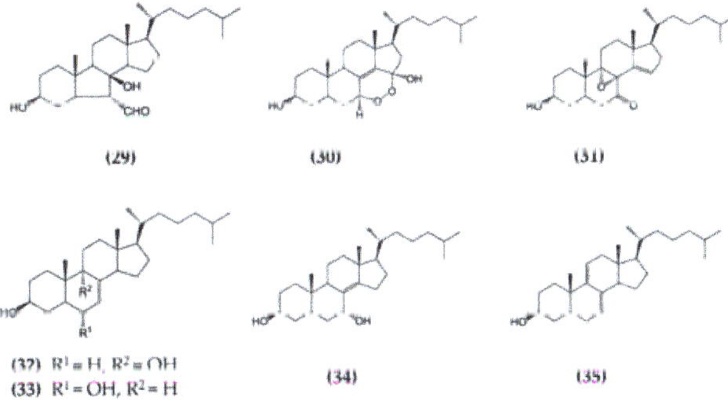

(29)   **(30)**   **(31)**

(32) R¹ = H, R² = OH
(33) R¹ = OH, R² = H   **(34)**   **(35)**

Figure 11. Structures of anti-inflammatory steroids derived from starfish *Astropecten polyacanthus* (structures (**29–35**) re-used from reference [111]).

Table 3. Anti-inflammatory bioactive compounds derived from starfish.

Species	Bioactive Compounds/Extracts	Model	Mechanism of Anti-Inflammatory Activity	Ref.
Astropecten monacanthus	Astrosteriosides A and D	LPS-stimulated BMDCs	Inhibits secretion of proinflammatory cytokines	[107]
Asterias amurensis	Fatty acids	LPS-stimulated RAW 264.7 macrophages	Downregulates expression of inflammatory genes via NF-κB and MAPK pathways	[108]
Marthasterias glacialis	cis 11-eicosenoic and cis 11,14 eicosadienoic acids	LPS-stimulated RAW 264.7 macrophages	Downregulates inflammatory gene expression: iNOS, COX-2, IKB-α and CHOP and NF-κB	[109]
Protoreaster nodosus	Oxygenated steroid Derivatives	LPS-stimulated BMDCs	Inhibits secretion of proinflammatory cytokines IL-12 p40, IL-6 and TNFα	[110]
Astropecten polyacanthus	Crude extracts and steroids	LPS-stimulated BMDCs	Inhibits production of IL-12 p40, IL-6 and TNFα	[111]
Protoreaster lincki	Protolinckiosides A-D (Figure 12: (**36–39**))	LPS-stimulated RAW 264.7 macrophages	Reduces ROS formation and NO production	[112]
Anthenea aspera	Anthenoside O (Figure 12: (**40**))	LPS-stimulated RAW 264.7 macrophages	Reduces ROS formation and NO production	[113]
Pentaceraster regulus	Pentareguloside C (Figure 13: (**41**)) Pentareguloside D (Figure 13: (**42**)) Pentareguloside E (Figure 13: (**43**))	LPS-stimulated RAW 264.7 macrophages	Reduces ROS formation and NO production	[114]
Acanthaster planci	Plancipyrrosides A and B (Figure 14.: (**44–45**))	LPS-stimulated RAW 264.7 macrophages	Reduces ROS formation and NO production	[115]
Asterina batheri	Astebatheriosides B-D (Figure 15: (**46–48**))	LPS-stimulated BMDCs cells	Inhibits IL-12 p40 production	[116]

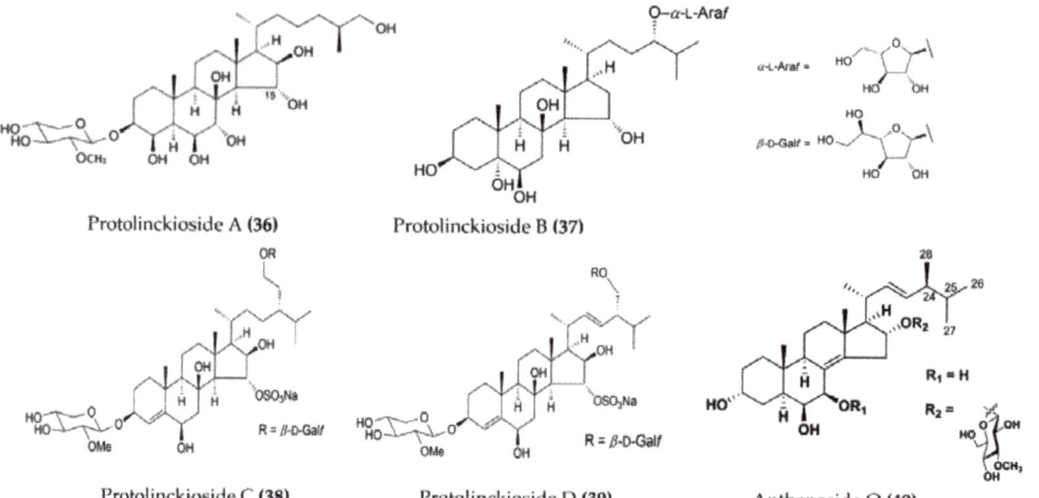

Figure 12. Structures of anti-inflammatory triterpenoid glycosides derived from starfish (structures (**36–39**) re-used with permission from reference [112], John Wiley and Sons, 2016; structure (**40**) re-used with permission from reference [113], ACS Publications, 2016).

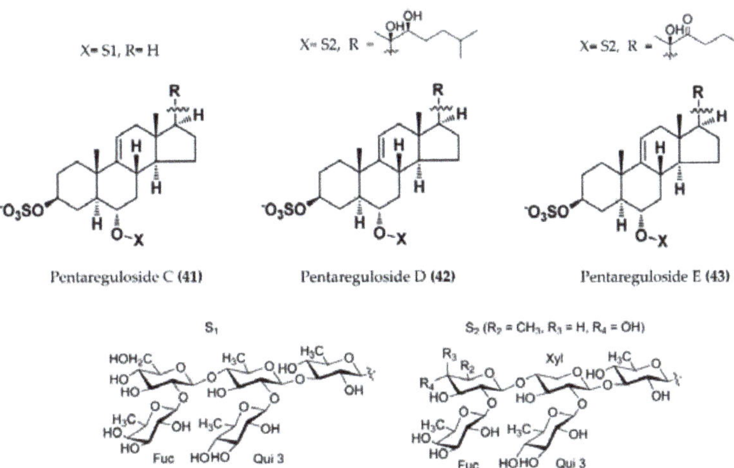

Pentareguloside C **(41)**   Pentareguloside D **(42)**   Pentareguloside E **(43)**

Figure 13. Structures of anti-inflammatory pentaregulosides (glycosides) derived from starfish *Pentaceraster regulus* (structures **(41–43)** re-used with permission from reference [114], ACS Publications, 2016).

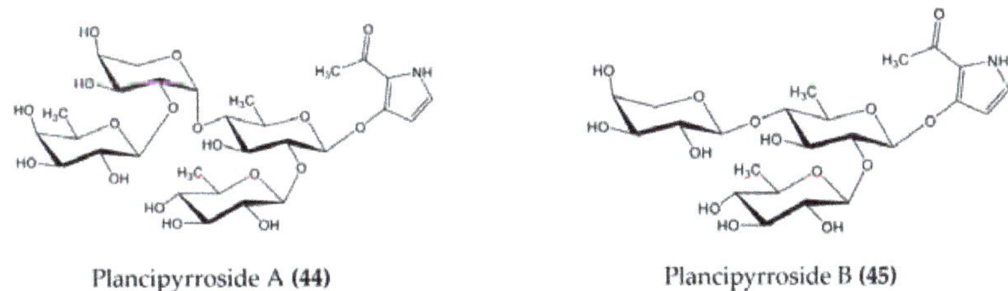

Plancipyrroside A **(44)**   Plancipyrroside B **(45)**

Figure 14. Structures of anti-inflammatory plancipyrrosides (glycosides) derived from starfish *Pentaceraster regulus* (structures **(44–45)** re-used from reference [115]).

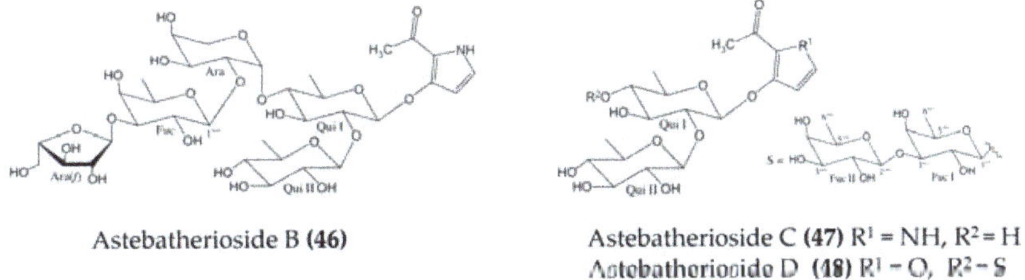

Astebatherioside B **(46)**   Astebatherioside C **(47)** R¹ = NH, R² = H
                                Astebatherioside D **(48)** R¹ = O, R² = S

Figure 15. Structures of anti-inflammatory astebatheriosides (glycosides) derived from starfish *Astorina batheri* (structures **(46–48)** re-used with permission from reference [116], Elsevier, 2016)

6. Application to the Pharmaceutical Industry

The drug discovery process is a very lengthy, time-consuming, and costly process for the pharmaceutical industry, and it includes target identification, lead compound discovery, the structure–activity relationship (SAR) study, in vitro and in vivo screening, and, finally, clinical trials on large human populations. More recently, the bioinformatics approach has been employed for target identification and the discovery of lead compounds, which has significantly reduced the length of the drug discovery process [117]. Lead compounds may come from combinational chemistry, computer-aided drug design, or from natural products [118,119]. However, lead compounds often produce suboptimal biological responses and require chemical modifications to improve their efficacy and potency. The majority of drugs available clinically are derived from natural sources. Indeed, many of the anticancer small molecules available on the market are either natural products or derived from natural products [120]. The search for novel or lead compounds was previously limited to plant-based natural products but has now been expanded to marine-derived natural products as well. There have been reports of a variety of marine natural products with exploitable properties, including those that treat cancer and inflammation and neurological, immunological, and metabolic disorders [121–123]. The global preclinical marine pharmacology pipeline, which is still producing significant preclinical data on numerous pharmacological classes, is what provides new leads [124]. In fact, some pharmaceutical companies are focusing on marine natural product research. However, there is a general trend that anticancer drugs have received more attention, resources, and efforts in terms of pharmacological research, discovery, and development than other drugs classes, such as anti-inflammatory drugs. For example, several marine organism-derived anticancer drugs (such as vidarabine (Ara-A) for Hodgkin's lymphoma and chronic large cell anaplastic lymphoma, cytarabine, Ara-C for acute non-lymphoblastic leukemia, and trabectedin vedotin for ovarian cancer and soft tissue sarcoma) have been approved by the FDA. Moreover, several anticancer molecules are in Phase I, II, or III clinical trials [125,126]. However, the discovery of several marine-derived anti-inflammatory molecules also has ignited the pharmaceutical industry's interest in developing them into lead compounds for the drug discovery process [127,128]. Unfortunately, to date, no marine-derived anti-inflammatory drug has been approved by the FDA, but a few promising anti-inflammatory compounds are under various phases of clinical trials: for example, pseudopterosin A (a diterpene glycoside obtained from soft coral) and IPL-576092 (a polyhydroxylated steroid obtained from a sponge) [129]. This suggests the notable involvement of marine-derived natural products in the potential pharmaceutical industry and encourages the pursuit of new anti-inflammatory lead compound discoveries. Productive teamwork among researchers from various universities and/or institutes and the leadership of the pharmaceutical industry is required to ensure the development of future therapeutic entities that will significantly contribute to the treatment of various inflammatory disorders.

7. Conclusions and Research Prospects

Chronic inflammation plays a crucial role in the development of various diseases, such as inflammatory bowel disease, rheumatoid arthritis, and asthma. Controlling the progression of inflammation is a critical step in the management of these diseases. The available steroidal and nonsteroidal anti-inflammatory drugs significantly reduce chronic inflammation, but many of them can have adverse effects, such as gastrointestinal distress and liver, heart, kidney, and endocrine dysfunction, when taken long-term. In this review, the PubMed, Scopus, Web of Science, ACS, ScienceDirect, SpringerLink, and MDPI databases were searched using various combinations of keywords for publications pertaining to the anti-inflammatory potential of compounds originating from the three echinoderms: sea cucumbers, sea urchins, and starfish. Due to the immense richness and diversity of marine organisms and their natural products, it is extremely difficult to cover all of the pertinent literature, even though a broad coverage was anticipated. The major bioactive compounds isolated from sea cucumbers are fucoidan, fucosylated chondroitin sulfate, triterpenoid glycosides, small peptides, lipids, and fatty acids such as the EPA derivatives (EPA-PC and EPA-PE) sphingolipids and frondanol. Similarly, sea urchins are well-documented to produce bioactive compounds such as EchA, spine and shell pigments, polysaccharides, stomopnolides, and small peptides. Starfish also produce a diverse range of bioactive compounds, including pentaregulosides, protolinckiosides, plancipyrroside, astebatherioside, and oxygenated steroid and fatty acids. These bioactive compounds from echinoderms suppress the expression and activation of major proinflammatory cytokines such as IL-6, TNFα, IL1β, IL-10, MIP-1, etc. by the inhibition of the NF-kB and MAPK signaling pathways. Moreover, the classical COX and LOX inflammation pathway inhibitions by these compounds are also documented in this review. In addition, compounds isolated from these echinoderms also inhibit ROS generation, as well as NO production.

Research into marine-derived anti-inflammatory lead compounds has received little consideration compared to anticancer leads; however, this is evolving very rapidly. In this review article, we presented anti-inflammatory compounds isolated from various species of sea cucumbers, sea urchins, and starfish, including their chemical structures. Many compounds, such as fucoidan, fucosylated chondroitin sulfate, eicosapentaenoic acid derivatives, and echinochrome A, have been investigated in detail for their anti-inflammatory activity and molecular mechanisms. Moreover, some novel compounds, such as glycosides from starfish, have been studied well in terms of their chemical structure and SAR with a target but only screened for preliminary anti-inflammatory activity (such as COX and 5-LOX inhibitory activity). These need further investigation to establish their molecular mechanisms. Marine pharmacology research faces many obstacles. For example, the isolation of bioactive compounds from marine organisms is extremely difficult, as they live in a complex and biodiverse environment, and it is difficult to mimic such an environment in the laboratory for their cultivation to obtain a large quantity of active substances. The future prospects in marine pharmacology should focus on following: (1) the reproduction of compounds by the chemical synthesis of established marine-derived anti-inflammatory leads to increase their production and overcome cultivation obstacles, (2) the chemical modification of existing marine-derived anti-inflammatory leads (analogs) to enhance their potency and efficacy, (3) develop lead compound libraries for large and rapid random high-throughput screening methods, (4) industry collaboration to translate preclinical leads into the clinical pipeline, and (5) establish comprehensive and efficient separation and purification techniques. The planet is gifted with vast and diverse coastlines by nature that are a treasure of bioactive compounds that have not been exploited. The scientific community should consider taking up further research to find other, potentially valuable marine drugs.

In conclusion, this review can serve as a well-documented reference for research progress on the development of potential drugs from marine sources against various chronic inflammatory conditions.

Author Contributions: H.G.: Conceptualization, Literature collection, Methodology, Investigation, and Writing—Original Draft. M.K.: Methodology, Investigation, and Writing—Original Draft. T.E.A.: Conceptualization, Resources, Methodology, Writing—Review and Editing, and Supervision. R.K.J.: Conceptualization, Resources, Methodology, Writing—Review and Editing, and Supervision. All authors have read and agreed to the published version of the manuscript.

Funding: This manuscript received publication fee support from Mohammed Bin Rashid University of Medicine and Health Sciences.

Acknowledgments: This work was supported in part by Mohammed Bin Rashid University of Medicine and Health Sciences (MBRU) and the Al Jalila Foundation for Post-Doctoral Research Fellowship awards to H.G. and M.K.

References

1. Medzhitov, R. Origin and physiological roles of inflammation. *Nature* **2008**, *454*, 428–435. [CrossRef] [PubMed]
2. Gerard, C.; Rollins, B.J. Chemokines and disease. *Nat. Immunol.* **2001**, *2*, 108–115. [CrossRef] [PubMed]
3. Galli, S.J.; Tsai, M.; Piliponsky, A.M. The development of allergic inflammation. *Nature* **2008**, *454*, 445–454. [CrossRef] [PubMed]
4. Barbu, E.; Popescu, M.R.; Popescu, A.C.; Balanescu, S.M. Inflammation as A Precursor of Atherothrombosis, Diabetes and Early Vascular Aging. *Int. J. Mol. Sci.* **2022**, *23*, 963. [CrossRef] [PubMed]
5. Kiss, A.L. Inflammation in Focus: The Beginning and the End. *Pathol. Oncol. Res.* **2022**, *27*, 1610136. [CrossRef]
6. Furman, D.; Campisi, J.; Verdin, E.; Carrera-Bastos, P.; Targ, S.; Franceschi, C.; Ferrucci, L.; Gilroy, D.W.; Fasano, A.; Miller, G.W.; et al. Chronic inflammation in the etiology of disease across the life span. *Nat. Med.* **2019**, *25*, 1822–1832. [CrossRef]
7. Netea, M.G.; Balkwill, F.; Chonchol, M.; Cominelli, F.; Donath, M.Y.; Giamarellos-Bourboulis, E.J.; Golenbock, D.; Gresnigt, M.S.; Heneka, M.T.; Hoffman, H.M.; et al. A guiding map for inflammation. *Nat. Immunol.* **2017**, *18*, 826–831. [CrossRef]

8. Bowie, A.G.; Unterholzner, L. Viral evasion and subversion of pattern-recognition receptor signalling. *Nat. Rev. Immunol.* **2008**, *8*, 911–922. [CrossRef]

9. Takeuchi, O.; Akira, S. Pattern recognition receptors and inflammation. *Cell* **2010**, *140*, 805–820. [CrossRef]

10. Zhao, H.; Wu, L.; Yan, G.; Chen, Y.; Zhou, M.; Wu, Y.; Li, Y. Inflammation and tumor progression: Signaling pathways and targeted intervention. *Signal Transduct. Target. Ther.* **2021**, *6*, 263. [CrossRef]

11. Yeung, Y.T.; Aziz, F.; Guerrero-Castilla, A.; Arguelles, S. Signaling Pathways in Inflammation and Anti-inflammatory Therapies. *Curr. Pharm. Des.* **2018**, *24*, 1449–1484. [CrossRef] [PubMed]

12. Hayden, M.S.; Ghosh, S. NF-κB in immunobiology. *Cell Res.* **2011**, *21*, 223–244. [CrossRef] [PubMed]

13. Oeckinghaus, A.; Hayden, M.S.; Ghosh, S. Crosstalk in NF-κB signaling pathways. *Nat. Immunol.* **2011**, *12*, 695–708. [CrossRef]

14. Mou, J.; Li, Q.; Qi, X.; Yang, J. Structural comparison, antioxidant and anti-inflammatory properties of fucosylated chondroitin sulfate of three edible sea cucumbers. *Carbohydr. Polym.* **2018**, *185*, 41–47. [CrossRef] [PubMed]

15. Olivera-Castillo, L.; Grant, G.; Kantun-Moreno, N.; Barrera-Perez, H.A.; Montero, J.; Olvera-Novoa, M.A.; Carrillo-Cocom, L.M.; Acevedo, J.J.; Puerto-Castillo, C.; May Solis, V.; et al. A Glycosaminoglycan-Rich Fraction from Sea Cucumber Isostichopus badionotus Has Potent Anti-Inflammatory Properties In Vitro and In Vivo. *Nutrients* **2020**, *12*, 1698. [CrossRef]

16. Subramanya, S.B.; Chandran, S.; Almarzooqi, S.; Raj, V.; Al Zahmi, A.S.; Al Katheeri, R.A.; Al Zadjali, S.A.; Collin, P.D.; Adrian, T.E. Frondanol, a Nutraceutical Extract from Cucumaria frondosa, Attenuates Colonic Inflammation in a DSS-Induced Colitis Model in Mice. *Mar. Drugs* **2018**, *16*, 148. [CrossRef]

17. Xiang, X.W.; Wang, R.; Yao, L.W.; Zhou, Y.F.; Sun, P.L.; Zheng, B.; Chen, Y.F. Anti-Inflammatory Effects of Mytilus coruscus Polysaccharide on RAW264.7 Cells and DSS-Induced Colitis in Mice. *Mar. Drugs* **2021**, *19*, 468. [CrossRef]

18. Palladino, M.A.; Bahjat, F.R.; Theodorakis, E.A.; Moldawer, L.L. Anti-TNF-alpha therapies: The next generation. *Nat. Rev. Drug Discov.* **2003**, *2*, 736–746. [CrossRef]

19. Costanzo, M.; Cesi, V.; Prete, E.; Negroni, A.; Palone, F.; Cucchiara, S.; Oliva, S.; Leter, B.; Stronati, L. Krill oil reduces intestinal inflammation by improving epithelial integrity and impairing adherent-invasive Escherichia coli pathogenicity. *Dig. Liver Dis.* **2016**, *48*, 34–42. [CrossRef]

20. Gómez-Lechón, M.J.; Donato, M.T.; Martínez-Romero, A.; Jiménez, N.; Castell, J.V.; O'Connor, J.E. A human hepatocellular in vitro model to investigate steatosis. *Chem. Biol. Interact.* **2007**, *165*, 106–116. [CrossRef]

21. Ye, J.; Zheng, J.; Tian, X.; Xu, B.; Yuan, F.; Wang, B.; Yang, Z.; Huang, F. Fucoxanthin Attenuates Free Fatty Acid-Induced Nonalcoholic Fatty Liver Disease by Regulating Lipid Metabolism/Oxidative Stress/Inflammation via the AMPK/Nrf2/TLR4 Signaling Pathway. *Mar. Drugs* **2022**, *20*, 225. [CrossRef] [PubMed]

22. Kapoor, S.; Nailwal, N.; Kumar, M.; Barve, K. Recent Patents and Discovery of Anti-inflammatory Agents from Marine Source. *Recent Pat. Inflamm. Allergy Drug Discov.* **2019**, *13*, 105–114. [CrossRef] [PubMed]

23. Tian, X.R.; Tang, H.F.; Tian, X.L.; Hu, J.J.; Huang, L.L.; Gustafson, K.R. Review of bioactive secondary metabolites from marine bryozoans in the progress of new drugs discovery. *Future Med. Chem.* **2018**, *10*, 1497–1514. [CrossRef] [PubMed]

24. Cheung, R.C.F.; Ng, T.B.; Wong, J.H.; Chen, Y.; Chan, W.Y. Marine natural products with anti-inflammatory activity. *Appl. Microbiol. Biotechnol.* **2016**, *100*, 1645–1666. [CrossRef] [PubMed]

25. Li, C.Q.; Ma, Q.Y.; Gao, X.Z.; Wang, X.; Zhang, B.L. Research Progress in Anti-Inflammatory Bioactive Substances Derived from Marine Microorganisms, Sponges, Algae, and Corals. *Mar. Drugs* **2021**, *19*, 572. [CrossRef]

26. Souza, C.R.M.; Bezerra, W.P.; Souto, J.T. Marine Alkaloids with Anti-Inflammatory Activity: Current Knowledge and Future Perspectives. *Mar. Drugs* **2020**, *18*, 147. [CrossRef]

27. Diederich, M. Chemical ecology and medicianl chemistry of marine Nf-kB inhibitors. In *Aquatic Ecosystem Research Trends*; Nairne, G., Ed.; Nova Science Publishers: Hauppauge, NY, USA, 2009.

28. Rubilar, T.; Barbieri, E.S.; Gazquez, A.; Avaro, M. Sea Urchin Pigments: Echinochrome A and Its Potential Implication in the Cytokine Storm Syndrome. *Mar. Drugs* **2021**, *19*, 267. [CrossRef]

29. Shikov, A.N.; Pozharitskaya, O.N.; Krishtopina, A.S.; Makarov, V.G. Naphthoquinone pigments from sea urchins: Chemistry and pharmacology. *Phytochem. Rev.* **2018**, *17*, 509–534. [CrossRef]

30. Dolmatova, L.S.; Dolmatov, I.Y. Different Macrophage Type Triggering as Target of the Action of Biologically Active Substances from Marine Invertebrates. *Mar. Drugs* **2020**, *18*, 37. [CrossRef]

31. Kumar, Y.; Tarafdar, A.; Kumar, D.; Badgujar, P.C. Effect of Indian brown seaweed Sargassum wightii as a functional ingredient on the phytochemical content and antioxidant activity of coffee beverage. *J. Food Sci. Technol.* **2019**, *56*, 4516–4525. [CrossRef]

32. Kalasariya, H.S.; Yadav, V.K.; Yadav, K.K.; Tirth, V.; Algahtani, A.; Islam, S.; Gupta, N.; Jeon, B.H. Seaweed-Based Molecules and Their Potential Biological Activities: An Eco-Sustainable Cosmetics. *Molecules* **2021**, *26*, 5313. [CrossRef] [PubMed]

33. Hossain, A.; Dave, D.; Shahidi, F. Northern Sea Cucumber (Cucumaria frondosa): A Potential Candidate for Functional Food, Nutraceutical, and Pharmaceutical Sector. *Mar. Drugs* **2020**, *18*, 274. [CrossRef] [PubMed]

34. Wen, J.; Hu, C.; Fan, S. Chemical composition and nutritional quality of sea cucumbers. *J. Sci. Food Agric.* **2010**, *90*, 2469–2474. [CrossRef] [PubMed]

35. Bordbar, S.; Anwar, F.; Saari, N. High-value components and bioactives from sea cucumbers for functional foods—A review. *Mar. Drugs* **2011**, *9*, 1761–1805. [CrossRef] [PubMed]

36. Wang, J.; Hu, S.; Jiang, W.; Song, W.; Cai, L.; Wang, J. Fucoidan from sea cucumber may improve hepatic inflammatory response and insulin resistance in mice. *Int. Immunopharmacol.* **2016**, *31*, 15–23. [CrossRef] [PubMed]

37. Yin, J.; Yang, X.; Xia, B.; Yang, Z.; Wang, Z.; Wang, J.; Li, T.; Lin, P.; Song, X.; Guo, S. The fucoidan from sea cucumber Apostichopus japonicus attenuates lipopolysaccharide-challenged liver injury in C57BL/6J mice. *J. Funct. Foods* **2019**, *61*, 103493. [CrossRef]

38. Hu, S.; Wang, J.; Wang, J.; Li, S.; Jiang, W.; Liu, Y. Renoprotective effect of fucoidan from Acaudina molpadioides in streptozotocin/high fat diet-induced type 2 diabetic mice. *J. Funct. Foods* **2017**, *31*, 123–130. [CrossRef]

39. Xu, X.; Chang, Y.; Xue, C.; Wang, J.; Shen, J. Gastric Protective Activities of Sea Cucumber Fucoidans with Different Molecular Weight and Chain Conformations: A Structure—Activity Relationship Investigation. *J. Agric. Food Chem.* **2018**, *66*, 8615–8622. [CrossRef]

40. Li, S.; Li, J.; Mao, G.; Yan, L.; Hu, Y.; Ye, X.; Tian, D.; Linhardt, R.J.; Chen, S. Effect of the sulfation pattern of sea cucumber-derived fucoidan oligosaccharides on modulating metabolic syndromes and gut microbiota dysbiosis caused by HFD in mice. *J. Funct. Foods* **2019**, *55*, 193–210. [CrossRef]

41. Ustyuzhanina, N.E.; Bilan, M.I.; Panina, E.G.; Sanamyan, N.P.; Dmitrenok, A.S.; Tsvetkova, E.A.; Ushakova, N.A.; Shashkov, A.S.; Nifantiev, N.E.; Usov, A.I. Structure and Anti-Inflammatory Activity of a New Unusual Fucosylated Chondroitin Sulfate from Cucumaria djakonovi. *Mar. Drugs* **2018**, *16*, 389. [CrossRef]

42. Zhu, Q.; Lin, L.; Zhao, M. Sulfated fucan/fucosylated chondroitin sulfate-dominated polysaccharide fraction from low-edible-value sea cucumber ameliorates type 2 diabetes in rats: New prospects for sea cucumber polysaccharide based-hypoglycemic functional food. *Int. J. Biol. Macromol.* **2020**, *159*, 34–45. [CrossRef] [PubMed]

43. Borsig, L.; Wang, L.; Cavalcante, M.C.; Cardilo-Reis, L.; Ferreira, P.L.; Mourão, P.A.; Esko, J.D.; Pavão, M.S. Selectin blocking activity of a fucosylated chondroitin sulfate glycosaminoglycan from sea cucumber. Effect on tumor metastasis and neutrophil recruitment. *J. Biol. Chem.* **2007**, *282*, 14984–14991. [CrossRef] [PubMed]

44. Stefaniak-Vidarsson, M.M.; Kale, V.A.; Gudjónsdóttir, M.; Marteinsdottir, G.; Fridjonsson, O.; Hreggvidsson, G.O.; Sigurjonsson, O.E.; Omarsdottir, S.; Kristbergsson, K. Bioactive effect of sulphated polysaccharides derived from orange-footed sea cucumber (*Cucumaria frondosa*) toward THP-1 macrophages. *Bioact. Carbohydr. Diet. Fibre* **2017**, *12*, 14–19. [CrossRef]

45. El Barky, A.R.; Hussein, S.A.; Alm-Eldeen, A.A.; Hafez, Y.A.; Mohamed, T.M. Anti-diabetic activity of Holothuria thomasi saponin. *Biomed. Pharmacother.* **2016**, *84*, 1472–1487. [CrossRef]

46. Chen, C.; Han, X.; Dong, P.; Li, Z.; Yanagita, T.; Xue, C.; Zhang, T.; Wang, Y. Sea cucumber saponin liposomes ameliorate obesity-induced inflammation and insulin resistance in high-fat-diet-fed mice. *Food Funct.* **2018**, *9*, 861–870. [CrossRef]

47. Ding, L.; Zhang, T.-T.; Che, H.-X.; Zhang, L.-Y.; Xue, C.-H.; Chang, Y.-G.; Wang, Y.-M. Saponins of sea cucumber attenuate atherosclerosis in ApoE$^{-/-}$ mice via lipid-lowering and anti-inflammatory properties. *J. Funct. Foods* **2018**, *48*, 490–497. [CrossRef]

48. Lu, Z.; Sun, N.; Dong, L.; Gao, Y.; Lin, S. Production of Bioactive Peptides from Sea Cucumber and Its Potential Health Benefits: A Comprehensive Review. *J. Agric. Food Chem.* **2022**, *70*, 7607–7625. [CrossRef]

49. Wan, H.; Han, J.; Tang, S.; Bao, W.; Lu, C.; Zhou, J.; Ming, T.; Li, Y.; Su, X. Comparisons of protective effects between two sea cucumber hydrolysates against diet induced hyperuricemia and renal inflammation in mice. *Food Funct.* **2020**, *11*, 1074–1086. [CrossRef]

50. Zhang, X.; Li, H.; Wang, L.; Zhang, S.; Wang, F.; Lin, H.; Gao, S.; Li, X.; Liu, K. Anti-inflammatory peptides and metabolomics-driven biomarkers discovery from sea cucumber protein hydrolysates. *J. Food Sci.* **2021**, *86*, 3540–3549. [CrossRef]

51. Song, J.; Li, T.; Cheng, X.; Ji, X.; Gao, D.; Du, M.; Jiang, N.; Liu, X.; Mao, X. Sea cucumber peptides exert anti-inflammatory activity through suppressing NF-kappaB and MAPK and inducing HO-1 in RAW264.7 macrophages. *Food Funct.* **2016**, *7*, 2773–2779. [CrossRef]

52. Ye, J.; Shen, C.; Huang, Y.; Zhang, X.; Xiao, M. Anti-fatigue activity of sea cucumber peptides prepared from Stichopus japonicus in an endurance swimming rat model. *J. Sci. Food Agric.* **2017**, *97*, 4548–4556. [CrossRef] [PubMed]

53. Mena-Bueno, S.; Atanasova, M.; Fernandez-Trasancos, A.; Paradela-Dobarro, B.; Bravo, S.B.; Alvarez, E.; Fernandez, A.L.; Carrera, I.; Gonzalez-Juanatey, J.R.; Eiras, S. Sea cucumbers with an anti-inflammatory effect on endothelial cells and subcutaneous but not on epicardial adipose tissue. *Food Funct.* **2016**, *7*, 953–963. [CrossRef] [PubMed]

54. Jo, S.-H.; Kim, C.; Park, S.-H. Novel Marine Organism-Derived Extracellular Vesicles for Control of Anti-Inflammation. *Tissue Eng. Regen. Med.* **2021**, *18*, 71–79. [CrossRef]

55. Feng, J.; Zhang, L.; Tang, X.; Hu, W.; Zhou, P. Major yolk protein from sea cucumber (*Stichopus japonicus*) attenuates acute colitis via regulation of microbial dysbiosis and inflammatory responses. *Food Res. Int.* **2022**, *151*, 110841. [CrossRef] [PubMed]

56. Chen, Z.; Liu, D.; Tang, X.; Cui, Y.; Hu, W.; Regenstein, J.M.; Zhou, P. Sea cucumber enzymatic hydrolysates relieve osteoporosis through OPG/RANK/RANKL system in ovariectomized rats. *Food Biosci.* **2022**, *46*, 101572. [CrossRef]

57. Zhang, L.; Ding, L.; Shi, H.; Wang, C.; Xue, C.; Zhang, T.; Wang, Y. Eicosapentaenoic acid-enriched phospholipids suppressed lipid accumulation by specific inhibition of lipid droplet-associated protein FSP27 in mice. *J. Sci. Food Agric.* **2020**, *100*, 2244–2251. [CrossRef]

58. Mao, L.; Wang, M.; Li, Y.; Liu, Y.; Wang, J.; Xue, C. Eicosapentaenoic acid-containing phosphatidylcholine promotes osteogenesis: mechanism of up-regulating Runx2 and ERK-mediated phosphorylation of PPARγ at serine 112. *J. Funct. Foods* **2019**, *52*, 73–80. [CrossRef]

59. Tian, Y.; Liu, Y.; Xue, C.; Wang, J.; Wang, Y.; Xu, J.; Li, Z. The exogenous natural phospholipids, EPA-PC and EPA-PE, contributes to ameliorate lipid accumulation and inflammation via activation of PPARα/γ. *Authorea* **2020**. [CrossRef]

60. Tian, Y.; Liu, Y.; Xue, C.; Wang, J.; Wang, Y.; Xu, J.; Li, Z. The exogenous natural phospholipids, EPA-PC and EPA-PE, contribute to ameliorate inflammation and promote macrophage polarization. *Food Funct.* **2020**, *11*, 6542–6551. [CrossRef]

61. Wang, X.; Lan, H.; Sun, T.; Cong, P.; Xue, C.; Xu, J. Serum metabolomics analysis reveals amelioration effects of sea cucumber ether phospholipids on oxidative stress and inflammation in high-fat diet-fed mice. *Food Funct.* **2022**, *13*, 10134–10146. [CrossRef]

62. Wen, M.; Ding, L.; Zhang, L.; Zhang, T.; Teruyoshi, Y.; Wang, Y.; Xue, C. Eicosapentaenoic Acid-Enriched Phosphatidylcholine Mitigated Aβ1-42-Induced Neurotoxicity via Autophagy-Inflammasome Pathway. *J. Agric. Food Chem.* **2019**, *67*, 13767–13774. [CrossRef] [PubMed]

63. Liu, X.; Xue, Y.; Liu, C.; Lou, Q.; Wang, J.; Yanagita, T.; Xue, C.; Wang, Y. Eicosapentaenoic acid-enriched phospholipid ameliorates insulin resistance and lipid metabolism in diet-induced-obese mice. *Lipids Health Dis.* **2013**, *12*, 109. [CrossRef] [PubMed]

64. Lee, D.I.; Kang, S.A.; Md, A.; Jeong, U.C.; Jin, F.; Kang, S.J.; Lee, J.Y.; Yu, H.S. Sea Cucumber Lipid-Soluble Extra Fraction Prevents Ovalbumin-Induced Allergic Airway Inflammation. *J. Med. Food* **2018**, *21*, 21–29. [CrossRef] [PubMed]

65. Collin, P.D. Sea Cucumber Carotenoid Lipid Fraction Products and Methods of Use. U.S. Patent 6,399,105B1, 4 June 2002.

66. Hu, S.; Wang, J.; Wang, J.; Xue, C.; Wang, Y. Long-chain bases from sea cucumber mitigate endoplasmic reticulum stress and inflammation in obesity mice. *J. Food Drug Anal.* **2017**, *25*, 628–636. [CrossRef]

67. Hu, S.; Wang, J.; Wang, J.; Yang, H.; Li, S.; Jiang, W.; Liu, Y.; Li, J. Long-chain bases from sea cucumber inhibits renal fibrosis and apoptosis in type 2 diabetic mice. *J. Funct. Foods* **2018**, *40*, 760–768. [CrossRef]

68. Yang, J.-Y.; Zhang, T.-T.; Dong, Z.; Shi, H.-H.; Xu, J.; Mao, X.-Z.; Wang, Y.-M.; Xue, C.-H. Dietary Supplementation with Exogenous Sea-Cucumber-Derived Ceramides and Glucosylceramides Alleviates Insulin Resistance in High-Fructose-Diet-Fed Rats by Upregulating the IRS/PI3K/Akt Signaling Pathway. *J. Agric. Food Chem.* **2021**, *69*, 9178–9187. [CrossRef]

69. Janakiram, N.B.; Mohammed, A.; Bryant, T.; Lightfoot, S.; Collin, P.D.; Steele, V.E.; Rao, C.V. Improved innate immune responses by Frondanol A5, a sea cucumber extract, prevent intestinal tumorigenesis. *Cancer Prev. Res.* **2015**, *8*, 327–337. [CrossRef]

70. Pranweerapaiboon, K.; Apisawetakan, S.; Nobsathian, S.; Itharat, A.; Sobhon, P.; Chaithirayanon, K. An ethyl-acetate fraction of Holothuria scabra modulates inflammation in vitro through inhibiting the production of nitric oxide and pro-inflammatory cytokines via NF-kappaB and JNK pathways. *Inflammopharmacology* **2020**, *28*, 1027–1037. [CrossRef]

71. Himaya, S.W.; Ryu, B.; Qian, Z.J.; Kim, S.K. Sea cucumber, Stichopus japonicus ethyl acetate fraction modulates the lipopolysaccharide induced iNOS and COX-2 via MAPK signaling pathway in murine macrophages. *Environ. Toxicol. Pharmacol.* **2010**, *30*, 68–75. [CrossRef]

72. Song, M.; Park, D.K.; Cho, M.; Park, H.-J. Anti-inflammatory and anti-allergic activities of sea cucumber (*Stichopus japonicus*) extract. *Food Sci. Biotechnol.* **2013**, *22*, 1661–1666. [CrossRef]

73. Mohd Heikal, M.Y.; Ahmad Nazrun, S.; Chua, K.H.; Norzana, A.G. Stichopus chloronotus aqueous extract as a chondroprotective agent for human chondrocytes isolated from osteoarthitis articular cartilage in vitro. *Cytotechnology* **2019**, *71*, 521–537. [CrossRef] [PubMed]

74. Kareh, M.; El Nahas, R.; Al-Aaraj, L.; Al-Ghadban, S.; Naser Al Deen, N.; Saliba, N.; El-Sabban, M.; Talhouk, R. Anti-proliferative and anti-inflammatory activities of the sea cucumber Holothuria polii aqueous extract. *SAGE Open Med.* **2018**, *6*, 2050312118809541. [CrossRef] [PubMed]

75. Saad, D.Y.; Baiomy, A.A.; Mansour, A.A. Antiseptic effect of sea cucumber (*Holothuria atra*) against multi-organ failure induced by sepsis: Molecular and histopathological study. *Exp. Ther. Med.* **2016**, *12*, 222–230. [CrossRef] [PubMed]

76. Olivera-Castillo, L.; Grant, G.; Kantún-Moreno, N.; Acevedo-Fernández, J.J.; Puc-Sosa, M.; Montero, J.; Olvera-Novoa, M.A.; Negrete-León, E.; Santa-Olalla, J.; Ceballos-Zapata, J.; et al. Sea cucumber (*Isostichopus badionotus*) body-wall preparations exert anti-inflammatory activity in vivo. *PharmaNutrition* **2018**, *6*, 74–80. [CrossRef]

77. Carletti, A.; Cardoso, C.; Juliao, D.; Arteaga, J.L.; Chainho, P.; Dionísio, M.A.; Sales, S.; Gaudêncio, M.J.; Ferreira, I.; Afonso, C.; et al. Biopotential of Sea Cucumbers (Echinodermata) and Tunicates (Chordata) from the Western Coast of Portugal for the Prevention and Treatment of Chronic Illnesses. *Proceedings* **2020**, *61*, 13.

78. Moreno-García, D.M.; Salas-Rojas, M.; Fernández-Martínez, E.; López-Cuellar, M.D.R.; Sosa-Gutierrez, C.G.; Peláez-Acero, A.; Rivero-Perez, N.; Zaragoza-Bastida, A.; Ojeda-Ramírez, D. Sea urchins: An update on their pharmacological properties. *PeerJ* **2022**, *10*, e13606. [CrossRef]

79. Park, G.-T.; Yoon, J.-W.; Yoo, S.-B.; Song, Y.-C.; Song, P.; Kim, H.-K.; Han, J.; Bae, S.-J.; Ha, K.-T.; Mishchenko, N.P.; et al. Echinochrome A Treatment Alleviates Fibrosis and Inflammation in Bleomycin-Induced Scleroderma. *Mar. Drugs* **2021**, *19*, 237. [CrossRef]

80. Oh, S.J.; Seo, Y.; Ahn, J.S.; Shin, Y.Y.; Yang, J.W.; Kim, H.K.; Han, J.; Mishchenko, N.P.; Fedoreyev, S.A.; Stonik, V.A.; et al. Echinochrome A Reduces Colitis in Mice and Induces In Vitro Generation of Regulatory Immune Cells. *Mar. Drugs* **2019**, *17*, 622.

81. Lennikov, A.; Kitaichi, N.; Noda, K.; Mizuuchi, K.; Ando, R.; Dong, Z.; Fukuhara, J.; Kinoshita, S.; Namba, K.; Ohno, S.; et al. Amelioration of endotoxin-induced uveitis treated with the sea urchin pigment echinochrome in rats. *Mol. Vis.* **2014**, *20*, 171–177.

82. Jeong, S.H.; Kim, H.K.; Song, I.-S.; Lee, S.J.; Ko, K.S.; Rhee, B.D.; Kim, N.; Mishchenko, N.P.; Fedoryev, S.A.; Stonik, V.A.; et al. Echinochrome A protects mitochondrial function in cardiomyocytes against cardiotoxic drugs. *Mar. Drugs* **2014**, *12*, 2922–2936.

83. Seol, J.E.; Ahn, S.W.; Seol, B.; Yun, H.R.; Park, N.; Kim, H.K.; Vasileva, E.A.; Mishchenko, N.P.; Fedoreyev, S.A.; Stonik, V.A.; et al. Echinochrome A Protects against Ultraviolet B-induced Photoaging by Lowering Collagen Degradation and Inflammatory Cell Infiltration in Hairless Mice. *Mar. Drugs* **2021**, *19*, 550. [CrossRef]

84. Yun, H.R.; Ahn, S.W.; Seol, B.; Vasileva, E.A.; Mishchenko, N.P.; Fedoreyev, S.A.; Stonik, V.A.; Han, J.; Ko, K.S.; Rhee, B.D.; et al. Echinochrome A Treatment Alleviates Atopic Dermatitis-like Skin Lesions in NC/Nga Mice via IL-4 and IL-13 Suppression. *Mar. Drugs* **2021**, *19*, 622. [CrossRef] [PubMed]

85. Hou, Y.; Carne, A.; McConnell, M.; Mros, S.; Bekhit, A.A.; El-Din A Bekhit, A. Macroporous resin extraction of PHNQs from Evechinus chloroticus sea urchin and their in vitro antioxidant, anti-bacterial and in silico anti-inflammatory activities. *LWT* **2020**, *131*, 109817. [CrossRef]

86. Hou, Y.; Carne, A.; McConnell, M.; Bekhit, A.A.; Mros, S.; Amagase, K.; Bekhit, A.E.A. In vitro antioxidant and antimicrobial activities, and in vivo anti-inflammatory activity of crude and fractionated PHNQs from sea urchin (Evechinus chloroticus). *Food Chem.* **2020**, *316*, 126339. [CrossRef]

87. Brasseur, L.; Hennebert, E.; Fievez, L.; Caulier, G.; Bureau, F.; Tafforeau, L.; Flammang, P.; Gerbaux, P.; Eeckhaut, I. The Roles of Spinochromes in Four Shallow Water Tropical Sea Urchins and Their Potential as Bioactive Pharmacological Agents. *Mar. Drugs* **2017**, *15*, 179. [CrossRef] [PubMed]

88. Niu, H.; Wang, X.; Wang, T.; Qin, L.; Sun, L.; Zhu, B. In vitro anti-inflammation and immune-modulating activities of pigment from spines and shells of sea urchin (*Strongylocentrotus nudus*). *J. Chin. Institue Food Sci. Technol.* **2016**, *16*, 39–43.

89. Salem, Y.B.; Amri, S.; Hammi, K.M.; Abdelhamid, A.; Cerf, D.L.; Bouraoui, A.; Majdoub, H. Physico-chemical characterization and pharmacological activities of sulfated polysaccharide from sea urchin, Paracentrotus lividus. *Int. J. Biol. Macromol.* **2017**, *97*, 8–15. [CrossRef] [PubMed]

90. Jiao, H.; Shang, X.; Dong, Q.; Wang, S.; Liu, X.; Zheng, H.; Lu, X. Polysaccharide Constituents of Three Types of Sea Urchin Shells and Their Anti-Inflammatory Activities. *Mar. Drugs* **2015**, *13*, 5882–5900. [CrossRef]

91. Han, R.; Blencke, H.M.; Cheng, H.; Li, C. The antimicrobial effect of CEN1HC-Br against Propionibacterium acnes and its therapeutic and anti-inflammatory effects on acne vulgaris. *Peptides* **2018**, *99*, 36–43. [CrossRef]

92. Björn, C.; Håkansson, J.; Myhrman, E.; Sjöstrand, V.; Haug, T.; Lindgren, K.; Blencke, H.-M.; Stensvåg, K.; Mahlapuu, M. Anti-infectious and anti-inflammatory effects of peptide fragments sequentially derived from the antimicrobial peptide centrocin 1 isolated from the green sea urchin, Strongylocentrotus droebachiensis. *AMB Express* **2012**, *2*, 67. [CrossRef]

93. Kim, A.T.; Kim, D.-O. Anti-inflammatory effects of vanadium-binding protein from Halocynthia roretzi in LPS-stimulated RAW264.7 macrophages through NF-κB and MAPK pathways. *Int. J. Biol. Macromol.* **2019**, *133*, 732–738. [CrossRef] [PubMed]

94. Francis, P.; Chakraborty, K. An anti-inflammatory salmachroman from the sea urchin Salmacis bicolor: A prospective duel inhibitor of cyclooxygenase-2 and 5-lipoxygenase. *Nat. Prod. Res.* **2021**, *35*, 5102–5111. [CrossRef] [PubMed]

95. Francis, P.; Chakraborty, K. Anti-inflammatory polyoxygenated furanocembranoids, salmacembranes A–B from the sea urchin Salmacis bicolor attenuate pro-inflammatory cyclooxygenases and lipoxygenase. *Med. Chem. Res.* **2020**, *29*, 2066–2076. [CrossRef]

96. Francis, P.; Chakraborty, K. Antioxidant and anti-inflammatory cembrane-type diterpenoid from Echinoidea sea urchin Stomopneustes variolaris attenuates pro-inflammatory 5-lipoxygenase. *Med. Chem. Res.* **2020**, *29*, 656–664. [CrossRef]

97. Chakraborty, K.; Francis, P. Stomopneulactone D from long-spined sea urchin Stomopneustes variolaris: Anti-inflammatory macrocylic lactone attenuates cyclooxygenase-2 expression in lipopolysaccharide-activated macrophages. *Bioorg. Chem.* **2020**, *103*, 104140. [CrossRef]

98. Francis, P.; Chakraborty, K. Stomopnolides A-B from echinoidea sea urchin Stomopneustes variolaris: Prospective natural anti-inflammatory leads attenuate pro-inflammatory 5-lipoxygenase. *Nat. Prod. Res.* **2021**, *35*, 4235–4247. [CrossRef]

99. Shikov, A.N.; Laakso, I.; Pozharitskaya, O.N.; Seppänen-Laakso, T.; Krishtopina, A.S.; Makarova, M.N.; Vuorela, H.; Makarov, V. Chemical Profiling and Bioactivity of Body Wall Lipids from Strongylocentrotus droebachiensis. *Mar. Drugs* **2017**, *15*, 365. [CrossRef]

100. Lee, D.S.; Cui, X.; Ko, W.; Kim, K.S.; Kim, I.C.; Yim, J.H.; An, R.B.; Kim, Y.C.; Oh, H. A new sulfonic acid derivative, (Z)-4-methylundeca-1,9-diene-6-sulfonic acid, isolated from the cold water sea urchin inhibits inflammatory responses through JNK/p38 MAPK and NF-κB inactivation in RAW 264.7. *Arch. Pharm. Res.* **2014**, *37*, 983–991. [CrossRef]

101. Shih, J.H.; Tsai, Y.F.; Li, I.H.; Chen, M.H.; Huang, Y.S. Hp-s1 Ganglioside Suppresses Proinflammatory Responses by Inhibiting MyD88-Dependent NF-κB and JNK/p38 MAPK Pathways in Lipopolysaccharide-Stimulated Microglial Cells. *Mar. Drugs* **2020**, *18*, 496. [CrossRef]

102. Castellano, I.; Di Tomo, P.; Di Pietro, N.; Mandatori, D.; Pipino, C.; Formoso, G.; Napolitano, A.; Palumbo, A.; Pandolfi, A. Anti-Inflammatory Activity of Marine Ovothiol A in an In Vitro Model of Endothelial Dysfunction Induced by Hyperglycemia. *Oxidative Med. Cell. Longev.* **2018**, *2018*, 2087373. [CrossRef]

103. Chamika, W.A.S.; Ho, T.C.; Roy, V.C.; Kiddane, A.T.; Park, J.-S.; Kim, G.-D.; Chun, B.-S. In vitro characterization of bioactive compounds extracted from sea urchin (*Stomopneustes variolaris*) using green and conventional techniques. *Food Chem.* **2021**, *361*, 129866. [CrossRef] [PubMed]

104. Sadek, S.A.; Hassanein, S.S.; Mohamed, A.S.; Soliman, A.M.; Fahmy, S.R. Echinochrome pigment extracted from sea urchin suppress the bacterial activity, inflammation, nociception, and oxidative stress resulted in the inhibition of renal injury in septic rats. *J. Food Biochem.* **2022**, *46*, e13729. [CrossRef] [PubMed]

105. Xia, J.-M.; Miao, Z.; Xie, C.-L.; Zhang, J.-W.; Yang, X.-W. Chemical Constituents and Bioactivities of Starfishes: An Update. *Chem. Biodivers.* **2020**, *17*, e1900638. [CrossRef]

106. Dong, G.; Xu, T.; Yang, B.; Lin, X.; Zhou, X.; Yang, X.; Liu, Y. Chemical constituents and bioactivities of starfish. *Chem. Biodivers.* **2011**, *8*, 740–791. [CrossRef] [PubMed]

107. Thao, N.P.; Cuong, N.X.; Luyen, B.T.; Thanh, N.V.; Nhiem, N.X.; Koh, Y.S.; Ly, B.M.; Nam, N.H.; Kiem, P.V.; Minh, C.V.; et al. Anti-inflammatory asterosaponins from the starfish Astropecten monacanthus. *J. Nat. Prod.* **2013**, *76*, 1764–1770. [CrossRef]

108. Chaiwat, M.; Seok Hyeon, G.; Il-shik, S.; SangGuan, Y.; Dae-ok, K.; SeokBeom, K. Anti-Inflammatory Effect of Asterias amurensis Fatty Acids through NF-κB and MAPK Pathways against LPS-Stimulated RAW264.7 Cells. *J. Microbiol. Biotechnol.* **2018**, *28*, 1635–1644.

109. Pereira, D.M.; Correia-da-Silva, G.; Valentao, P.; Teixeira, N.; Andrade, P.B. Anti-inflammatory effect of unsaturated fatty acids and Ergosta-7,22-dien-3-ol from Marthasterias glacialis: Prevention of CHOP-mediated ER-stress and NF-kappaB activation. *PLoS ONE* **2014**, *9*, e88341. [CrossRef]

110. Thao, N.P.; Luyen, B.T.; Koo, J.E.; Kim, S.; Koh, Y.S.; Cuong, N.X.; Nam, N.H.; Van Kiem, P.; Kim, Y.H.; Van Minh, C. Anti-inflammatory components of the Vietnamese starfish Protoreaster nodosus. *Biol. Res.* **2015**, *48*, 12. [CrossRef]

111. Thao, N.P.; Cuong, N.X.; Luyen, B.T.; Quang, T.H.; Hanh, T.T.; Kim, S.; Koh, Y.S.; Nam, N.H.; Van Kiem, P.; Van Minh, C.; et al. Anti-inflammatory components of the starfish Astropecten polyacanthus. *Mar. Drugs* **2013**, *11*, 2917–2926. [CrossRef]

112. Malyarenko, T.V.; Kicha, A.A.; Kalinovsky, A.I.; Ivanchina, N.V.; Popov, R.S.; Pislyagin, E.A.; Menchinskaya, E.S.; Padmakumar, K.P.; Stonik, V.A. Four New Steroidal Glycosides, Protolinckiosides A—D, from the Starfish Protoreaster lincki. *Chem. Biodivers.* **2016**, *13*, 998–1007. [CrossRef]

113. Malyarenko, T.V.; Kharchenko, S.D.; Kicha, A.A.; Ivanchina, N.V.; Dmitrenok, P.S.; Chingizova, E.A.; Pislyagin, E.A.; Evtushenko, E.V.; Antokhina, T.I.; Minh, C.V.; et al. Anthenosides L-U, Steroidal Glycosides with Unusual Structural Features from the Starfish Anthenea aspera. *J. Nat. Prod.* **2016**, *79*, 3047–3056. [CrossRef]

114. Kicha, A.A.; Kalinovsky, A.I.; Ivanchina, N.V.; Malyarenko, T.V.; Dmitrenok, P.S.; Kuzmich, A.S.; Sokolova, E.V.; Stonik, V.A. Furostane Series Asterosaponins and Other Unusual Steroid Oligoglycosides from the Tropical Starfish Pentaceraster regulus. *J. Nat. Prod.* **2017**, *80*, 2761–2770. [CrossRef] [PubMed]

115. Vien, L.T.; Hanh, T.T.; Huong, P.T.; Dang, N.H.; Thanh, N.V.; Lyakhova, E.; Cuong, N.X.; Nam, N.H.; Kiem, P.V.; Kicha, A.; et al. Pyrrole Oligoglycosides from the Starfish Acanthaster planci Suppress Lipopolysaccharide-Induced Nitric Oxide Production in RAW264.7 Macrophages. *Chem. Pharm. Bull.* **2016**, *64*, 1654–1657. [CrossRef] [PubMed]

116. Thao, N.P.; Dat, L.D.; Ngoc, N.T.; Tu, V.A.; Hanh, T.T.; Huong, P.T.; Nhiem, N.X.; Tai, B.H.; Cuong, N.X.; Nam, N.H.; et al. Pyrrole and furan oligoglycosides from the starfish Asterina batheri and their inhibitory effect on the production of pro-inflammatory cytokines in lipopolysaccharide-stimulated bone marrow-derived dendritic cells. *Bioorg. Med. Chem. Lett.* **2013**, *23*, 1823–1827. [CrossRef] [PubMed]

117. Xia, X. Bioinformatics and Drug Discovery. *Curr. Top. Med. Chem.* **2017**, *17*, 1709–1726. [CrossRef]

118. Liu, R.; Li, X.; Lam, K.S. Combinatorial chemistry in drug discovery. *Curr. Opin. Chem. Biol.* **2017**, *38*, 117–126. [CrossRef]

119. Sliwoski, G.; Kothiwale, S.; Meiler, J.; Lowe, E.W., Jr. Computational methods in drug discovery. *Pharmacol. Rev.* **2014**, *66*, 334–395. [CrossRef]

120. Newman, D.J.; Cragg, G.M. Natural Products as Sources of New Drugs over the Nearly Four Decades from 01/1981 to 09/2019. *J. Nat. Prod.* **2020**, *83*, 770–803. [CrossRef]

121. Mayer, A.M.S.; Rodríguez, A.D.; Taglialatela-Scafati, O.; Fusetani, N. Marine Pharmacology in 2009–2011: Marine Compounds with Antibacterial, Antidiabetic, Antifungal, Anti-Inflammatory, Antiprotozoal, Antituberculosis, and Antiviral Activities; Affecting the Immune and Nervous Systems, and other Miscellaneous Mechanisms of Action. *Mar. Drugs* **2013**, *11*, 2510–2573.

122. Villa, F.A.; Gerwick, L. Marine natural product drug discovery: Leads for treatment of inflammation, cancer, infections, and neurological disorders. *Immunopharmacol. Immunotoxicol.* **2010**, *32*, 228–237. [CrossRef]

123. Blunt, J.W.; Copp, B.R.; Keyzers, R.A.; Munro, M.H.G.; Prinsep, M.R. Marine natural products. *Nat. Prod. Rep.* **2015**, *32*, 116–211. [CrossRef] [PubMed]

124. Jekielek, K.; Le, H.; Wu, A.; Newman, D.; Glaser, K.; Mayer, A. The Marine Pharmacology and Pharmaceuticals Pipeline in 2020. *FASEB J.* **2021**, *35*. [CrossRef]

125. Saeed, A.F.U.H.; Su, J.; Ouyang, S. Marine-derived drugs: Recent advances in cancer therapy and immune signaling. *Biomed. Pharmacother.* **2021**, *134*, 111091. [CrossRef] [PubMed]

126. Ruiz-Torres, V.; Encinar, J.A.; Herranz-López, M.; Pérez-Sánchez, A.; Galiano, V.; Barrajón-Catalán, E.; Micol, V. An Updated Review on Marine Anticancer Compounds: The Use of Virtual Screening for the Discovery of Small-Molecule Cancer Drugs. *Molecules* **2017**, *22*, 1037. [CrossRef]

127. Vasarri, M.; Degl'Innocenti, D. Antioxidant and Anti-Inflammatory Agents from the Sea: A Molecular Treasure for New Potential Drugs. *Mar. Drugs* **2022**, *20*, 132. [CrossRef]

128. Bilal, M.; Nunes, L.V.; Duarte, M.T.S.; Ferreira, L.F.R.; Soriano, R.N.; Iqbal, H.M.N. Exploitation of Marine-Derived Robust Biological Molecules to Manage Inflammatory Bowel Disease. *Mar. Drugs* **2021**, *19*, 196. [CrossRef]

129. Ghareeb, M.A.; Tammam, M.A.; El-Demerdash, A.; Atanasov, A.G. Insights about clinically approved and Preclinically investigated marine natural products. *Curr. Res. Biotechnol.* **2020**, *2*, 88–102. [CrossRef]

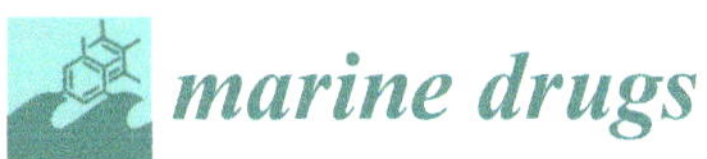 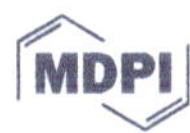

Review

Phytochemical and Potential Properties of Seaweeds and Their Recent Applications: A Review

Hossam S. El-Beltagi [1,2,*], Amal A. Mohamed [3,4,*], Heba I. Mohamed [5,*], Khaled M. A. Ramadan [6,7], Aminah A. Barqawi [3] and Abdallah Tageldein Mansour [8,9]

[1] Agricultural Biotechnology Department, College of Agriculture and Food Sciences, King Faisal University, Al-Ahsa 31982, Saudi Arabia
[2] Biochemistry Department, Faculty of Agriculture, Cairo University, Giza 12613, Egypt
[3] Chemistry Department, Al-Leith University College, Umm Al-Qura University, Makkah 24831, Saudi Arabia; aabbarqawi@uqu.edu.sa
[4] Plant Biochemistry Department, National Research Centre, Cairo 12622, Egypt
[5] Biological and Geological Science Department, Faculty of Education, Ain Shams University, Cairo 11757, Egypt
[6] Central Laboratories, Department of Chemistry, King Faisal University, Al-Ahsa 31982, Saudi Arabia; kramadan@kfu.edu.sa
[7] Biochemistry Department, Faculty of Agriculture, Ain Shams University, Cairo 11566, Egypt
[8] Animal and Fish Production Department, College of Agricultural and Food Sciences, King Faisal University, Al-Ahsa 31982, Saudi Arabia; amansour@kfu.edu.sa
[9] Fish and Animal Production Department, Faculty of Agriculture (Saba Basha), Alexandria University, Alexandria 21531, Egypt
* Correspondence: helbeltagi@kfu.edu.sa (H.S.E.-B.); aaaydeyaa@uqu.edu.sa (A.A.M.); hebaibrahim79@gmail.com (H.I.M.)

Citation: El-Beltagi, H.S.; Mohamed, A.A.; Mohamed, H.I.; Ramadan, K.M.A.; Barqawi, A.A.; Mansour, A.T. Phytochemical and Potential Properties of Seaweeds and Their Recent Applications: A Review. *Mar. Drugs* **2022**, *20*, 342. https://doi.org/10.3390/md20060342

Academic Editors: Donatella Degl'Innocenti and Marzia Vasarri

Received: 11 April 2022
Accepted: 21 May 2022
Published: 24 May 2022

Publisher's Note: MDPI stays neutral with regard to jurisdictional claims in published maps and institutional affiliations.

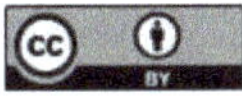

Abstract: Since ancient times, seaweeds have been employed as source of highly bioactive secondary metabolites that could act as key medicinal components. Furthermore, research into the biological activity of certain seaweed compounds has progressed significantly, with an emphasis on their composition and application for human and animal nutrition. Seaweeds have many uses: they are consumed as fodder, and have been used in medicines, cosmetics, energy, fertilizers, and industrial agar and alginate biosynthesis. The beneficial effects of seaweed are mostly due to the presence of minerals, vitamins, phenols, polysaccharides, and sterols, as well as several other bioactive compounds. These compounds seem to have antioxidant, anti-inflammatory, anti-cancer, antimicrobial, and anti-diabetic activities. Recent advances and limitations for seaweed bioactive as a nutraceutical in terms of bioavailability are explored in order to better comprehend their therapeutic development. To further understand the mechanism of action of seaweed chemicals, more research is needed as is an investigation into their potential usage in pharmaceutical companies and other applications, with the ultimate objective of developing sustainable and healthier products. The objective of this review is to collect information about the role of seaweeds on nutritional, pharmacological, industrial, and biochemical applications, as well as their impact on human health.

Keywords: antioxidant activity; functional foods; health benefits; seaweeds; secondary metabolites

1. Introduction

Seaweeds have received lot of attention in recent years because of their incredible potential. Seaweeds are essential nutritional sources and traditional medicine components [1]. Marine macroalgae, sometimes known as seaweeds, are microscopic, multicellular, photosynthetic eukaryotic creatures. Based on their coloration and depending on their taxonomic classification, they can be classified into three groups: Rhodophyta (red), Phaeophyceae (brown), and Chlorophyta (green). The global variety of all algae (micro and macro) is estimated to consist of over 164,000 species with roughly 9800 of them being seaweeds, just 0.17% of which have been domesticated for commercial exploitation [2]. In recent years, seaweed has gained in popularity, making it a more versatile food item that may be used directly or indirectly in preparation of dishes or beverages [3]. Many types of seaweed are edible, they provide the body with a different variety of vitamins and critical minerals (including iodine) when consumed as food, and some are also high in protein and polysaccharides [4].

Seaweeds are now used in several industrial products as raw materials such as agar, algin, and carrageenan, but they are still widely consumed as food in several nations [5]. Seaweeds are frequently subjected to harsh environmental conditions with no visible damage; as a result, the seaweed generates a wide variety of metabolites (xanthophylls, tocopherols, and polysaccharides) to defend itself from biotic and abiotic factors such as herbivory or mechanical aggression at sea [6]. Please note that the content and diversity of seaweed metabolites are influenced by abiotic and biotic factors such as species, life stage, nutrient enrichment, reproductive status, light intensity exposure, salinity, phylogenetic diversity, herbivory intensity, and time of collection; thus, fully exploiting algal diversity and complexity necessitates knowledge of environmental impacts as well as a thorough understanding of biological and biochemical variability [7,8].

Seaweeds and their products are particularly low in calories but high in vitamins A, B, B2, and C, minerals, and chelated micro-minerals (selenium, chromium, nickel, and arsenic), as well as polyunsaturated fatty acids, bioactive metabolites, and amino acids [9]. Although current research revealed that the amount of specific secondary metabolites dictates the effective bioactive potential of seaweeds, phenolic molecules are prevalent among these secondary metabolites [10]. Furthermore, integrating seaweed into one's daily diet has been linked to a lower risk of a range of disorders, including digestive health and chronic diseases such as diabetes, cancer, or cardiovascular disease, according to research mentioned by [11]. As a result, incorporating seaweed components into the production of novel natural drugs is one of the goals of marine pharmaceuticals, a new discipline of pharmacology that has evolved in recent decades.

The $4.7 billion worldwide algae products market is predicted to increase at a compound yearly growth rate of 6.3% to $6.4 billion by 2026. North America has the highest proportion of the algae market [6]. Functional and nutritional attributes, as well as the potential sustainability benefits of algae, are driving demand and positioning it as a promising food of the future. The potential uses of different algae are numerous: generation of energy [12], the biodegradation of urban, industrial and agricultural wastewaters [13,14], the production of biofuels [15], the exclusion of carbon dioxide from gaseous emissions via algae biofixation [16], the manufacturing of ethanol or methane, animal feeds [17], raw material for thermal treatment [18], organic fertilizer or biofertilizer in farming [17]. The high protein content and health advantages have fueled an interest in foods derived from entire algae biomass [19]. Algae can be used as functional ingredients to boost food's nutritional value [20]. In cosmeceuticals, marine algae have received a lot of interest [21]. Seaweeds are one of the most abundant and harmless marine resources, with little cytotoxicity effects on people. Marine algae are high in bioactive compounds, which have been demonstrated to have significant skin advantages, especially in the treatment of rashes, pigmentation, aging, and cancer [22]. The use of algal bioactive components in cosmeceuticals is growing quickly since they contain natural extracts that are deemed harmless, resulting in fewer adverse effects on humans. Marine algae were used as a medicine in ancient times to treat skin problems such as atopic dermatitis and matrix metalloproteinase (MMP)-related sickness [22]. In summary, marine algae represent a promising resource for cosmeceutical production.

This review aimed to study the bioactive compounds in seaweeds and the role of these compounds as antioxidants, anti-inflammatory, anti-cancer, antimicrobial and anti-diabetic activities.

2. Seaweed Resources

The word "seaweed" has no taxonomic importance; rather, it is a popular term for the common large marine algae.

2.1. Brown Seaweeds

Phaeophyceae have not been well investigated, despite the fact that they have been shown to offer several health benefits. Fucoxanthin (Fuco), the principal marine carotenoid (Car), is a commercially important component of brown seaweeds, in addition to sodium alginate. Fuco contains anti-inflammatory properties. The presence of the xanthophyll pigment fucoxanthin, which is higher than chlorophyll-a, chlorophyll-c, -carotene, and other xanthophylls, gives these seaweeds their brown color [23]. Because of its bigger size and ease of collecting, brown seaweed is used in animal feed more often than other algae species. Brown algae are the largest seaweeds, with some species reaching up to 35–45 m in length and a wide range of shapes. *Ascophyllum*, *Laminaria*, *Saccharina*, *Macrocystis*, *Nereocystis*, and *Sargassum* are the most prevalent genera. Sargassum as a member of brown seaweeds is low in protein, but high in carbs and easily accessible minerals. They are high in beta-carotene and vitamins, and they are free of anti-nutrients [24].

2.2. Red Seaweeds

These algae are red because of the pigments phycoerythrin and phycocyanin. The walls are made of carrageenan and cellulose agar. Both of these polysaccharides with a lengthy chain are commonly employed in the industry. Coralline algae, which secrete calcium carbonate on the surface of their cells, are an important category of red algae. *Chondrus*, *Porphyra*, *Pyropia*, and *Palmaria* are some of the most common red algae genera. The antioxidant activity of Phaeophyta (brown seaweeds) is higher than that of green and red algae [25].

2.3. Green Seaweeds

The majority of the species are aquatic, living in both freshwater and marine habitats. The green color of these algae is due to chlorophyll-a or chlorophyll-b. Some of them are terrestrial, meaning they grow in soil, trees, or rocks. Ulva is one of the most common green seaweeds. *Ulva*, *Cladophora*, *Enteromorpha*, and *Chaetomorpha* are the most common genera. Green algae thrive in regions with lots of light, including shallow waterways and tide pools. *Ulva* sp. has a high protein content (typically > 15%) and a low energy content and is abundant in both soluble and insoluble dietary fiber (glucans) [26]. The main types of seaweeds are shown in Figure 1.

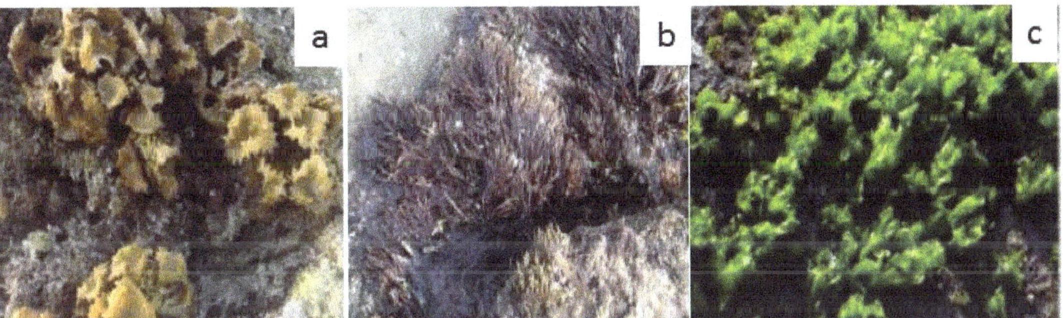

Figure 1. Three example species of brown (a) red (b) and green (c) seaweeds. Adapted from ref. [14] obtained from mdpi journals.

3. Bioactive Compounds

The chemical composition of algae varies depending on the species, cultivation location, meteorological conditions, and harvesting period. Because of the broad diversity of compounds produced by seaweeds, they are currently considered to be prospective organisms for contributing new physiologically active chemicals for the production of novel food (nutraceutical), cosmetic (cosmeceutical), and medical compounds. Polyphenolic compounds, carotenoids, minerals, vitamins, phlorotannins, peptides, tocotrienols, proteins, tocopherols, and carbohydrates (polysaccharides) are considered to be a great variety of bioactive compounds (Figure 2).

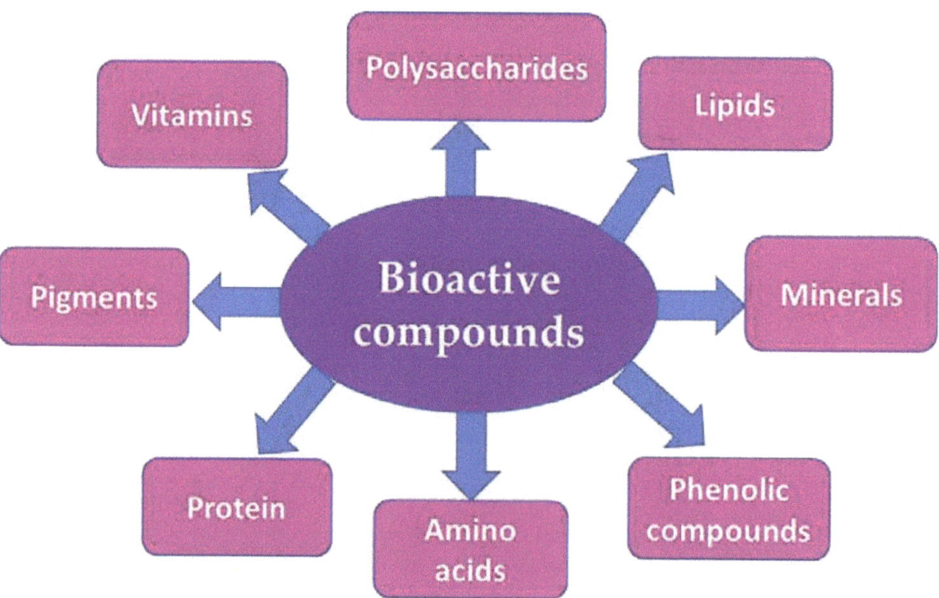

Figure 2. Main bioactive compounds from marine seaweeds.

3.1. Polysaccharides

Seaweeds have a significant carbohydrate component in their cell membranes, or these polysaccharides are unique to every variety from algae: Brown alginate contains fucoidan; green Ulvan or red agar contains carrageenan. Polysaccharides are becoming increasingly popular as a result of their physicochemical properties [27]. Polysaccharides are biopolymers created from natural resources that have developed as a sustainable and environmentally friendly alternative to typical polymers and plastics. They are also known as an energy store and structural molecules in a variety of species, including plants and marine organisms. Polysaccharides are the major macromolecule in seaweed, accounting for more than 80% of its weight. Polysaccharides are classified into two types based on where they are found in seaweeds: cell-membrane polysaccharides or storage polysaccharides. With the exception of accumulating carbohydrates found in cell plastids, the majority of seaweed polysaccharides are cell-membrane polysaccharides. At present, they can be classed as food-grade or non-food-grade polysaccharides, depending on how they are used [28].

3.1.1. Role of Polysaccharides in Medicine

Algal polysaccharides differ from those found in terrestrial plants because they include unique poly-uronides, some of which are pyruvylated, methylated, sulfated, or acetylated. Sulfated polysaccharides including fucan sulfate, ulvan, and carrageenan have received the most interest because of their biological features [29]. Some of polysaccharide's structures are presented in Figure 3. Sulfated polysaccharides (SPS) are found in edible seaweeds such as ulvan (Chlorophyta), fucoidan (Phaeophyta), or carrageenan (Rhodophyta), and have numerous applications in pharmaceutical, nutraceutical, and cosmeceutical sectors. Antioxidant, anticancer, anti-inflammatory, anti-diabetic, anticoagulant, immunomodulatory, or anti-HIV activities have been discovered in SPS. The interaction between polysaccharide or intestinal microbes is widely credited with these actions, indicating functional or therapeutic feature of sulfated polysaccharides [30]. In most circumstances, smaller molecular weight SPS has more antioxidant activity than high molecular weight SPS because proton donor action occurs in cells in low molecular weight SPS. Furthermore, this antioxidant property is vital in preventing generation of free radicals in cell, which prevents oxidative cell wall damage [31]. The antigenotoxic property of alginate oligosaccharide in form of nanocomposites extracted from brown alga has received significant attention [32]. Table 1 shows some of the activities and qualities of polysaccharides from seaweeds that are useful as antioxidants and anticancer agents.

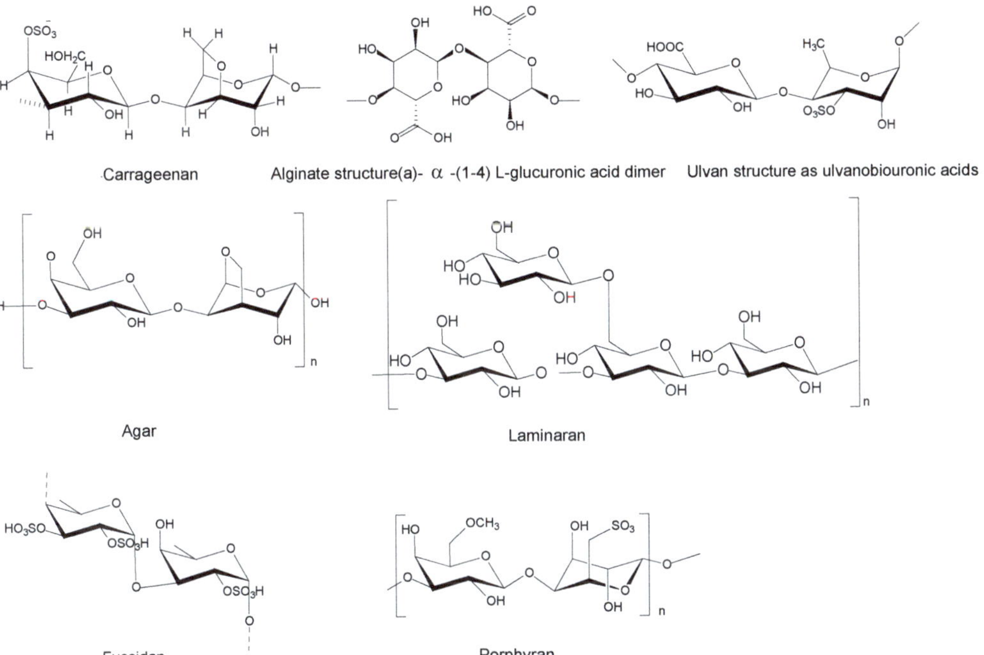

Figure 3. Chemical structures of different types of polysaccharides in seaweeds.

Table 1. Seaweeds polysaccharides and their roles in medicine.

Component	Species	Molecular Weight	Chemical Composition	Doses	Properties/Activities	References
Carrageenan	*Tribonema minus*	197 kDa	Heteropolysaccharide composed mainly of galactose	250 μg mL^{-1}	Anticancer activity	[33]
Porphyran	*Chondrus armatus*	f 9.7–34.6 kDa	Mainly composed of 3,6-anhydro-L-galactose	327.3 μg mL^{-1}	Anticancer activity	[34]
Fucoidans	*Cladosiphon okamuranus*	75.0 kDa	5.01 mg mL^{-1} of l-fucose, 2.02 mg mL^{-1} of uronic acids and 1.65 ppm of sulfate	1 mg mL^{-1}	Anticancer activities	[35]
	Fucus vesiculosus	-	Fucose and Xylose	-	Antioxidant activity	[36]
Agar	*Gelidium amansii*	1.21 × 104 Da and 1.85 × 105 Da	(1–4)-linked 3,6-anhydro-α-L-galactose alternating with (1–3)-linked β-D-galactopyranose	25.6 mg L^{-1}	Antioxidant activity	[37]
Laminaran	*Laminaria digitata*	-	β-(1,3)-glucan	10 μg mL^{-1}	Antioxidant protection	[38]
Ulvan	*Ulva pertusa*	83.1 from 143.2 kDa	Rhamnose, and xylose	500 mg kg^{-1}	Antioxidant and antihyperlipidemic activity	[39]
		143.47 kDa	Rhamnose and xylose	1.5 mg mL^{-1}	Antioxidant Activity	[40]

Carrageenans are polysaccharides present in cell walls of red algae that are classified into three categories based on their sulfation level: iota, kappa, or lambda [41]. Carrageenans, galactan, or xylomannan sulfates discovered in red seaweeds have antimicrobial effects that prevent viruses from interacting with cells by inhibiting the formation of structurally similar complexes [42]. Carrageenans derived from Hypnea spp. (including green alga *Ulva lactuca*) have antioxidant and antiviral characteristics, as well as strong hypocholesterolemic capabilities, by lowering cholesterol or sodium uptake whereas raising potassium absorption [43]. Agar is polysaccharide made up of agaropectin or agarose, which are both derived from red seaweeds and have structural or functional characteristics that are comparable to carrageenans [41]. Porphyran, a polysaccharide produced from red Porphyra spp., was shown to have anticancer, immunoregulatory, and antioxidant effects [44].

Sulfated polysaccharides such as galactose, glucose, rhamnose, glucuronic acid, or arabinose isolated from the microalgae *Spirulina platensis*, as well as those speculated from red algae *Gracilariopsis lemaneiformis* (i.e., 3,6-anhydro-l-galactose or d-galactose) demonstrated antiviral and antitumor action [44]. Fucoidan polysaccharides, usually manufactured by brown algae, such as *Ascophyllum nodosum, Laminaria japonica, Viz fucusvesiculosus, Fucus evanescens, Sargassum thunbergi,* or *Laminaria cichorioides*, were shown to reduce blood cholesterol levels and deter metabolic syndrome [43]. Antiproliferative, antiviral, anti-peptic, antioxidant, anticanceranti-coagulant, antithrombotic, anti-inflammatory, or antiadhesive characteristics are all found in algae fucoidans. They also have potent anticancer properties or can prevent lung cancer metastasis through hindering matrix metalloproteinases (MMPs) or Vascular Endothelial Growth Factor (VEGF) [45]. Fucoidans may have a synergistic impact on currently used anticancer drugs [46]. To improve the efficacy of existing conventional treatments, these polysaccharides can be added into or mixed with them. *Caulerpa lentilifera, Eucheuma cottonii, Ahnfeltiopsis concinna, Chondrus ocellatus, Sargassum polycystum, Ulva fasciata, Gayralia oxysperma,* or *Sargassum obtusifolium* soluble dietary fibers have been found to prevent metabolic syndrome or lower blood cholesterol levels [43].

Alginate (β-d-mannuronic acid, α-l-guluronic acid, d-guluronic, or d-mannuronic) is non-sulfated polysaccharide isolated from dark brown seaweed *Laminaria digitata* that is commercially accessible (in acid and salt forms) [41]. Alginates isolated from brown have a nutritional function or are beneficial to gut health, donating to water binding, fecal bulking, or reduction in colon transfer time that is an important indicator through colon cancer prevention, according to previous studies [47]. Furthermore, because of their binding nature, alginates alter mineral bioabsorption, aid in maintaining body weight, discourage overweight and obesity, and lower hypertension [41].

3.1.2. Role of Polysaccharides in Food Industry

While the global market for healthy ingredients expands, there is significant interest in the identification of new functional food ingredients from various natural sources [48]. As a result, the prospect of employing algae-derived molecules to create novel functional food products has piqued the interest of many people in recent years. The largest and most often used hydrocolloids from marine algae in the food industry include agars, alginates, and carrageenans, as illustrated in Table 2.

Table 2. Seaweeds polysaccharides and their roles in foods and cosmeceuticals.

Component	Species	Models	Doses	MW	Activity	Results	References
Carrageenan	*Padina tetrastromatic*	Paw edema in rats	20 mg kg^{-1}	25 kDa	Anti-inflammation	COX-2 and iNOS inhibitions	[49]
Fucoidan	*Fucus vesiculosus*	Human malignant melanoma cells	100–400 µg mL^{-1}	60 kDa	Anticancer activity	Inhibit cell proliferation	[50]
		B16 murine melanoma cells	550 µg mL^{-1}	-	Anti-melanogenic	Inhibit tyrosinase and melanin	[51]
Ulvans	*Ulva* sp.	*Human dermal fibroblast*	100 and 500 µg mL^{-1}	4–57 kDa	Anti-aging	Increase hyaluronan production	[52]
Laminaran	*Laminaria japonica*	In vitro	15 mg mL^{-1}	250 kDa	antioxidant activity	ROS scavenging potential	[53]
Fucoidan	*Chnoospora minima*	RAW macrophages	27.82 µg mL^{-1}	60 kDa	Anti-inflammation	Inhibition of LPS-induced NO production, iNOS, COX-2, and PGE2 levels	[54]
Fucoidan	*Sargassum hemiphyllum*	RAW 264.7 macrophage cells	dose-dependent manner	-	Anti-inflammation	Inhibit LPS-induced inflammatory response	[55]
Fucoidan	*Sargassum hemiphyllum*	B16 melanoma cells	dose-dependent manner	-	Anticancer	Activation of caspase-3	[56]

Agar is a type of phycocolloid formed of agarose (a linear polysaccharide) and a heterogeneous combination of smaller molecules (agaropectin). Agar is a widely recommended food additive in the USA and in Europe (E406), and cannot be digested into the gastrointestinal system in humans due to the lack of α/β-agarases [57]. Furthermore, gut bacteria can convert it to d-galactose [58]. At low doses, agar is an excellent gelling agent, capable of forming a brittle, stiff, and thermally reversible gel [59].

Surprisingly, agarose is the primary gelling agent in agar. In this manner, hydrogen bonding between nearby D-galactose and 3,6-anhydro-L-galactose create agar gel along its linear chains of agarose with repeating units. The food sector uses 90% of the agar produced for its gellifying characteristics. It is used as a gelling agent in the culinary, food, and confectionery sectors to produce Asian traditional foods, canned meats, confectionery jellies, and aerated items such as marshmallows, nougat, and toffees [60]. Agar is commonly used as a food additive in the production of dishes that require warming before consumption, such as cake, sausage, roast pig, and bacon [61]. Agar fluid gels can be used to make foams with excellent stability to replace fat in whipped desserts [61].

Alginates, such as agar, are commonly used in the food manufactures for gelling, thickening, stabilizing, and film formation. In contrast to other hydrocolloids, alginates are unique in their cold solubility, allowing the creation of heat/temperature-independent non-melting gels, cold-setting gels, and freeze–thaw-stable gels [62].

Carrageenan is commonly used in dairy products such as cheese and chocolate milk to provide thickening, gelling, stabilizing, and strong protein-binding characteristics [63]. Carrageenan was used in dairy products at low doses due to its exceptional ability to link milk proteins. This hydrocolloid was capable of keeping milk solids suspended and therefore stabilize them. The meat industry is another area where carrageenan (mostly manufactured by Eu-cheuma) is used. It is commonly used in the manufacture of hamburgers, ham, seafood, and poultry preparations, due to its water retention properties. Carrageenan is also found in aqueous gels such jelly, fruit gels, juices, and marmalade [61]. Carrageenans, as cryoprotecting agents, play an important role in the structural and textural stability of frozen foods. Additionally, k-carrageenan was used as a supplementary stabilizer in an ice cream mix [64].

3.1.3. Role of Polysaccharides in Cosmeceuticals

In algal tissues, there are numerous forms of bioactive polysaccharides. These chemicals are often moisturizing and antioxidant substances that are employed in cosmeceuticals as shown in Table 2. They are also commonly employed in emulsions as gelling agents and stabilizers [65]. Agar is a common ingredient in creams, used as an emulsifier and stabilizer, and to control the moisture content in cosmetic products such as hand lotions, deodorants, foundations, exfoliant/scrub, cleansers, shaving creams, anti-aging treatments, facial moisturizer/lotions, liquid soaps, acne treatments, body washes, and face powder [66]. Alginates are commonly used as gelling agents in drugs and cosmetics, as thickeners, protective colloids, or emulsion stabilizers, and are effective for hand gels and lotions, ointment bases, pomades and other hair products, toothpastes, and other products due to their chelating characteristics. Alginates can also be used to make a skin-protecting barrier lotion to avoid dermatitis. This type of cream produces flexible films with increased skin adhesion and is an appropriate component in beauty masks or facial packs [67,68].

Carrageenans are derived from several carrageenophytes, including *Betaphycus gelatinum, Chondrus crispus, Eucheuma denticulatum, Gigartina skottsbergii, Kappaphycus alvarezii, Hypnea musciformis, Mastocarpus stellatus, Mazzaella laminaroides, Sarcothalia crispata*, from the order Gigartinales (Rhodophyta). This phycocolloid is found in dentifrices, lotions, hair products, lotions, medications, sunscreens, shaving creams, shampoos, deodorants sticks, sprays, and foams. Over 20% of carrageenan manufacture is used in the pharmaceutical and cosmetic industries [69].

The usage of laminarin in cosmetics is based on its bioactive qualities rather than its physical characteristics. In terms of use, laminarin is commonly found in anticellulite cosmetics [70]. Fucoidan can be effectively "cooked" out of edible seaweed by heating it in water for 20–40 min. It appears to lower the strength of the inflammatory process and facilitate speedier tissue repair after injuring or surgical trauma when ingested. As a result, it is recommended for muscle and joint injuries (such as sports injuries), falls, bruises, deep wounds, and surgery [71]. These sulfated polysaccharides are gaining popularity due to their numerous bioactivities, which include anticoagulant, antithrombotic, anti-inflammatory, skin protection against ultraviolet radiation, tyrosinase receptor, anticancer, antimicrobial, anti-obesity, antidiabetic, antioxidative, and antihyperlipidemic properties [72,73].

According to an ulvans patent, rhamnose and fucose have synergistic skin protecting and therapeutic benefits against skin aging [74]. The technique of ulvan gel production is complex, involving the development of spherically shaped ulvan molecules in the presence of boric acid and calcium ions [75]. Ulvans have moisturizing, protecting, anticancer, and antioxidative effects in addition to their ability to form gels [76]. The chemical and physicochemical features of ulvan make it an appealing choice for innovative functional and biologically useful polymers in the pharmaceutical, cosmeceutical, agriculture, and food industries [75].

3.2. Protein and Amino Acids

Protein content in seaweed varies by species, season, and geographic location, and can be as high as 45% DW. The contents of peptides, proteins, or amino acids in seaweed are affected by seasonal fluctuations and habitat; in general, red algae have larger concentrations (up to 47%) than green algae (around 9 and 26%), while brown algae have low amounts (3–15%) [77]. The difference in the amounts of proteinas and amino acids in some seaweeds are illustrated in Tables 3 and 4. All essential and non-essential amino acids are found in the proteins of the three macroalgae groups [78]. Seaweed protein and bioactive peptides have a variety of health benefits as well as significant antioxidant activity, especially through compounds with low molecular weight compounds that are far secure than produced substances or have less adverse impacts [79,80].

Table 3. Different proteins accumulation of some seaweeds.

Seaweed	Species	Name of the Protein	Protein Yield %	References
Ulva sp.	Green algae	Glycoproteins (GP)	"UvGP-1" (0.54) "UvGP-2 DA"(0.52) "UvGP-2-DS"(1.98)	[81]
Ulva lactuca	Green algae	GP fraction G	ND	[82]
Saccharina japonica	Brown algae	Glycoprotein	0.27	[83]
Solieria filiformis	Red algae	Lectins "SfL-1" "SfL-2"	ND	[84]
Solieria filiformis	Red algae	Lectin "SfL"	ND	[85]
Capsosiphon fulvescens	Green algae	"Cf-hGP"	ND	[86]
Undaria pinnatifida	Brown algae	"UPGP"	ND	[87]

ND: Not detected; SfL: *Solieria filiformis* lectin; Cf-hGP: *Capsosiphon fulvescens* hydrophilic glycoproteins; UPGP: *Undaria pinnatifida* glycoprotein.

Table 4. Amino acid composition accumulation of some seaweeds (g amino acid 100 g^{-1} protein).

No.	Amino Acids (AA)	*Caulerpa lentillifera* (Green Algae) [88]	*Ulva reticulate* (Green Algae) [88]	*Kappaphycus alvarezii* (Red Algae) [89]	*Gracilaria salicornia* (Red Algae) [89]	*Turbinaria ornata* (Brown Algae) [90]	*Durvillaea antarctica* (Brown Algae) [91]
	Essential AA						
1	Threonine	6.38	5.41	2.49	2.25	0.15	5.84
2	Valine	7.03	6.30	2.49	2.20	0.23	9.97
3	Lysine	6.63	6.02	1.51	-	0.20	4.22
4	Isoleucine	5.01	4.23	2.14	1.98	0.18	8.05
5	Leucine	8.00	7.90	2.34	2.16	0.26	15.88
6	Phenylalanine	4.93	5.26	2.11	1.79	0.19	9.97
7	Methionine	-	-	1.69	1.61	0.05	3.89
	Non essential AA						
8	Aspartic	11.56	12.50	3.33	-	0.53	4.17
9	Serine	6.14	6.39	2.68	2.90	0.10	5.38
10	Glutamic	14.39	12.98	11.67	2.79	0.58	17.87
11	Glycine	6.87	6.49	2.97	2.18	0.22	18.36
12	Arginine	7.03	8.65	2.40	2.40	0.19	4.83
13	Histidine	0.65	1.08	1.60	2.29	0.07	2.26
14	Alanine	6.87	8.09	2.93	2.51	0.23	9.57
15	Tyrosine	3.88	3.62	1.81	1.74	0.05	4.45
16	Proline	4.61	5.08	-	-	0.17	7.95
17	Cystin	-	-	-	-	0.00	0.78

Various seaweeds contain amino acids such as valine, leucine, isoleucine, or taurine which have potential biological action as antioxidants [92,93]. Acidic amino acids aspartic acid or glutamic acid is abundant in most seaweed species, and they comprise most essential amino acids [94]. While algal proteins were being thought to consist of threonine, tryptophan, sulfur amino acids (cysteine and methionine), lysine, or histidine-limiting amino acids, their overall levels are larger than in terrestrial plants [95]. Furthermore, amino acids are required for the production of hormones and nitrogenous low molecular weight compounds, both of which are important biologically. Amino acids can be used to help treat some disorders since they have distinct physiological roles. Supplementing with methionine, for example, can help people with multiple sclerosis [96]. Despite the fact that seaweed proteins contain low amounts of some essential amino acids, these seaweeds could be introduced to cereal foods such as pasta to enhance the amino acid composition [97].

Macroalgal species such as *Chlorella* sp., *Dunaliella tertiolecta*, *Aphanizomenon flosaquae* and *Spirulina plantensis*, due to their high protein content or nutritive quality, are often used as human food sources [98]. Endogenous (threonine, serine, aspartic acid, proline, glutamic acid, or glycine) and exogenous (histidine, lysine, isoleucine, methionine, phenylalanine, leucine, valine or threonine) amino acids are abundant in some algae species [43]. Ulva spp. has glutamic or aspartic acid (26–32% amino acid), *Ulva australis* has taurine or histidine, *Himanthalia elongata* (sea spaghetti) *Palmaria palmata* (Dulse) and have a lot of glutamic acid, serin or alanine, and *Sargassum vulgare* has lot of methionine [99]. Several applications of seaweeds protein are illustrated in Table 5.

Table 5. Seaweeds proteins and their roles in medicinal.

Component	Properties/Activities	Seaweed	Doses	Molecular Weight	References
Peptide PPY1	Anti-aging	*Pyropia yezoensis*	250–1000 ng mL^{-1}	532 Da	[100]
Peptides PYP1-5 and porphyra 334	Boost synthesis of elastin	*Porphyra yezoensis* f. *coreana Ueda*	0–200 μM	1622 kDa	[101]
Lactate and progerin	Reduce synthesis, anti-elastase, anti-collagenase	*Alaria esculenta*	-	112 KDa	[102]
Phycobiliproteins	Antioxidant	*Gracilaria gracilis*	0.5–30 mg mL^{-1}	240 KDa	[103]
Deoxygadusol, palythene and usujirene	Antioxidant	*Rhodymenia pseudopalmata*	-	-	[104]
Palythine, palythinol, porphyra-334, asterina-330, shinorine, or usujirene	Antioxidant, antiproliferative	*Palmaria palmate*, *Mastocarpus stellatus*, *Chondrus crispus*	2.0–4.0 mg mL^{-1}	244.24 KDa	[105]
Porphyra-334, shinorine, palythine and asterina-330	Antioxidant; UV-protective effect	*Gracilaria vermiculophylla*	-	346.33 KDa	[106]

3.2.1. Role of Proteins and Amino Acid in Medicine

Furthermore, mycosporine-like amino acids (MAAs) were revealed in a variety of species, most notably Rhodophyta: *Chondrus crispus* spp., *Grateloupia lanceola*, *Porphyra/Pyropia* spp., *Solieria chordalis*, *Asparagopsis armata*, *Palmaria palmata*, *Gracilaria cornea*, Gelidium, or *Curdiea racovit* [106–108]. Phycobiliproteins are made up of phycobilins, which are proteins that are covalently attached to chromophores [43]. Such water-soluble proteins have antioxidant properties and could be used as a natural food colorant [26]. PC, blue-colored phycobiliprotein derived mostly from cyanobacteria Arthrospira spp., or PE (pink-colored protein pigment) derived from cyanobacteria Lyngbya spp., both demonstrated anticancer activity upon A549 lung cancer cells [22]. Glycoproteins were also proteins found in marine algae which are made up from proteins linked to carbohydrates. Rhamnose, galactose, glucose, and mannose make up 36.24% of glycoproteins, with a mole ratio of 38:30:26:6 [109].

Protein concentrations are high in *Rhizoclonium riparium*, *Dictyota caylinica*, *Enteromorpha intestinalis*, *Catenella repens*, *Gelidiella acerosa*, *Polysiphonia mollis*, *Capsosiphon fulvescens*,

Osmundea pinnatifida, *Sphaerococcus coronopifolius*, *Ulva lactuca*, *Gelidium microdon*, *Fucus spiralis*, *Pterocladium capillacea*, or *Ulva compressa* [110]. Anti-aging, antioxidant, anti-tumor, anti-inflammatory or protective qualities of proteins make them valuable in the prevention and treatments of neurological illnesses, DNA replication, gastric ulcers, improve response, molecule transfer, or biochemical reaction catalysis [45]. According to Cicero et al. [111], bioactive peptides can increase biological defenses against oxidative stress and inflammatory illnesses, hence boosting the real frame of nutraceutical and functional meals. As a result, MAAs have wide range of properties, such as ability to act like natural sunscreens, anti-inflammatory, antioxidants or anti-aging agents, skin renewal stimulators, cell proliferation activators, and so on, making it attractive or secure option for cosmetic industries or pharmaceutical [112].

3.2.2. Role of Proteins and Amino Acid in Cosmeceuticals

Because several amino acids are components of the natural moisturizing factor (NMF) in human skin, they are commonly used as moisturizing agents in cosmetic preparations [113,114]. MAA content is higher in the summer and at a mild depth (0–1 m). MAAs have the ability to be used in cosmetic products and uses as ultraviolet protectors and cell proliferation stimulators [115].

Algae protein concentration differs significantly among the different algae groups (brown, red, and green). Brown algae have a lower protein concentration (5–24%) of dry weight, while red and green algae have a greater protein concentration (10–47%) of dry weight [116]. Holdt and Kraan [107] show that protein, peptide, and amino acid concentration, like other bioactive components of algae, is affected by a variety of circumstances, including seasonal change. During the months from February to May, for example, brown algae Saccharina and Laminaria had the highest protein content [107]. A similar trend was observed in red algae species, with a high concentration of protein in the summer and a significant decrease in the winter [116]. Algae proteins are high in glycine, arginine, alanine, and glutamic acid, and they include essential amino acids at amounts comparable to FAO/WHO needs. Lysine and cystine are their limiting amino acids [117]. Taurine, laminin, kainoids, kainic and domoic acids, and several mycosporin-type amino acids are also found in algae [118]. Taurine is involved in several physiological activities in the human body, including immunomodulation, membrane stabilization, ocular development, and nervous system function [119]. Furthermore, kainic and domoic acids play a role in the control of neurophysiological functions [120].

3.3. Fatty Acids

Fatty acids (FAs) are required for all organisms to function normally. FAs are components of plasma membranes that serve as energy storage materials as well as signal molecules that control cell development and differentiation as well as gene expression. Elongation and desaturation can change the structure of FAs [121,122]. The quantity of unsaturated bonds in FA molecules determines their biological effects. Additionally, lipids are essential to transport and absorb fat-soluble vitamins (i.e., A, E, D or K), PUFAs (25–60% of total lipids), glycolipids, phytosterols, phospholipids, or fat-soluble vitamins are all found in low concentrations (1–5% of dry weight) in seaweed lipids (vitamin A, D, E or K, carotenoids) [1]. Several seaweeds have a greater total lipid concentration above 10% of dry weight; however, 50% of these lipids are in the form of extractable fatty acids in the brown alga *Spatoglossum macrodontum*. In addition, *S. macrodontum* showed the maximum fatty acid concentration (57.40 mg g^{-1} DW) and a fatty acid profile rich in saturated fatty acids with a higher concentration of C18:1, making it an excellent biofuel feedstock. Similarly, the green seaweed *Derbesia tenuissima* possesses significant quantities of fatty acids (39.58 mg g1 DW), but with a greater amount of PUFA (n-3) (31% lipid) that can be used as nutraceuticals or fish oil substitutes [123]. The lipid algae concentration is low (1–5%), with neutral lipids and glycolipids dominating. Because algae generate long-chain polyunsaturated fatty acids, including eicosapentaenoic acid (EPA) and docosahexaenoic acid (DHA), the amount of essential fatty acids in algae is greater than in terrestrial plants [124]. In general, red algae have higher concentrations of EPA, palmitic acid, oleic acid, and arachidonic acid than brown algae, which have greater amounts of oleic acid, linoleic acid, and α-linolenic acid but lower amounts of EPA. Green algae have more linoleic acid and α-linolenic acid, as well as palmitic, oleic, and DHA [125]. Both red and brown algae contain omega-3 and omega-6 fatty acids [126]. The different in the amounts of lipid in different seaweeds are illustrated in Table 6.

Table 6. Lipids accumulation of some seaweeds.

Seaweed	Species	Lipids g/100 g	EPA (%)	DHA (%)	References
Caulerpa lentillifera	Green algae	1.11 ± 0.05	0.86	-	[127]
Codium fragile	Green algae	1.5 ± 0.0	2.10 ± 0.00	-	[128]
Ulva lactuca	Green algae	1.27 ± 0.11	0.87 ± 0.16	0.8 ± 0.01	[129]
Agarophyton chilense	Red algae	1.3 ± 0.0	1.3 ± 0.01	-	[128]
Porphyra/Pyropia spp. (China)	Red algae	1.0 ± 0.2	10.4 ± 7.46	-	[128]
Ascophyllum nodosum	Brown algae	3.62 ± 0.17	7.24 ± 0.08	-	[130]
Bifurcaria bifurcata	Brown algae	6.54 ± 0.27	4.09 ± 0.08	11.10 ± 1.13	[130]
Durvillaea antarctica	Brown algae	0.8 ± 0.1	4.95 ± 0.11	1.66 ± 0.02	[129]
Fucus vesiculosus	Brown algae	3.75 ± 0.20	9.94 ± 0.14	-	[130]
Himanthalia elongata	Brown algae	<1.5	7.45	-	[131]
Laminaria spp.	Brown algae	1.0 ± 0.3	16.2 ± 8.9	-	[132]
Macrocystis pyrifera	Brown algae	0.7 ± 0.1	0.47 ± 0.01	-	[128]
Sargassum fusiforme	Brown algae	1.4 ± 0.1	42.4 ± 11.9	-	[132]
Undaria pinnatifida	Brown algae	4.5 ± 0.7	413.2 ± 0.66	-	[132]

EPA: eicosapentaenoic acid; DHA: docosahexaenoic acid.

3.3.1. Role of Fatty Acids in Medicine

There is an increasing need to assess new food sources that do not involve overexploitation of terrestrial ecosystems [133]. Seaweeds have a lipid output of 0.61% to 4.15% dry weight (DW) on average. Some seaweed species, on the other hand, can have greater levels since they are a strong source of unsaturated fatty acids. Although seaweed has lower lipid content than marine fish, their abundance in coastal areas makes it a viable source of functional lipid. Recent studies indicated that the levels of total lipid (TL) or omega-polyunsaturated fatty acids in seaweeds vary seasonally, reaching up to 15% TL per DW or more than 40% omega-3 PUFAs per total fatty acids [134]. Brown seaweed lipids, on the other hand, contain up to 5% fucoxanthin. Anti-obesity activities of fucoxanthin have been demonstrated. It also reduces insulin resistance and lowers blood glucose levels significantly. Brown seaweed lipids are found in brown seaweed, according to a study. Excess fat builds up in abdomen white adipose tissue (WAT) is dramatically decreased, or glucose levels are regained to average limits in obesity/diabetes model mice due to presence of fucoxanthin in lipids [135].

On the other hand, the group of lipid bioactive chemicals known as sterols is another appealing lipid bioactive substance found in marine sources. Sterols extracted from macro- or microalgae, as well as other marine invertebrates, were researched extensively by [136]. Previously, it was discovered that sterols and several of their derivatives have a key role in decreasing low-density lipoproteins (LDL) cholesterol levels in vivo. Anti-inflammatory and antiaterogenic action are two further bioactivities linked to sterols. Phytosterols (C28 and C29 sterols) are also key precursors of a wide range of chemicals, including vitamins. Ergosterol, for example, is a precursor to vitamin D2 and cortisone [137].

Omega-3 (eicosapentaenoic acid, docosahexanoic acid, stearidonic acid, -linolenic acid) and omega-6 (arachidonic acid, -linoleic acid, -linoleic acid) are the most common polyunsaturated fatty acids (PUFAs) [1]. Essential fatty acids (EFAs) are nutraceuticals that are combined with nutritional supplements or used as part of healthy food [41]. Food and Drug Administration (FDA) declared in 2004 which foods including PUFA omega-3 substances are medicinally essential, as they provide therapeutic properties byregulating blood pressure, membrane fluidity, or blood clotting; (ii) lowering risk of cardiovascular disease, osteoporosis, or diabetes; (iii) correcting brain or nervous system development and function [138]. Marine algae were found to have elevated high levels from PUFAs (α-linolenic acid, γ-linoleic, α-linoleic acid, stearidonic acid, arachidonic acid, and icosapentaenoic acid) [1]. Moreover, a previous study asserted that green seaweeds such as *Ulva pertusa* possess a high concentration of hexadecatetraenoic, oleic, and palmitic acids [139]. Additionally, *Undaria pinnatifida* contains significant levels of eicosapentaenoic acid, docosahexanoic acid, and monounsaturated fatty acids (C12:1 (lauroleic acid), C14:1 (myristoleic acid), C16:1 (palmitoleic acid), C17:1 (cis-10-heptadecenoic acid), and C18:1 (cis-10-hepta (oleic acid) [140].

Upwards of 200 phytosterols (662–2320 mg/g dry weight) were discovered through marine algae. Phytosterol derivatives are abundant in brown algae such as *Laminaria japonica*, *Agarum cribosum*, or *Undaria pinnatifida* (for example, fucosterol, which accounts for 83–97 percent of total phytosterol content) [141,142]. Phospholipids in seaweed contain about 10–20% total lipids which seem to be more resistant to oxidation and contain elevated concentration from FAs such as eicosapentaenoic or docosahexanoic acid [43]. Glycolipids make up more than half of all algal material and are characterized by high levels of n-3 PUFAs (e.g., monogalactosyldiacylglycerides, digalactosyldiacylglycerides or sulfoquinovosyldiacylglycerides) [41]. Carotenoids are a group of lipophilic colorful chemicals found in nature that include lutein, lycopene, canthaxanthin, β-carotene, or astaxanthin [143]. Furthermore, these properties make algal lipids more bioavailable or provide a variety of health benefits to people or animals [109].

3.3.2. Role of Fatty Acids in Foods

Microalgae have a high PUFA content. They are fatty acids with many double bonds in the carbon chain and have numerous useful qualities. Microalgae may produce members of the PUFAs ω-6 family, such as linoleic acid (LA), γ-linolenic acid (GLA), and arachidonic acid (ARA), as well as members of the PUFAs ω-6 family, such as α-linolenic acid (ALA), eicosapentaenoic acid (EPA), and docosahexaenoic acid (DHA) [144,145]. Many microalgae manufacture the long chain of -3 PUFAs, with yields exceeding 20% of total lipids. The microalgae most commonly employed for the formation of algal oil rich in ω-3 and biomass are marine members of the Thraustochytriacea and Crythecodiniacea families [146].

Because of their obvious benefits to tissue integrity and health, they are vital ingredients for food additives and feeds. Microalgae such as *Chlorella vulgaris*, *Arthrospira platensis*, *Haematococcus pluvialis*, and *Dunaliella salina* have been identified as safe or permitted as human and animal food additives. *Scenedesmus almeriensis* and *Nannocholoropsis* sp. are two more species that have been investigated but have not yet been commercialized [147].

Crypthecodinium, *Schizochytrium*, *Thraustochytrids*, and *Ulkenia* microalgal species are employed in the manufacture important fatty acids [148]. DHA rich oil derived from *Crypthecodinium cohnii* is commercially accessible and contains 40–50% DHA with no EPA or other longchain PUFAs [149]. Schizochytrium species that synthesize DHA and EPA are currently employed as an adult dietary supplement in food and drinks, health foods, animal feeds, and foodstuffs products such as cheeses, yogurts, spreads and sauces, and breakfast cereals. This microalga's essential fatty acids are used as supplements in diets for pregnant and nursing women, as well as cardiovascular patients [149].

3.3.3. Role of Fatty Acids in Cosmeceuticals

Algae fatty acids and other lipophilic chemicals are also anti-allergic, antioxidant, and anti-inflammatory [150]. Furthermore, lipids can act as moisturizing ingredients substances, protecting the skin from water loss [151]. Many fatty acids, including lauric acid, myristic acid, palmitic acid, and stearic acid, can be used as raw materials. Furthermore, FAs are skin components that play a crucial role in the maintenance of skin integrity [152].

Waxes are classified as fatty esters, which are a type of fatty acyl [153]. *Euglena gracilis* is a microalga that produces a large quantity of wax-ester as a byproduct of the biodegradation of storage polysaccharides. These wax-esters are now used in biofuel generation but could possibly be useful in cosmetics [154]. Waxes, for example, are important components in lipsticks because they give the stick sufficient rigidity, hardness, stability, and texture. Today's lipsticks can be made with a range of waxes. Alkenones are a class of lipids, long-chain ketones that are produced by haptophyte microalgae such as *Isochrysis* sp. and employed as structuring agents in some cosmetic preparations in place of animal-derived and petroleum-derived waxes. They are a vegan and recyclable marine-based component that will meet customer demands. Because alkenones can be made in a variety of locales, their supply is not as limited as that of some other waxes. Given their waxy structure and relatively high melting point, alkenones may offer an appealing class of natural chemicals with potential applications in a wide range of cosmetic and skin care products [155]. Table 7 highlights the applications of lipids.

Table 7. The seaweeds lipids and their apllications.

Component	Molecular Mass	Properties/Activities	Seaweed	References
E-9-oxooctadec-10-enoic acid E-10-oxooctadec-8-enoic acid	282.46 g mol^{-1}	Anti-inflammatory	*Gracilaria verrucosa*	[156]
Essential oil (tetradeconoic acid, hexadecanoic acid, (9Z)-hexadec-9-enoic acid) (9Z,12Z)-9,12-octadecadienoic acid	280.447 g mol^{-1}	Antioxidant: radical scavenging Antibacterial activity upon *Staphylococcus aureus* and *Bacillus cereus*	*Laminaria japonica*	[157]
Fucosterol	412.69 g mol^{-1}	Antioxidant: increased antioxidative enzymes (glutathione peroxidase, superoxide dismutase, catalase)	*Pelvetia siliquosa*	[158]
Fucosterol	412.69 g mol^{-1}	Anti-inflammatory, Ati-photodamage: decreased UVB-induced MMPs	*Hizikia fusiformis*	[159]
Palmitic acid	256.430 g mol^{-1}	Enzyme inhibition, Antioxidant	*Ulva rigida, Gracilaria* sp., *Saccharina latissima, Fucus vesiculosus*	[160]
Omega 3 fatty acids	909.4 g mol^{-1}	Antioxidant	Brown algae	[161]
Arachidonic acid (ARA)	-	Improves growth and development of neonates	*P. purpureum, P. cruentum*	[162]
Eicosapentaenoic acid (EPA)	500 mg/day	Cognition, heart health, protection against arthrosclerosis, anti-inflammatory	*Nannochloropsis, P. tricornutum, P. cruentum*	[163,164]
Docosahexaenoic acid (DHA)	500 mg/day	Brain and eye health, cardiovascular benefits, nervous system development	*C. cohnii, Schizochytrium* sp., *Ulkenia* sp.	[162–164]
Fucosterol	1 and 10 μg mL^{-1}	Anti-aging Inhibit MMP expression	*Hizikia fusiformis*	[165]
Polyunsaturated fatty acid	10.3 mg mL^{-1}	Anti-inflammation	*Undaria pinnatifida*	[166]

3.4. Pigments

Natural pigments are necessary for photosynthesizing algal metabolism, or macroalgae are divided into three groups depending on pigment content: Phaeophyceae (brown algae), Chlorophyceae (green algae), or Rhodophyceae (red algae) are three families of algae (red algae) [139]. Macroalgae can produce three fundamental types of organic pigments: chlorophylls, carotenoids, or phycobilins [140]. Macroalgae that are wealthy in chlorophylls a or b seem green, whereas algae appear greenish-brown owing to a combination of fucoxanthin (carotenoid), and algae appear red owing to combination of chlorophylls a, c, or d, and phycobilins. Chlorophylls are natural lipid-soluble greenish pigments with porphyrin ring [139]. The chemical structures of different types of pigments in seaweeds are presented in Figure 4.

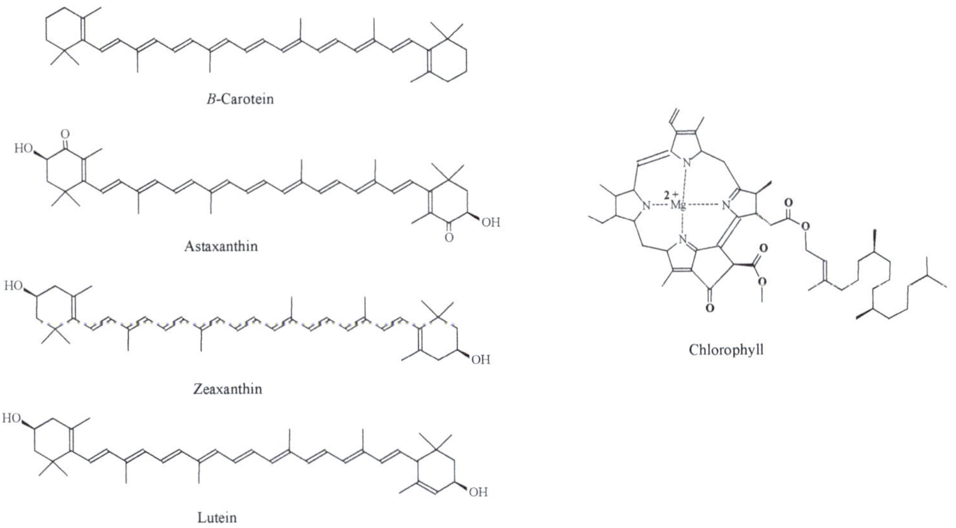

Figure 4. Chemical structures of different types of pigments in seaweeds.

Carotenoids have received much interest and are used in nutritional supplements, fortified foods, animal feed, pharmaceuticals, or cosmetics because of their antioxidant and antimicrobial characteristics, which assist to decrease the prevalence of cardiovascular diseases, ophthalmologic diseases, or cancer [138]. Carotenoids are lipophilic, linear polyenes in two categories: (i) carotenoids, carotenoids, and lycopene; (ii) xanthophylls (e.g., antheraxanthin, zeaxanthin, lutein, fucoxanthin, violaxanthin) [167]. *Ascophyllum nodosum, Cladosiphon okamuranus, Fucus serratus, Chaetoseros* sp., *Ishige okamurae, Ecklonia stolonifera, Himanthalia elongata,* and *Fucus vesiculosus* all contain carotenoid. It is more efficient upon Gram-positive bacteria (like, *Streptococcus agalactiae, Staphylococcus aureus, Proteus mirabilis, Pseudomonas aeruginosa, Staphylococcus epidermidis,* or *Serratia marcescens*) and Gram-negative bacteria (like, *Klebsiella pneumoniae, Klebsiella oxytoca, Serratia marcescens, Acinetobacter lwoffii, Pseudomonas aeruginosa* or *Escherichia coli*) [139].

Phycobiliproteins are naturally fluorescent, water-soluble proteins classified as PC (blue pigment), PE (red pigment), and allophycocyanins (light-blue pigment), with PE being most common in several red macroalgae species [139]. Algae rich in phycobiliproteins include *Spirulina, Botryococcus, Chlorella* and *Nostoc.* These pigments were discovered to have anti-obesity, anti-inflammatory, anti-angiogenic, antioxidant, anti-carcinogenic or neuroprotective activities in a recent study [168]. Table 8 illustrates the role of different carotenoids in human health.

Table 8. Summarizes the key activities of carotenoids in human health.

Carotenoid	Seaweed Source	Effect	Model	Bioactive Concentration	Target	Reference
Astaxanthin	*Hematococcus pluvialis*	Antioxidant	Human monocytes (U-937)	10 μM	SHP-1	[168]
			Mice brain	2 mg/kg/day	MDA, NO, APOP, GSH.	[169]
			Leydig cells	10 μg/mL	StAR	[170]
		Antiproliferative	human prostatic adenocarcinoma (LNCaP)	10 μM	prostate specific antigen (PSA)	[171]
		immune system stimulation	transplantable methylcholanthrene-induced fibrosarcoma (Meth-A tumor)	40 mg/kg/day	interferon-g (IFN-γ)	[172]
		anti-obesity	Humans	0, 6, 12 and 18 mg/day	adiponectin	[173]
		Cardiovascular protective	spontaneously hypertensive rats (SHR)	50 mg/kg	blood pressure (BP)	[174]
Fucoxanthin	*Sargassum horneri*	antioxidant and protective	Vero cells	5, 50, 100 and 200 μM (50 μM H_2O_2)	DNA	[175]
		UV protection	Human fibroblasts	5, 50 and 100 μM (50 mJ/cm2 UV-B)	DNA	[176]
		Antioxidant	Retinol deficiency rats	0.83 μM	CAT, GST and Na^+K^+ATPase activity	[177]
		Antiproliferative	leukemia cells (HD-60)	11.3 and 45.2 μM	DNA fragmentation	[178]
			colorectal adenocarcinoma cells (Caco-2)	15.2 μM	DNA fragmentation	[178]
			colorectal adenocarcinoma cells (DLD-1)	15.2 μM	DNA fragmentation	[178]
			colorectal adenocarcinoma cells (CHT-29)	15.2 μM	DNA fragmentation	[178]
			human colorectal carcinoma (HCT116)	5 and 10 μM	Bcl-xL, PARP and caspase 3 and 7	[179]
		Antiproliferative	human urinary bladder cancer cells (EJ-1)	20 μM		[180]
		anti-obesity	Rats	2 mg	absorption of triglycerides, pancreatic lipase	[181]

Table 8. *Cont.*

Carotenoid	Seaweed Source	Effect	Model	Bioactive Concentration	Target	Reference
Fucoxanthinol	*Corbicula fluminea*	Antiproliferative	human prostate cancer (PC-3)	2.0 µM	Bcl-xL, PARP and caspase 3 and 7	[179]
		anti-obesity	Rats	2 mg	absorption of triglycerides, pancreatic lipase	[181]
Halocynthia-xanthin	*Mastocarpus stellatus*	Antiproliferative	human neuroblastoma cells (GOTO)	5 µg/mL		[182]
β-carotene	*Kappaphycus alvarezii*	Antioxidant	Smokers	20 mg	Breath pentane	[183]
		Cure of erythema	Humans	30 to 90 mg/day		[184]
		Antiproliferative	murine osteosarcoma (LM8)	30 µM		[185]
		Antiinfiammatory	human umbilical vein endothelial cells (HUVECs)	0.02 µmol/L	VCAM-1, ICAM-1 and E-Selectin	[186]
Lutein	*Zostera noltii*	ADM prevention	Human Dermal Lymphatic Endothelial Cells (HLEC)	5 µM	DNA, lipid and protein level	[187]
		Cardiovascular protective	Human monocytes	0.1, 1, 10 and 100 nM	LDL associated with artery wall	[182]
Zeaxanthin	*Pyropia yezoensis*	ADM prevention	Human Dermal Lymphatic Endothelial Cells (HLEC)	5 µM	DNA, lipid and protein level	[187]

Abbreviations: SHP-1: protein tyrosine phosphatase non-receptor type 6; MDA: Malondialdehyde; NO: nitric oxide; APOP: protein oxidation product; GSH: glutathione; CAT: catalase; GST: glutathione S-transeferase; Bcl-xL: antiapoptotic factor; PARP: poly-ADP-ribose polymerase; (VCAM-1, ICAM-1): genes coding for vascular adhesion proteins.

3.5. Phenolic Compounds

Phenolic acids, tannins, flavonoids, and catechins are some of the phenolic compounds found in marine algae. The method of phenolic chemical extraction and the yield are strongly dependent on seaweed species. Brown seaweeds (Pheophyceae: P) are known for their high content of phlorotannins, complicated polymers made up of oligomers of phloroglucinol (1,3,5-trihydroxybenzene), while red or green seaweeds (Rhodophyceae: R) are known for their phenolic acids, flavonoids or bromophenols [10]. Polyphenols extracted from seaweeds were linked to variety of biological functions, containing antimicrobial, anticancer, antiviral, anti-obesity, antitumor, antiproliferative, antidiabetic, anti-inflammatory, or antioxidant effects [10]. Previous studies [101,188] demonstrated the anti-inflammatory activity of polyphenol-rich fraction derived from Rhodophyceae. Furthermore, phlorotannins and bromophenols derived from green or red algae possess strong inhibitory activity upon in vitro cancer cell proliferation or in vivo tumor growth, as well as antidiabetic and antithrombotic activities in vitro.

The phenolic active ingredients in seaweeds differ depending on whether they are red, green, or brown. Different phyla create different chemicals; for example, brown seaweeds produce phlorotannins, but red seaweeds produce a greater range of mycosporine-like amino acids (MAAs) than green species [189,190]. As a result of cellular mechanisms and genetic codification, the synthesis and diversity of phenolic chemicals are intimately tied to the seaweed taxonomic group and individual species [191]. Furthermore, phenolic acids such as benzoic acid, p-hydroxybenzoic acid, salicylic acid, gentisic acid, protocatechuic acid, vanillic acid, gallic acid, and syringic acid have been found in the genus Gracilaria (Rhodophyta, red alga) [192,193]. Phlorotannins are well-known phenolic chemicals that brown seaweeds produce [194]. Flavonoids such as rutin, quercitin, and hesperidin were detected in many Chlorophyta, Rhodophyta, and Phaeophyceae species [195]. Chondrus crispus and *Porphyra/Pyropia* spp. (Rhodophyta), as well as *Sargassum muticum* and *Sargassum vulgare* (Phaeophyceae), may synthesis isoflavones, as can daidzein and genistein [196]. Furthermore, several flavonoid glycosides were found in the brown seaweeds *Durvillaea antarctica*, *Lessonia spicata*, and *Macrocystis pyrifera* (also known as *Macrocystis integrifolia*) [195].

Terpenoids are belonging to secondary metabolites discovered in seaweeds [190]. Meroditerpenoids (such as plastoquinones, chromanols, and chromenes) were discovered in brown seaweeds, primarily from the Sargassaceae family (Phaeophyceae). These compounds are produced in part from terpenoids and are distinguished by the presence of a polyprenyl chain connected to a hydroquinone ring moiety [197]. In Rhodomelaceae, red seaweeds manufacture phenolic terpenoids such as diterpenes and sesquiterpenes. *Callophycus serratus*, for example, synthesizes a particular diterpene called bromophycolide [198]. Some studies revealed the existence of phenolic and flavonoids acids in marine algae as seen in Figure 5 and the chemical structure of phenolics also presented in Figure 6.

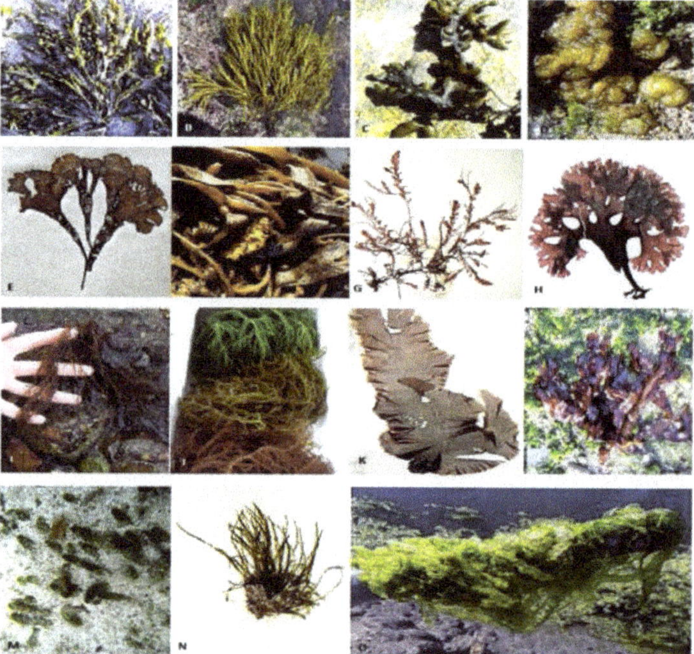

Figure 5. Several seaweeds synthesize phenolic substances. Adapted from ref [194] obtained from mdpi journals. (**A**)—*Ascophyllum nodosum* (P); (**B**)—*Bifurcaria bifurcata* (P); (**C**)—*Fucus vesiculosus* (P); (**D**)—*Leathesia marina* (P); (**E**)—*Lobophora variegata* (P); (**F**)—*Macrocystis pyrifera* (P); (**G**)—*Asparagopsis armata* (R); (**H**)—*Chondrus crispus* (R); (**I**)—*Gracilaria* sp. (R); (**J**)—*Kappaphycus alvarezii* (R); (**K**)—*Neopyropia* sp. (R); (**L**)—*Palmaria palmata* (R); (**M**)—*Dasycladus vermicularis* (Chl); (**N**)—*Derbesia tenuissima* (Chl); (**O**)—*Ulva intestinalis* (Chl); P—Phaeophyceae, R—Rhodophyta; Chl—Chlorophyta.

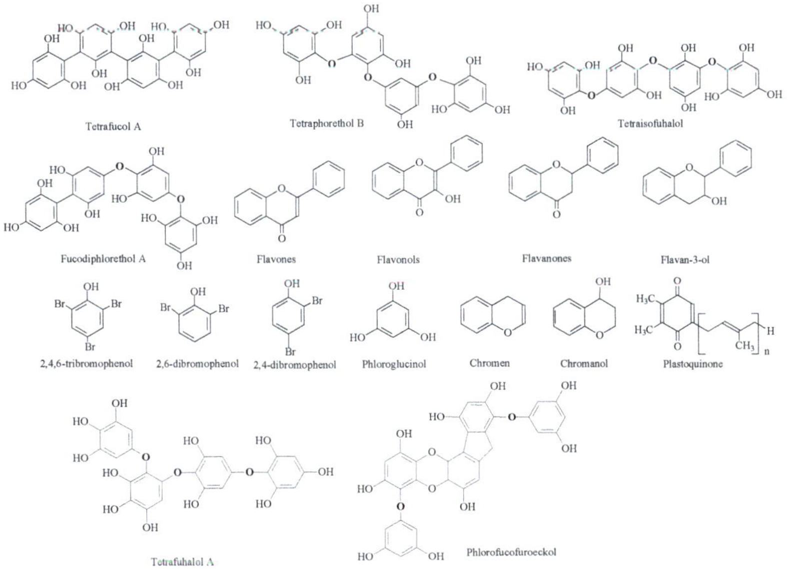

Figure 6. Chemical structures of different types of phenols in seaweeds.

3.6. Minerals

Seaweeds comprise greater numbers of important minerals, such as macroelements (e.g., Na, Ca, P, Mg, K) and trace minerals (like, Fe, Zn, Mn, Cu) due to their marine environment [118]. Minerals and cell wall polysaccharides (such as agar, alginic acid, alginate, or cellulose) play critical roles in the formation of human tissues or the regulation of crucial reactions as cofactors of some enzymes as cofactors among some enzymes [107]. As a result, seaweeds are important source of minerals and, when consumed regularly, have been recognized as advantageous functional foods (i.e., food supplements) [98]. It is worth noting that brown algae have greater mineral content than red algae [118].

Furthermore, elements such as Fe or Cu are found in higher concentrations in seaweeds than in meats and spinach [43]. Seaweeds were identified to be a promising supplier of iodine, which occurs at different chemical components, or brown algae, which contains more than 1% moisture content; its buildup in seaweed tissues may be 30,000 times greater than its concentration in sea water [45]. Iodine, which comes in a variety of forms, is anti-goiter, anticancer, antioxidant agent or a key nutrient in metabolic control. However, excessive intake may result in some unfavorable effects [43].

Green seaweeds have a Na^+/K^+ ratio of 0.9 to 1, red seaweeds have a ratio of 0.1 to 1.8, and brown seaweeds have a ratio of 0.3 to 1.5. This ratio was found to be especially low in *Palmaria palmata* (0.1) and Laminaria spp. (0.3–0.4) from Spain [199]. Because the World Health Organization (WHO) recommends a Na^+/K^+ ratio close to one, consumption of food products with this proportion or lower should be examined for healthy cardiovascular purposes [199]. In contrast, using seaweeds as NaCl replacements in processed meals could be a useful technique for reducing overall Na+ consumption while boosting intake of K^+ and other lacking components that would otherwise not be present in NaCl salted foods. In addition to Na^+ and K^+, Ca^{2+} and Mg^{2+} intake is linked to cardiovascular health. Indeed, it was proposed that enough Mg^{2+} intake may lower blood pressure by acting as a calcium antagonist on smooth muscle tone, inducing vasorelaxation [200].

Green seaweeds accumulate Mg^{2+} more than Ca^{2+}, whereas brown seaweeds do the opposite. In turn, with the exception of *Phymatolithon calcareum*, which can accumulate exceptionally high concentrations of Ca^{2+} [201], red seaweeds generally have lower, but balanced, amounts of these two minerals compared to the two other macroalgae types. It should be noted that the Ca/Mg ratio is also important in terms of calcium absorption because a lack of magnesium can result in a buildup of calcium in soft tissues, resulting in the production of kidney stones and the formation of arthritis [202].

Finally, phosphorus (P) levels appear to be similar in the three macroalgae groups, with values ranging from 0.5 to 7 g/kg DW. Notably, Fe is prevalent in all three macroalgae types, while Chlorophyta has a greater rate than Rhodophyta and Phaeophyta. However, at low doses, some species from the chlorophyta phylum (e.g., *Alaria esculenta*, *Saccharina latissima*, and *Fucus* spp.) might also be proposed to be a good source of Fe, as accumulation in some cases can exceed 1 g/kg DW [203]. In turn, the maximum Mn concentrations were found in red seaweeds, specifically *Chondrus crispus*, *Palmaria palmata*, and *Gracilaria* spp. [204]. Dawczynski et al. [205] also described the preferential deposition of Mn by red macroalgae over brown macroalgae.

The production of seaweed-fortified foods with the goal of reducing NaCl consumption and increasing nutritive value has been notably emphasized in meat-based products. López-López et al. [206] conducted outstanding work in the reformulation of many meat products, partially replacing the application of sodium chloride with diverse species of edible seaweeds while retaining their textural and sensory qualities. This research group created meat emulsions, meat patties, and frankfurters enriched with *Undaria pinnatifida*, *Himanthalia elongata*, or *Porphyra umbilicalis* that were both low in Na+ and rich in K^+, presenting Na^+/K^+ ratios below 1, which is much smaller than the ratios above 3 observed in their traditional recipes [207,208].

Furthermore, increasing the mineral content of meat, fish, and other animal-derived products can be accomplished by providing algae-supplemented diets to animals. Similarly, supplementing fish with seaweed-fortified meals has been shown to be an efficient way of increasing the iodine content of their fillets. Milk, dairy products, and, more recently, plant "milks" (e.g., soy, almond, oat, and rice) are another category of food products that play a critical role in the dietary routines of specific geographical areas of the world and, as such, are ideal candidates for macroalgae supplementation [209].

3.7. Vitamins

Vitamins are needed for a variety of skin functions and can be obtained from food or by topical application. Supplementation is indicated for skin protection against dryness and premature aging, aesthetic UV protection, and sebaceous gland secretory activity modulation. Vitamins are frequently found in skin care products or cosmetics. Vitamins A, C, E, K, or vitamin complex B seem to be the most essential or medically proven vitamins for skin photoaging treatment or prevention [77], as well as most abundant vitamins through algae have been vitamins A, B, C, or E [210].

Some seaweeds contain vitamins with several health benefits and antioxidant activity, which help to lower a variety of health issues such as high blood pressure, cardiovascular illnesses, and the risk of cancer [211]. Various seaweeds have been found to include water-soluble vitamins B1, B2, B12, and C, as well as fat-soluble vitamins E and β-carotene with vitamin A activity [212].

Vitamin A (β-carotene), in the form of retinol, has antioxidant and anti-wrinkle qualities [213] and is used in cosmetics to reduce hyperpigmentation or fine wrinkles on the face [214]. Vitamin B complex is found with higher concentrations in green or red seaweeds (B1, B2, B3 or niacine, B6, B9, B12, or folic acid) [215]. Active forms of vitamin B3 found in skincare products contain nicotinate esters, niacinamide, or nicotinic acid. Niacinamide is antioxidant that lowers hyperpigmentation (also caused by blue light) and enhances epidermal features by lowering trans-epidermal water loss [216]. Red algae or other species are good sources of vitamin B12, which has anti-aging characteristics or is required for hair, nail growth, or health in vegetarians [217].

Vitamin C is employed in cosmeceutical production because it contains L-ascorbic acid, the bioactive version of which is most well-known [213]. In this context, Ceramium rubrum and *Porphyr leucosticta* are red algae with elevated vitamin C content. This vitamin possesses antioxidant, antiviral, anti-inflammatory, antibacterial, detoxifying, or anti-stress properties when applied topically and could be used to improve tissue growth, repair blood vessels, teeth or bones [218]. A previous study found that if it is present in optimum concentration in cosmetic product, it can improve complexion, reduce pigmentation, and inflammation [219]. Vitamin C suppresses tyrosinase by interacting to copper ions that reduces melanogenesis, according to several studies [213].

Water-soluble vitamins, such as vitamin C, are abundant in *Ulva lactuca*, *Eucheuma cottonii*, *Caulerpa lentillifera*, *Sargassum polycstum*, and *Gracilaria* spp. and aid in the inhibition of low-density lipoprotein (LDL) oxidation and the creation of thrombosis/atherosclerosis [220]. Red algae have significantly higher levels of dried carotene (e.g., 197.9 mg/g in Codium fragile and 113.7 mg/g in *Gracilaria chilensis*) than other vegetables (e.g., 17.4 mg/g in *Macrocystis pyrifera*) [98], while brown seaweeds (e.g., *Undaria pinnatifida*) have greater concentrations of a-tocopherol/vitamin E (99% vitamins) than green and red seaweeds [107].

The primary fat-soluble vitamins (A and E) boost nitric oxide (NO) and nitric oxide synthase (NOS) activity, which aids in the prevention of CVDs [220]. Furthermore, vitamin E has antioxidant properties that can limit the oxidation of LDL [211]. Many disorders, such as chronic fatigue syndrome (CFS), anemia, and skin problems, are caused by a lack of water-soluble vitamins such as B12. Most terrestrial plants do not synthesize vitamin B_{12}, but numerous prokaryotes that can synthesize vitamin B_{12} interact with seaweeds, and this interaction enhances vitamin levels in macroalgae [221]. Arthrospira (previously *Spirulina*) (Cyanobacteria) contains four times more vitamin B12 than raw liver [222]. Brown and green seaweeds are high in vitamin A, with 500–3000 mg/kg dry weight on average, but red algae have 100–800 mg/kg dry weight [223]. When compared to terrestrial plants, seaweeds such as *Crassiphycus changii* (previously *Gracilaria changii*), *Porphyra umbilicalis* (Rhodophyta), and *Himanthalia elongata* (Ochrophyta, Phaeophyceae) are high in vitamins [224]. Vitamins (A, B, C, D, and E) are found in seaweeds and are widely used in skincare [225].

Vitamin C minimizes the severity of allergic reactions to infection, boosts the immune system, regulates the creation of conjunctive tissue, and aids in the removal of free radicals. It also plays an important role in many diseases and disorders such as diabetes, atherosclerosis, cancer, and neurodegenerative problems [226]. The brown seaweeds Ascophyllum and *Fucus* sp. have higher levels of vitamin E (α-tocopherols) than other red and green seaweeds [227]. The seaweed *Macrocystis pyrifera* (Ochrophyta, Phaeophyceae) is high in vitamin E, similar to plant oils recognized for their vitamin E content, such as soybean oil (*Glycine max*), sunflower seed oil (*Helianthus annuus*), and palm oil (*Elaeis guineensis*) [227]. Vitamin E prevents the oxidation of low-density lipoprotein and is also effective in reducing the risk of cardiovascular disease [228].

4. Biological Activities

4.1. Antioxidant Activity

An imbalance in the creation and neutralization of free radicals causes oxidative stress, which leads to a variety of degenerative illnesses [229]. Several free radicals, particularly reactive oxygen species (ROS), were created in living organisms as a result of metabolic activity, and hence have an impact on health (Figure 7). ROS were formed in form of hydrogen peroxide (H_2O_2), superoxide radical (O_2^-), hydroxyl radical ($\cdot OH$), or nitric oxide (NO). Oxidative stress causes unconscious or prominent enzyme activation, as well as oxidative damage for cellular systems [230]. ROS attack or damage important macromolecules including lipids membrane, proteins, or DNA, resulting in a variety of conditions include inflammatory or neurodegenerative diseases, diabetes mellitus, cancer, or severe tissue injuries [231,232] (Figure 7).

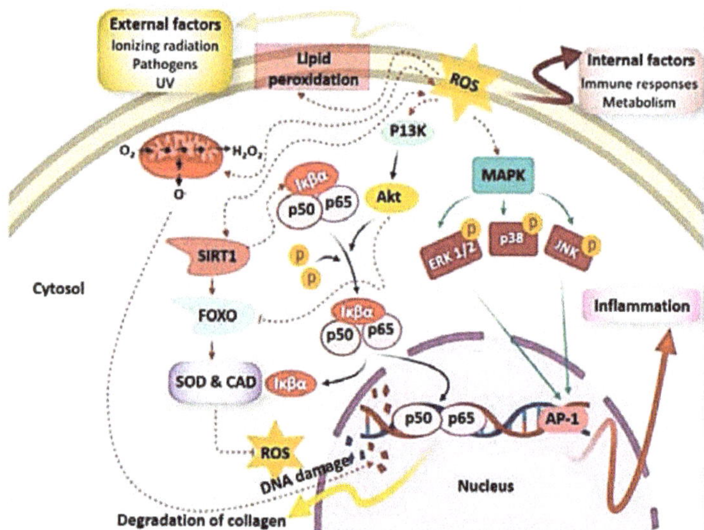

Figure 7. Damage caused via reactive oxygen species (ROS). Adapted from ref. [233] obtained from mdpi journals.

Antioxidants may have a favorable impact on human health because they may protect the body from damage caused via reactive oxygen species (ROS) [234]. To determine the antioxidant activity of marine derived bioactive peptides, researchers used electron spin resonance spectroscopy as well as intracellular free-radical scavenging assays.

ROS can produce several detrimental biological events, such as DNA oxidative lesions, membrane peroxidation, structural changes in proteins and functional carbohydrate, and so on. All of these structural and functional changes have direct clinical effects, speed up the aging process while also causing pathological phenomena, such as increased capillary permeability and impaired blood cell function [235]. All of these antioxidant systems behave differently depending on their structure and characteristics, whether hydrophilic or lipophilic, and where they are located (intracellular or extracellular, in cell or organelles membrane, in the cytoplasm, etc.). All of the above processes work in concert to establish a network that protects live cells from the damaging impacts of reactive oxygen species (ROS).

Figure 8 represents reactive oxygen species and neutralization with several biomolecules [236]. Hydrophobic amino acids in peptide chain contribute to their possible antioxidant effect [237]. Seaweeds also include nutraceutical and medicinal chemicals such phenols that have antioxidant activity. Polyphenols generated by seaweeds received special attention because their pharmacological action and broad range of health-promoting advantages, as polyphenols play a vital role in a variety of seaweed biological activities. Seaweed phenolic compounds are metabolites with hydroxylated aromatic rings that are chemically defined as molecules. In this context, Al-Amoudi et al. [25] stated that sulfated polysaccharides from three marine algae (Phaeophyta *Sargassum crassifolia* (S), Chlorophyta *Ulva lactuca* (U) and Rhodophyta *Digenea simplex* (D) exert antioxidant activity.

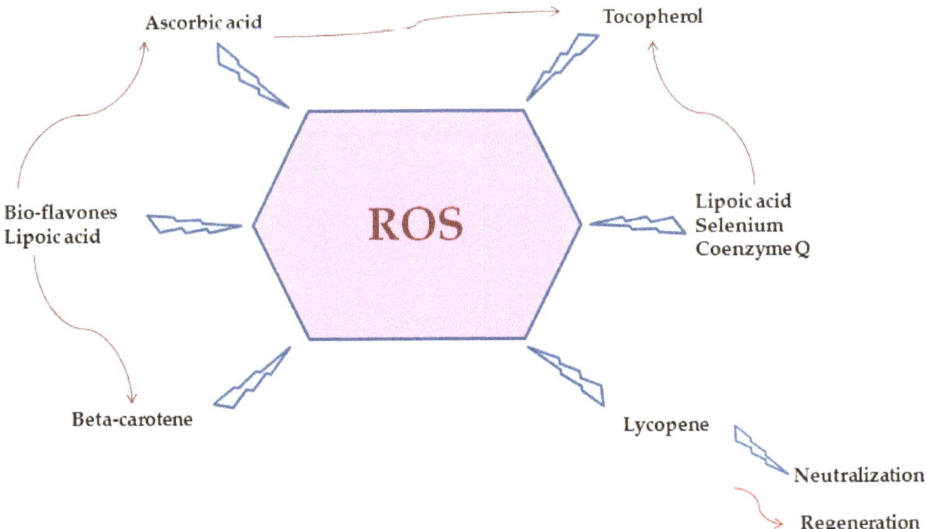

Figure 8. Reactive oxygen species and neutralization by several biomolecules.

4.2. Antimicrobial Activity

Susceptibility testing of harmful microorganisms (e.g., bacteria and fungi) in the presence of possible compounds of interest is the focus of antimicrobial activity assays. Microbial infections can cause life-threatening illnesses, resulting in millions of deaths each year. Despite the fact that the discovery of penicillin pushed many aggressive pathogenic bacteria back, many strains evolved and developed remarkable resistance mechanisms to most antibiotics [238]. Variable solvents have different antibacterial action depending on their solubility and polarity. As a result, chemical compounds isolated from various seaweeds should be optimized for antibacterial activity by selecting the optimal solvent system [239]. Micro-algal cell-free extracts are already being studied as food and feed additives in an attempt to replace synthetic antibacterial chemicals currently in use. According to Tuney et al. [240], the antibacterial action of the extract is attributable to various chemical agents found in the extract, such as flavonoids, triterpenoids, and other phenolic compounds or free hydroxyl groups. Extraction procedures, solvents used, and the time window in which samples were collected all have the potential to alter antibacterial activity [241]. A variety of organic solvents had previously been recommended for screening algae for antibacterial activity.

Pérez et al. [242] demonstrated that seaweed extracts are effective at suppressing a variety of pathogens, including *E. coli* and *Salmonella*. The majority of the research looked at crude seaweed extracts of the chemicals in ethanol or methanol crude extract. It is unclear from these investigations whether the antibacterial activity is due to a single molecule or a combination of chemicals working together. Phytochemicals were shown in several investigations to produce significant bacterial cell-membrane damage by disrupting membrane integrity [243]. The active phytochemical substances can penetrate the bacterium after the membrane has been disrupted and interfere with DNA, RNA, protein, or polysaccharide formation, resulting in bacterial cell inactivation [244]. Two of the most common types of seaweeds, namely, the total phenolic, total flavonoid, and antibacterial properties of *Padina boryana* Thivy and *Enteromorpha* sp. marine algae were extensively examined, and the authors revealed that both seaweeds show antimicrobial activity against multiple pathogens [245].

4.3. Anticancer Activity

Cancers are life-threatening diseases that are considered to be a major public health issue around the world [246,247]. Uncontrolled cell development spreads into the surrounding tissues, resulting in the formation of a tumor mass [248]. Much research has looked into the anticancer potential of natural compounds derived from seaweeds, as well as the signaling pathways involved in anticancer activity [249]. Because those secondary metabolites have no hazardous effects, they have seen a lot of progress in the treatment of numerous diseases, including cancer. Thymoquinone (TQ) is one of the most important bioactive elements of black seeds, and it has been found to have numerous health advantages, including cancer prevention and treatment. Following on this, Algotiml et al. [250] studied the effect of biosynthesized Red Sea marine algal silver nanoparticles AgNPs on anticancer and antibacterial properties and the authors stated that due to their relatively moderate side effects, marine resources are currently being increasingly examined for antibacterial and anticancer medication prospects.

According to Palanisamy et al. [251], Fucoidans derived from Sargassum polycystum show antiproliferative characteristics at 50 g/mL. Additionally, Usoltseva et al. [252] also showed that native and deacetylated fucoidans (at 200 g/mL) from the brown seaweeds *Sargassum duplicatum*, *Sargassum feldmannii*, impeded colony formation in human colon cancer cells (DLD-1, HCT-116 or HT-29). According to findings of previous study [253], fucoidan extracted from the Brown seaweed Sargassum cinereum displays potent anticancer or apoptotic effects via preventing metastasis. In B-16 (mouse melanoma), CT-26 (murine colon cancer), HL-60 (human promyelocytic leukemia), or U-937 (human leukemic monocyte lymphoma) cell lines, polysaccharides produced through Pheophyceae *Ecklonia cava* show putative antiproliferative properties [254].

In addition, kappa-carrageenan extracted from *Hypnea musciformis* (Hm-SP) decreased proliferation of MCF-7 or SH-SY5Y cancer cell lines [255]. Additionally, polysaccharides derived from *Sargassum fusiforme* (SFPS) reduced SPC-A-1 cell proliferation in vitro and tumor formation in vivo [256]. Additionally, Ji and Ji [257] found that commercial laminaran (400–1600 g/mL) inhibited the growth of human colon cancer LoVo cells through stimulating mitochondrial or DR pathways. Additionally, Fucoidans isolated from *Undaria pinnatifida* have anticancer potential comparable to commercial fucoidans in cell lines Hela (human cervical), PC-3 (human prostate), HepG2 (human hepatocellular liver carcinoma), or A549 (carcinomic human alveolar basal epithelial) [258]. Moreover, previous study reported that fucoidan isolated from *Sargassum hemiphyllum* may increase miR-29b expression in human hepatocellular carcinoma cells, which aids in the lowering of DNA methyltransferase 3B expression [259]. Moreover, Fucoidans from *Fucus vesiculosus* were revealed to have anticancer potential, inducing apoptosis in MC3 human mucoepidermoid carcinoma cells via caspase-dependent apoptosis signaling cascade [260] (Figure 9).

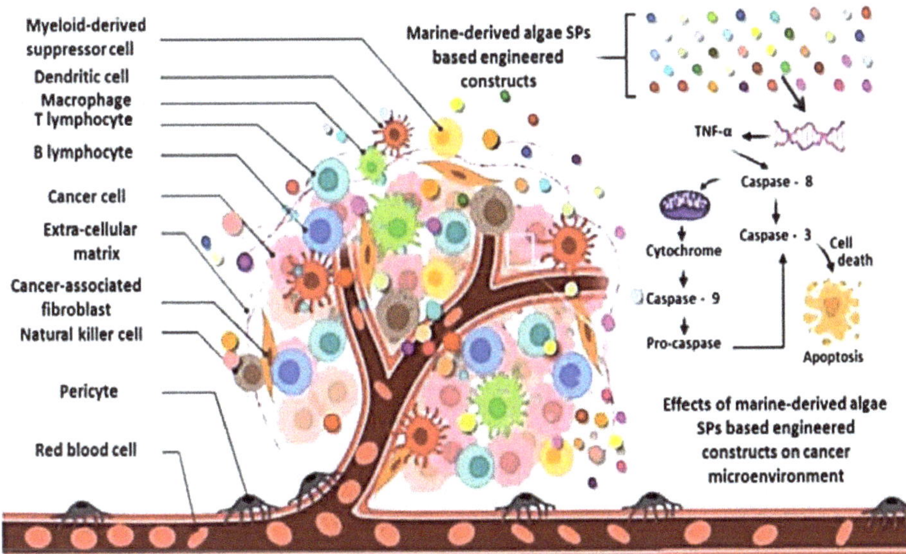

Figure 9. Demonstrate the ability of algal polysaccharide (SP)-based customized signals produced from sea algae to cause tumor cell death (apoptosis). Adapted from ref. [233] obtained from mdpi journals.

4.4. Antidiabetics Activity

As a result of an unhealthy lifestyle, obesity, and stress, diabetes is becoming a global illness. Additionally, obesity has been on the rise in Saudi Arabia as a result of changing lifestyles and socioeconomic status [260,261]. There is a close association between obesity and type 2 diabetes. Drugs that suppress the enzymes α-glucosidase and α-amylase, which break down starch into glucose before it is absorbed into the bloodstream, could be used to treat diabetes [262]. It is necessary to look for effective therapeutic natural medications with less side effects. Garcimartn et al. [263] showed that a α-glucosidase inhibitory effect on restructured pork treated with seaweeds such as *Undaria pinnatifida*, *Himanthalia elongata*, and *Porphyra umbilicalis* caused a reduction in the blood glucose absorption. *Padina tetrastromatica* phenolic extracts inhibited both α-glucosidase and α-amylase, with higher inhibition linked with a higher phenolic concentration in the extracts. The extracts inhibited α-glucosidase (IC$_{50}$ value of 28.8 g mL^{-1}) and -amylase (IC$_{50}$ value of 47.2 g mL^{-1}) by 38.9 and 26.8%, respectively [264]. Similarly, α-glucosidase inhibitory action was observed in methanol, ethanol, and acetone extracts of *Durvillea antarctica*, methanol extracts of *Ulva* sp., and acetone extracts of *Lessonia spicata* [265]. Methanol extracts of *Padina tenuis* (400 µg mL^{-1}) and ethanol extract of *Eucheuma denticulatum* (10 mg mL^{-1}) and *Sargassum polycystum* (10 mg mL^{-1}) significantly inhibited α-amylase by 60%, 67%, and 46%, respectively [266]. Recently, the acetone extract (80%) of brown seaweed *Turbinaria decurrens* was studied for its antihyperglycemic effects in alloxan induced diabetic wistar male rats [267]. The results showed a significant reduction in postprandial blood glucose levels of seaweed extracts treated rats to 180.33 mg dL^{-1} and 225.33 mg dL^{-1} at the dose of 300 mg/kg body weight and 150 mg/kg body weight, respectively, compared to diabetic control (565.0 mg dL^{-1}) and positive control (115.33 mg dL^{-1}). The bioactive compounds derived from algae and their application is illustrated in Table 9.

Table 9. Bioactive compounds derived from algae and their applications.

Algae Species	Bioactive Compound/Extract	Beneficial Activity	Mechanism of Action	Experimental Model	Reference
Brown algae					
Ascophyllum nodosum	Ascophyllan	Anticancer	Inhibit MMP expression	B16 melanoma cells	[268]
Bifurcaria bifurcata	Eleganonal	Antioxidant	DPPH inhibition	In vitro	[269]
Chnoospora implexa	Ethanol extract	Antimicrobial	Bacterial growth inhibition	*Staphylococcus aureus, Staphylococcus pyogenes*	[270]
Chnoospora minima	Fucoidan	Anti-inflammation	Inhibition of LPS-induced NO production, iNOS, COX-2, and PGE2 levels	RAW macrophages	[53]
Cladosiphon okamuranus	Fucoxanthin	Antioxidant	DPPH inhibition	In vitro	[271]
Colpomenia sinuosa	Ethanol extract	Antimicrobial	Bacterial growth inhibition	*S. aureus, S. pyogenes*	[270]
Cystoseira barbata	Fat-soluble vitamin and carotenoids	Antioxidant	High fat-soluble vitamin and carotenoid content	In vitro	[272]
Dictyopteris delicatula	Ethanol extract	Antimicrobial	Bacterial growth inhibition	*S. aureus, S. pyogenes*	[270]
Dictyota dichotoma	Algae extract	Antimicrobial	Inhibit the synthesis of the peptidoglycan layer of bacterial cell walls	*Penicillium purpurescens, Candida albicans, Aspergillus flavus*	[273]
Eisenia arborea	Phlorotannin	Anti-inflammation	Inhibit release of histamine	Rat basophile leukemia cells (RBL-2HE)	[274]
Fucus evanescens	Fucoidan	Anticancer	Inhibit cell proliferation	Human malignant melanoma cells	[50]
Halopteris scoparia	Ethanol extract	Anti-inflammation	COX-2 inhibition	COX inhibitory screening assay kit	[275]
Laminaria japonica	Fucoxanthin	Anti-melanogenic	Suppress tyrosinase activity	UVB-irradiated guinea pig	[276]
Padina concrescens	Ethanol extract	Antimicrobial	Bacterial growth inhibition	*S. aureus, S. pyogenes*	[270]
Saccharina latissima	Phenol	Antioxidant	High total phenolic content, DPPH scavenging activity and FRAP	In vitro	[277]
Red algae					
Alsidium corallinum	Methanol extract	Antimicrobial	Bacterial growth inhibition	*Escherichia coli, Klebsiella pneumoniae, Staphylococcus aureus*	[278]
Ceramium rubrum	Methanol extract	Antimicrobial	Bacterial growth inhibition	*Escherichia coli, Enterococcus faecalis, Staphylococcus aureus*	[278]
Ganonema farinosum	Ethanol extract	Antimicrobial	Bacterial growth inhibition	*S. aureus, S. pyogenes*	[270]
Gelidium robustum	Ethanol extract	Antimicrobial	Bacterial growth inhibition	*S. aureus, S. pyogenes*	[270]
Jania rubens	Glycosaminoglycan	Anti-aging	Collagen synthesis	Unknown	[279]
Laurencia luzonensis	Sesquiterpenes	Antimicrobial	Bacterial growth inhibition	*Bacillus megaterium*	[280]
Palisada flagellifera	Methanol extract	Antioxidant	β-carotene bleaching activity	In vitro	[281]
Porphyra haitanensis	Sulfated Polysaccharide	Antioxidant	ROS scavenging potential	Mice	[282]
Schizymenia dubyi	Phenol	Anti-melanogenic	Inhibit tyrosinase activity	In vitro	[283]

Table 9. *Cont.*

Algae Species	Bioactive Compound/Extract	Beneficial Activity	Mechanism of Action	Experimental Model	Reference
Green algae					
Bryopsis plumose	Polysaccharide	Antioxidant	ROS scavenging potential	In vitro	[54]
Cladophora sp.	Ethanol extract	Antimicrobial	Bacterial growth inhibition	*S. aureus, S. pyogenes*	[270]
Entromorpha intestinalis	Chloroform and methanol extract	Antioxidant	SOD activity is reduced	*Labidochromis caeruleus*	[284]
Gayralia oxysperma	Fucoxanthin	Antioxidant	High FRAP value (>6 µM/µg of extract)	In vitro	[285]
Ulva dactilifera	Ethanol extract	Antimicrobial	Bacterial growth inhibition	*S. aureus, Streptococcus pyogenes*	[270]
Ulva fasciata	Fucoxanthin	Antioxidant	DPPH inhibition (83.95%)	In vitro	[286]
Ulva pertusa	Polysaccharide	Antioxidant	ROS scavenging potential	In vitro	[54]
Microalgae/Cyanobacteria					
Anabaena vaginicola	Lycopene	Antioxidant Anti-aging	N/A	In vitro	[287]
Arthrospira platensis	Methanol extracts of exopolysaccharides	Antioxidant	N/A	In vitro	[287]
Chlorella fusca	Sporopollenin	Anti-aging	Protect cells from UV radiation	N/A	[288]
Chlorella minutissima	MAA	Anti-aging	Protect cells from UV radiation	N/A	[288]
Chlorella sorokiniana	MAA	Anti-aging	Protect cells from UV radiation	N/A	[288]
	Lutein	Anti-aging	Reduce UV induced damage	N/A	[289]
Chlorella vulgaris	Hot water extract	Anti-aging	Reduced activity of SOD	Human diploid fibroblast	[290]
		Anti-inflammation	Down-regulated mRNA expression levels of IL-4 and IFN-γ	NC/Nga mice	[291]
Dunaliella salina	β-carotene	Antioxidant	Protect against oxidative stress	Rat	[292]
	β-cryptoxanthin	Anti-inflammation	Reduced the production of IL-1β, IL-6, TNF-α, the protein expression of iNOS and COX-2	LPS-stimulated RAW 264.7 cells	[293]
Haematococcus pluvialis	Astaxanthin (carotenoid)	Anti-aging	Inhibit MMP expression	Mice and human dermal fibroblasts	[294]
		Anticancer	ROS scavenging potential	Mice	[295]
Nannochloropsis granulata	Carotenoid	Antioxidant	DPPH inhibition	In vitro	[296]
Nannochloropsis oculata	Zeaxanthin	Anti-melanogenic	Inhibit tyrosinase	In vitro	[297]
Nitzschia sp.	Fucoxanthin	Antioxidant	Reduced oxidative stress	Human Glioma Cells	[298]
Nostoc sp.	MAA	Antioxidant	ROS scavenging potential	In vitro	[299]
Odontella aurita	EPA	Antioxidant	Reduce oxidative stress	Rat	[300]
Planktochlorella nurekis	Fatty acid	Antimicrobial	Bacterial growth inhibition	*Campylobacter jejuni, E. coli, Salmonella enterica var.*	[301]
Porphyridium sp.	Sulfated polysaccharide	Anti-inflammation Antioxidant	Inhibit proinflammatory modulator Inhibited oxidative damage	Unknown 3T3 cells	[282]

Table 9. *Cont.*

Algae Species	Bioactive Compound/Extract	Beneficial Activity	Mechanism of Action	Experimental Model	Reference
Rhodella reticulata	Sulfated polysaccharide	Antioxidant	ROS scavenging potential	In vitro	[282]
Skeletonema marinoi	Polyunsaturated aldehyde and fatty acid	Anticancer	Inhibit cell proliferation	Human melanoma cells (A2058)	[302]
Spirulina platensis	β-carotene and phycocyanin	Antioxidant Anti-inflammation	Inhibit lipid peroxidation Inhibit TNF-α and IL-6 expressions	Mouse Human dermal fibroblast cells (CCD-986sk)	[303]
	Ethanol extract	Antimicrobial	Bacterial growth inhibition	*E. coli, Pseudomonas aeruginosa, Bacillus subtilis,* and *Aspergillus niger*	[304]
Synechocystis spp.	Fatty acids and phenols	Antimicrobial	Bacterial growth inhibition	*E. coli, S. aureus*	[305]

5. Seaweeds in Bio-Manufacturing Applications

Modern consumers are well aware of the nutritional value of food and the negative impact that synthetic preservatives may have worse effect on their health, so it is unsurprising that they prefer fresh and lightly preserved foods that are free of chemical preservatives, but contain natural compounds that may benefit their health [306].

5.1. Fertilizer and Soil Conditioners

Seaweed extracts have been frequently employed in agriculture in recent years to increase crop yield. This improvement is achieved by stimulating various physiological processes involved in plant growth and development, as well as improving final product quality (Figure 10). The use of traditional chemical fertilizers has expanded dramatically as result of world's fast-growing population or ever-increasing food demand [307]. The usage of these chemical fertilizers, as well as their impacts, notably on environment, has become major source of worry [308]. As a result, farmers began to switch to organic farming rather than using synthetic agricultural fertilizers. Seaweeds are abundant or long-lasting resources discovered along the world's coastlines, and they are important sources of food, feed, biofuels, cosmetics, fertilizers, nutraceuticals, and pharmaceuticals [309,310]. Due to their commercial importance or potential applications, seaweeds are used as fodder, cosmetics, human food, or biofertilizers [311]. Because of availability of various trace elements, vitamins, growth regulators, or amino acids, macroalgae extracts are currently being used as foliar sprays or presoaking for boosting growth or production of variety of plants, particularly crops [312]. Each year, more than 15 million tons of seaweed is produced, with much of it used as biofertilizers in agriculture or horticulture industries [313,314].

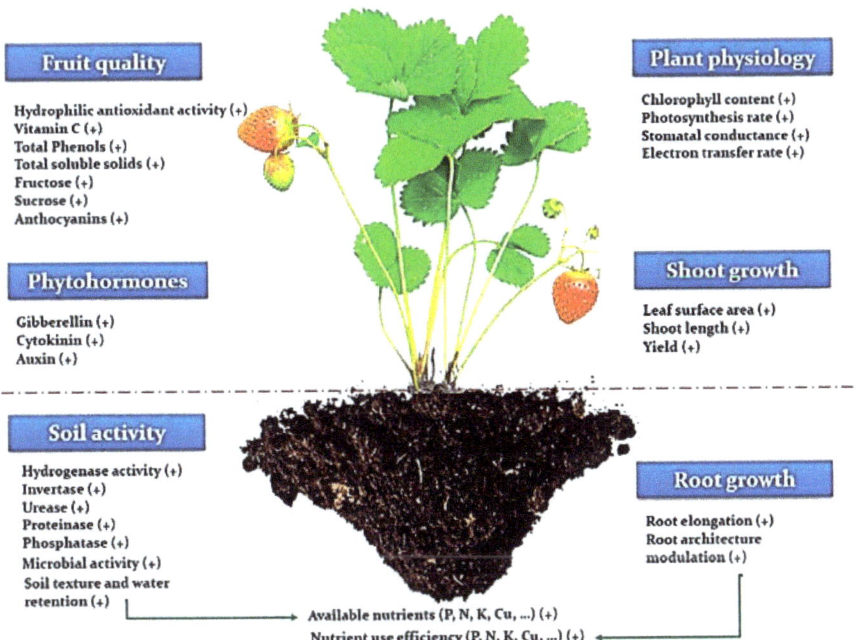

Figure 10. Illustration demonstrating beneficial effects of seaweed extracts on the entire soil-plant system. Such impacts include increased fruit quality and phytohormone content in plants, increased soil enzymatic activity, improved roots system, and overall physiological properties of plants. Adapted from ref. [315] obtained from mdpi journals.

5.2. Medical and Pharmaceutical Use

5.2.1. Biomedical Applications of Seaweeds

Bioactive chemicals found in seaweeds have features that make them appealing for biomedical applications. Many species of seaweeds have been employed in traditional medicine for a long time, notably in Asian nations, against goiter, nephritic disorders, anthelmintic, catarrh, and a few other ailments as medicaments or pharmaceutical auxiliaries, long before scientific study information [316]. *Fucus vesiculosus* has been used as a medicinal drug, primarily due to its iodine content, for obesity defects and goiters [316], for the treatment of sore knees [317], healing wounds [318], and also as herbal teas for their laxative effects [319]. The application of different seaweeds is presented in Table 10.

Table 10. Biomedical effects of seaweed bioactive compounds.

Seaweed	Compound Extracted	Cell Lines/Animals Surveyed	Route of Administration	Dosage (µg/mL)	Effect	Reference
Laminaria cichorioides (Phaeophyceae)	Sulfated fucan	Human plasma	The lyophilized crude polysaccharide was dissolved in human plasma	10, 30, 50	In vitro anticoagulant activity	[320]
Fucus evanescens (Phaeophyceae)	Fucoidans	Human plasma Rat plasma	Intravenous Injection	125, 250, 500, 1000	In vitro and in vivo anticoagulant activity	[321]
Gracilaria edulis (Rhodophyceae)	Phenolic, Flavonoid and Alkaloid compounds	Bovine serum albumin (protein)	The extracts were tested on the protein	20, 40, 60, 80, 100, 120	Hypoglycemic activity	[322]

Table 10. *Cont.*

Seaweed	Compound Extracted	Cell Lines/Animals Surveyed	Route of Administration	Dosage (µg/mL)	Effect	Reference
Sargassum fulvellum (Phaeophyceae)	Phlorotannins, grasshopper ketone, fucoidan and polysaccharides	Mice	Oral administration	Based on weight of mice	Antioxidant, anticancer, antiinflammatory, antibacterial, and anticoagulant activities	[323]
Griffithsia sp. (Rhodophyceae)	Griffithsin (protein)	MERS-CoV and SARS-CoV glycoproteins	The extracts were tested on the proteins	0.125, 0.25, 0.5, 1, 2	Antiviral activity against MERS-CoV virus and SARS-CoV glycoprotei	[324]
Ulva rigida (Chlorophyceae)	Ethanolic extract	Twenty-four male Wistar rats	Oral administration	500 mL of water with extracts in 2% wt/vol as drinking water for exposed groups per each day (from 3 to 30 days).	In vivo antihyperglycaemic, antioxidative and genotoxic/ antigenotoxic activities	[325]
Saccharina japonica (Phaeophyceae)	polysaccharides	SARS-CoV-2 S-protein	The extracts were tested on the proteins	50–500	In vitro inhibition to SARS-CoV-2	[326]

Chondrus crispus (Rhodophyta) carrageens have been used as mucilage against diarrhea, dysentery, gastric ulcers, and as a component of several health teas, such as for colds, for a long time. *Gelidium cartilagineum* (Rhodophyta) has been used in pediatric medicine in Japan for colds and scrofula [284]. *Ulva lactuca* (Chlorophyta) has been used for gout and as an astringent in folk medicine [284]. Rhodophyta extracts are very promising natural chemicals that could be used in biomedicine. Many species of Asian seaweeds are employed in traditional medicine, including *Gracilaria* spp. (Rhodophyta), which is used as a laxative, *Sargassum* spp. (Phaeophyceae), which is used to treat Chinese influence, and *Caloglossa* spp., *Codium* spp., *Dermonema* spp., and *Hypnea* spp. (Rhodophyta) [327].

Carrageenans' biological actions make them attractive candidates for future antitumoral therapeutics since they activate antitumor immunity [328]. Kappaphycus species (Rhodophyta), for example, are used to treat ulcers, headaches, and tumors [327]. Antitumoral efficacy of carrageenans derived from Kappaphycus striatum against human nasopharyngeal carcinoma, human gastric carcinoma, and cervical cancer cell lines [329]. The bioactivity of chemicals from various Laurencia species (Rhodophyta) was investigated. In vitro, certain halogenated metabolites of *Laurencia papillosa* showed action against Jurkat (acute lymphoblastic leukemia) human tumor cells [330]. Laurencia obtuse extracts, specifically three sesquiterpenes, have been extracted and tested against Ehrlich ascites cancer cells. The sesquiterpenes were found to have antitumoral action against Ehrlich ascites cells [331]. *Gracilaria edulis* ethanol extracts showed antitumor efficacy in mice with ascites tumors [332].

Undaria pinnatifida (Phaeophyceae) has anti-inflammatory qualities and can be used to treat postpartum depression in women. This alga can also be used to treat edema and as a diuretic. Celikler et al. [333] investigated the antigenotoxic effect of *Ulva rigida* extracts in human cells in vitro (Chlorophyta).

Seaweeds have been suggested as a way to avoid neurogen-erative illnesses in investigations over the last decade [334]. Alzheimer's disease (AD), Parkinson's disease (PD), Huntington's disease (HD), and Amyotrophic Lateral Sclerosis (ALS) are the most frequent [334]. According to Bauer et al., several studies highlighted the use of algal polysaccharides for the treatment of neurodegenerative illnesses [335]. Park et al. [336] found that mice treated with fucoidan extracts from Ecklonia cava had better memory and learning; consequently, the study implies favorable results in future human trials. In comparison to the control group, mice treated with polysaccharide isolated from *Sargassum fusiforme* demonstrated enhanced memory and cognition [337]. Dieckol and phlorofucofuroeckol, two phlorotannins from Ecklonia cava, are linked to an increase in the main central neurotransmitters in the brain, particularly Acetylcholine (ACh) [338]. Ahn et al. [339] investigated *Eisenia bicyclis* phlorotannins and found that 7-phloroeckol and phlorofucofuroeckol A were powerful neuroprotective agents against induced cytotoxicity, while eckol had a weaker impact.

5.2.2. Pharmaceutical Applications of Seaweeds

Bioactive chemicals from seaweeds are used in the pharmaceutical industry to help develop new formulations for revolutionary treatments and to replace synthetic components with natural ones. Bioactive chemicals found in seaweeds have important pharmacological properties, including anticoagulant, antioxidant, antiproliferative, antititumoral, anti-inflammatory, and antiviral effects [340] (Table 11).

Table 11. The potential pharmacological activity of brown, red and green seaweeds.

Component	Properties/Activities	Seaweed	Doses	Models	References
Fucoxanthins	Antitumoral activity on lung cancer cells	*Laminaria japonica*	12.5–100 µM	Female and male (1:1 ratio) BALB/c nude mice (18–20 g; 6–8 weeks of age)	[341]
	Antitumoral activity on MCF-7, HepG-2, HCT-116 cells	*Colpomenia sinuosa, Sargassum prismaticum*	100 and 200 mg/kg	Paracetamol-administered rats (one dose of 1 g/kg)	[342]
	Antitumoral activity on SiHa, Malme-3M cells	*Undaria pinnatifida*	1.5625, 6.25, 12.5, 25, 50, 80, 100 µM	Human cell lines	[343]
	Antimicrobial activity	*Cladosiphon okamuranus*	2–2000 µg/mL.	*Helicobacter pylori*	[344]
	Antimicrobial activity	*Laminaria japonica*	2, 3, 4, 5, 6, 7, and 7.5 mg/mL	*Staphylococcus aureus, Escherichia coli*	[345]
	Antimicrobial activity	*Fucus vesiculosus*	2, 4, 6, 8 and 10 mg/mL	*Staphylococcus aureus, Bacillus licheniformis, Escherichia coli, Staphylococcus epidermidis*	[346]
	Antiviral activity against ECHO-1, HIV-1, HSV-1, HSV-2	*Fucus evanescens*	200 µg/mL	Female outbred mice (16–20 g)	[347]
Sulfate polysaccharide	Antiviral activity against HSV-1, HVS-2	*Sargassum patens*	0.78–12.5 µg/mL	Vero cells (African green monkey kidney cell line)	[348]
	Anti-obesity, antidiabetic activities	*Gracilaria lemaneiformis*	5–10% Seaweed powder	Dawley laboratory rats (4 to 5 months old, 250–300 g)	[349]
Phloroglucinol	Anti-inflammatory activity	*Ecklonia cava*	1, 5, 10, 50 100 µM	HT1080 and RAW264.7 cells	[350]

Fucoidans extracted from *Laminaria cichorioides* (Phaeophyceae) [351] and Fucus evanescens [352] behave like heparin in both in vitro and in vivo experiments, demonstrating anticoagulant activity by accelerating the development of antithrombin III to inhibit the effect against thrombin.

Fucoidans have a variety of characteristics. Pozharitskaya et al. [353] investigated the antioxidant, anti-inflammatory, anti-hyperglycaemic, and anticoagulant bioactivities of fucoidans isolated from *Fucus vesiculosus*. Even though their free-radical scavenging activity was lower than that of synthetic antioxidants, it was comparable to that of the natural antioxidant quercetin, which is found in plants. Furthermore, inhibition of both isoforms of the pro-inflammatory cyclooxygenase (COX-1) enzymes has been demonstrated, making fucoidans isolated from *Fucus vesiculosus* interesting substances for anti-inflammatory natural medicines [353]. Fucoidans from *Fucus vesiculosus* also have a role in fucoidan's suppression of the enzyme DPP-IV. This enzyme is involved in the breakdown of incretin hormones, which prevents greater levels of glucose in the blood (postprandial hyperglycemia); a new pharmaceutical company is developing DPP-IV inhibitors to lower blood glucose levels and ensure anti-hyperglycaemic effects. As a result, according to Pozharitskaya et al. [353], fucoidans may be engaged in anti-hyperglycaemic activity via DPP-IV inhibition. *Sargassum fulvellum* (Phaeophyceae) has been found to contain a variety of bioactive compounds, including phlorotannins, grasshopper ketone, fucoidan, and polysaccharides, according to previous research. For years, *Sargassum fulvellum* extracts have been researched for their various pharmacological effects, including antioxidant, anticancer, anti-inflammatory, antibacterial, and anticoagulant properties [354].

Sargassum fulvellum extracts were studied for disorders such a lump, swelling, testicular discomfort, and urinary tract infections [355]. Agar made from red algae is frequently used in biomedicine as a suspension component in medicinal solutions and prescription goods, as well as anticoagulant and laxative agents in capsules [356]. The red algae *Gracilaria edulis* is well-known around the world for its biological and medicinal qualities. *Gracilaria edulis* extract exhibited antidiabetic, antioxidant, antibacterial, anticoagulant, anti-inflammatory, and antiproliferative characteristics [357]; consequently, these compounds could be used in new pharmaceutical formulations. Furthermore, Gunathilaka et al. [358] investigated the in vitro hypoglycemic efficacy of *Gracilaria edulis* phenolic, flavonoid, and alkaloid extracts. The suppression of carbohydrate-digesting enzymes, glucose absorption, and the generation of antiglycation end products demonstrated the red alga's hypoglycemic potential. In vivo, *Ulva rigida* (Chlorophyta) has been shown to have a hypoglycemic impact [359].

Seaweeds' antiviral qualities make them an excellent alternative for improving the health of infected persons; also, their use in pharmaceuticals will provide new and natural antiviral drugs that can replace synthetic chemicals. Furthermore, when compared to the creation of synthetic antivirals, the use of bioactive components from seaweeds is less expensive [360]. Antiviral activity of macroalgae has been discovered to protect against a variety of viruses, including HIV, Herpes Simplex Virus (HSV), genital warts [361], and hepatitis C (HCV) [362]. HSV [363], Encephalomyocarditis virus, Influenza "A" virus [364], and human metapneumovirus [365] are only a few of the viruses that Chlorophyta species have been shown to be effective against. The antiviral action of macroalgae is linked to a variety of substances such as as fatty acids and diterpenes, but most notably to the presence of Seaweed bioactive compounds [366], which can inhibit virus multiplication or help the immune system combat viral infection.

5.3. Cosmetic Industry

Cosmetics and cosmeceuticals are commonplace therapies for improving the skin's appearance and treating several dermatological problems. Seaweeds are a valuable component in product development because of their wide range of functional, sensory, and biological properties. Consumer demand for green or eco-friendly products has risen in recent years. This pattern can be seen in the globally competitive cosmetics industry, in need of natural, secure, or effective ingredients to make innovative skin care products [367]. The usage of seaweed-isolated compounds in cosmetic products rose steadily as a result of various scientific studies revealing prospective skincare properties of seaweed bio-actives. Biologically active substances include carotenoids, polysaccharides, phlorotannins, fatty acids, sterols, tocopherol, vitamins, phycocyanins, or phycobilins [368–372]. In this context, a *Sargassum plagyophyllum* extract was shown to have antioxidant and anti-collagenase that can considered to be potent pharmaceutical ingredient for anti-wrinkle cosmetics action [373–376]. As a form of polyphenol, phlorotannins contain a group of heterogeneous polymeric molecules with substantial chemical modifications and various chemical structures [377]. These molecules can play a key role in the interaction between the skin and UVR, such as preventing radiation from penetrating the skin and lowering inflammation, oxidative stress, DNA damage, and maintaining signaling pathways intact. They also attracted a lot of interest because of their participation in several phototoxic pathways and mechanisms [378]. Brown algae *Sargassum fusiforme* [379], *Halidrys siliquosa* [380], *Padina australis* [381], *Sargassum coreanum* [382], and *Polycladia myrica* [383] have been explored for using in cosmetic products.

6. Materials and Methods

Literature Search

The preferred reporting items for systematic reviews were used for the collection, identification, screening, selection, and analysis of the studies reviewed. A literature search was performed using different databases, including Scopus, Web of Science, Google Scholar, Wiley, MDPI, and PubMed. The search criteria included scientific articles on seaweeds published between 1989 and 2022. The keywords used in the literature search were "seaweeds" and "bioactivites OR "biological activities" OR "safety" OR "toxicity" OR "characteristics" OR "structure" OR "anticancer" OR "antidiabitics" OR "lipids" OR "polysaccarides" OR "phenolic compounds" OR "vitamines" OR "cosometics" OR "foods" OR "human" OR "minerals" OR "pigments and carotenoids" OR "protein" OR "amino acids". The total number of articles found was 650. Studies focusing on the above keywords were selected, as well as those addressing the biological activity of seaweeds and the different applications of seaweeds. The figures were obtained from MDPI journals, and the chemical structure of compounds was designed by Chem windo 6 ver.4.1.1 Biorad edition.

7. Conclusions

Seaweeds include a wealth of bioactive compounds that could be used to develop novel functional ingredients for food as well as a therapy or prevention strategy for chronic diseases. Seaweeds could be an alternative source for synthetic substances that may help to increase consumer well-being via being incorporated into new functional foods or medications, as consumers have recently paid a lot of attention to natural bioactive compounds as functional ingredients in foods (Figure 11). However, because of the probable presence of hazardous pollutants such as heavy metals or their high iodine content, seaweed eating must be accompanied with an understanding of the hazards to human health. Because of the presence of numerous of innovative bioactive substances with potential anti-disease activities, using green extraction or purification processes of compounds from complex seaweed matrix is a viable or logical strategy for avoiding these health-related issues or creating added-value functional products.

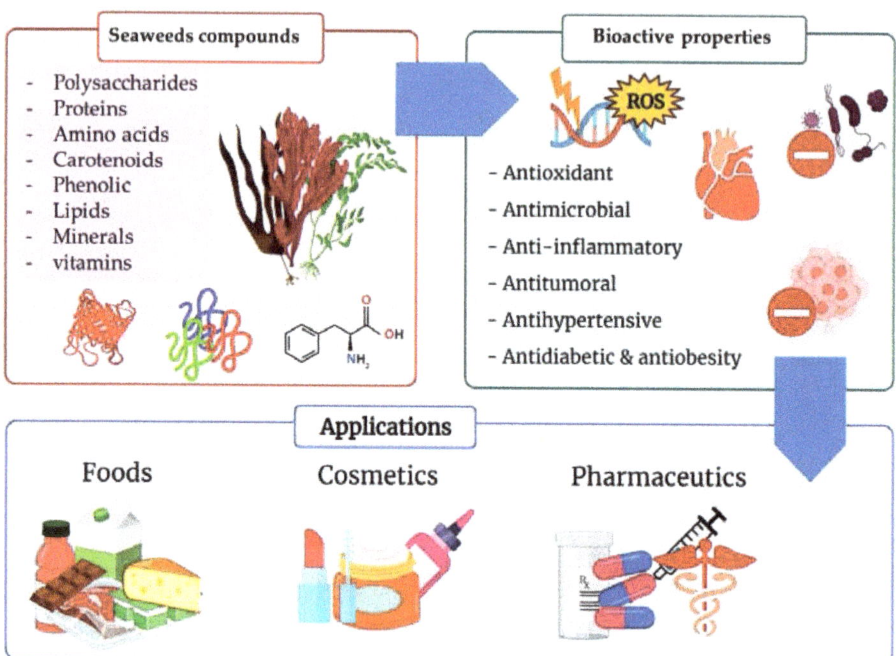

Figure 11. A summary for the bioactive compounds that have different biological activities and used in different applications. Adapted from ref. [384] obtained from mdpi journals.

Author Contributions: Conceptualization, H.S.E.-B., A.A.M., H.I.M., K.M.A.R., A.A.B. and A.T.M.; software, H.S.E.-B., A.A.M., H.I.M., K.M.A.R., A.A.B. and A.T.M.; validation, H.S.E.-B., A.A.M., H.I.M., K.M.A.R., A.A.B. and A.T.M.; investigation, H.S.E.-B., A.A.M., H.I.M., K.M.A.R., A.A.B. and A.T.M.; resources, H.S.E.-B., A.A.M., H.I.M., K.M.A.R., A.A.B. and A.T.M.; data curation, H.S.E.-B., A.A.M., H.I.M., K.M.A.R., A.A.B. and A.T.M.; writing—original draft preparation, H.S.E.-B., A.A.M., H.I.M., K.M.A.R., A.A.B. and A.T.M.; writing—review and editing, H.S.E.-B., A.A.M., H.I.M., K.M.A.R., A.A.B. and A.T.M.; visualization, H.S.E.-B., A.A.M., H.I.M., K.M.A.R., A.A.B. and A.T.M.; supervision, H.S.E.-B., A.A.M.; project administration, H.S.E.-B. and A.A.M.; funding acquisition, H.S.E.-B. and A.A.M. All authors have read and agreed to the published version of the manuscript.

Funding: 1—Deanship of Scientific Research, Vice Presidency for Graduate Studies and Scientific Research, King Faisal University, Saudi Arabia (Grant 402). 2—Deanship of Scientific Research at Umm Al-Qura University, Saudi Arabia (Grant Code: 22UQU4361052DSR01).

Data Availability Statement: All data available in the review.

Acknowledgments: The authors acknowledge the Deanship of Scientific Research, Vice Presidency for Graduate Studies and Scientific Research, at King Faisal University, for the financial support, under (Grant 402). Furthermore, we thank Deanship of Scientific Research at Umm Al-Qura University for supporting this work by Grant Code: 22UQU4361052DSR01.

Conflicts of Interest: The authors declare no conflict of interest.

References

1. Menaa, F.; Wijesinghe, P.A.U.I.; Thiripuranathar, G.; Uzair, B.; Iqbal, H.; Khan, B.A.; Menaa, B. Ecological and Industrial Implications of Dynamic Seaweed-Associated Microbiota Interactions. *Mar. Drugs* **2020**, *18*, 641. [CrossRef] [PubMed]
2. Duarte, C.M.; Marbá, N.; Holmer, M. Rapid domestication of marine species. *Science* **2007**, *316*, 382–383. Available online: https://www.science.org/doi/10.1126/science.1138042 (accessed on 20 April 2007). [CrossRef] [PubMed]
3. Irkin, L.C.; Yayintas, Ö. Pharmacological Properties and Therapeutic Benefits of Seaweeds (A Review). *Int. J. Trend Sci. Res. Dev.* **2018**, *2*, 1126–1131. [CrossRef]

4. Chapman, V.J.; Chapman, D.J. *Seaweeds and Their Uses*, 3rd ed.; Chapman and Hall in Associate with Methuen: London, UK, 1980; p. 334. [CrossRef]

5. Vieira, E.F.; Soares, C.; Machado, S.; Correia, M.; Ramalhosa, M.J.; Oliva-Teles, M.T.; Paula Carvalho, A.; Domingues, V.F.; Antunes, F.; Oliveira, T.A.C.; et al. Seaweeds from the Portuguese coast as a source of proteinaceous material: Total and free amino acid composition profile. *Food Chem.* **2018**, *269*, 264–275. [CrossRef]

6. Cotas, J.; Leandro, A.; Pacheco, D.; Gonçalves, A.M.M.; Pereira, L. A comprehensive review of the nutraceutical and therapeutic applications of red seaweeds (Rhodophyta). *Life* **2020**, *10*, 19. [CrossRef]

7. Singh, I.P.; Sidana, J. Phlorotannins. In *Functional Ingredients from Algae for Foods and Nutraceuticals*; Domínguez, H., Ed.; Woodhead Publishing: Cambridge, UK, 2013; pp. 181–204.

8. Alshehri, M.A.; Al Thabiani, A.; Alzahrani, O.; Ibrahim, A.A.S.; Osman, G.; Bahattab, O. DNA-barcoding and Species Identification for some Saudi Arabia Seaweeds using rbcL Gene. *J. Pure Appl. Microbiol.* **2019**, *13*, 2035–2044. [CrossRef]

9. Francavilla, M.; Franchi, M.; Monteleone, M.; Caroppo, C. The Red Seaweed Gracilaria gracilis as a Multi Products Source. *Mar. Drugs* **2013**, *11*, 3754–3776. [CrossRef]

10. Gómez-Guzmán, M.; Rodríguez-Nogales, A.; Algieri, F.; Gálvez, J. Potential role of seaweed polyphenols in cardiovascular-associated disorders. *Mar. Drugs* **2018**, *16*, 250. [CrossRef]

11. Misurcová Cao, J.; Wang, J.; Wang, S.; Xu, X. Porphyra species: A mini-review of its pharmacological and nutritional properties. *J. Med. Food* **2016**, *19*, 111–119. [CrossRef]

12. Dolganyuk, V.; Belova, D.; Babich, O.; Prosekov, A.; Ivanova, S.; Katserov, D.; Patyukov, N.; Sukhikh, S. Microalgae: A promising source of valuable bioproducts. *Biomolecules* **2020**, *10*, 1153. [CrossRef]

13. Renuka, N.; Guldhe, A.; Prasanna, R.; Singh, P.; Bux, F. Microalgae as multi-functional options in modern agriculture: Current trends, prospects and challenges. *Biotechnol. Adv.* **2018**, *36*, 1255–1273. [CrossRef] [PubMed]

14. Mantri, V.A.; Kavale, M.G.; Kazi, M.A. Seaweed biodiversity of India: Reviewing current knowledge to identify gaps, challenges, and opportunities. *Diversity* **2020**, *12*, 13. [CrossRef]

15. Kumar, M.; Sun, Y.; Rathour, R.; Pandey, A.; Thakur, I.S.; Tsang, D.C. Algae as potential feedstock for the production of biofuels and value-added products: Opportunities and challenges. *Sci. Total Environ.* **2020**, *716*, 137116. [CrossRef]

16. Saratale, R.G.; Kumar, G.; Banu, R.; Xia, A.; Periyasamy, S.; Saratale, G.D. A critical review on anaerobic digestion of microalgae and macroalgae and co-digestion of biomass for enhanced methane generation. *Bioresour. Technol.* **2018**, *262*, 319–332. [CrossRef] [PubMed]

17. Chiaiese, P.; Corrado, G.; Colla, G.; Kyriacou, M.C.; Rouphael, Y. Renewable sources of plant biostimulation: Microalgae as a sustainable means to improve crop performance. *Front. Plant Sci.* **2018**, *9*, 1782. [CrossRef]

18. Lee, X.J.; Ong, H.C.; Gan, Y.Y.; Chen, W.H.; Mahlia, T.M.I. State of art review on conventional and advanced pyrolysis of macroalgae and microalgae for biochar, bio-oil and bio-syngas production. *Energy Convers. Manag.* **2020**, *210*, 112707. [CrossRef]

19. Eppink, M.H.; Olivieri, G.; Reith, H.; van den Berg, C.; Barbosa, M.J.; Wijffels, R.H. From current algae products to future biorefinery practices: A review. *Biorefineries* **2017**, *166*, 99–123. Available online: https://link.springer.com/chapter/10.1007/10_2016_64 (accessed on 7 March 2017).

20. Ariede, M.B.; Candido, T.M.; Jacome, A.L.M.; Velasco, M.V.R.; de Carvalho, J.C.M.; Baby, A.R. Cosmetic attributes of algae—A review. *Algal Res.* **2017**, *25*, 483–487. [CrossRef]

21. Pulz, O.; Broneske, J.; Waldeck, P. IGV GmbH experience report, industrial production of microalgae under controlled conditions: Innovative prospects. In *Handbook of Microalgal Culture: Applied Phycology and Biotechnology*; Wageningen University: Wageningen, The Netherlands, 2013; pp. 445–460. [CrossRef]

22. Thiyagarasaiyar, K.; Goh, B.H.; Jeon, Y.J.; Yow, Y.Y. Algae metabolites in cosmeceutical: An overview of current applications and challenges. *Mar. Drugs* **2020**, *18*, 323. [CrossRef]

23. Ghosh, R.; Banerjee, K.; Mitra, A. Seaweeds in the Lower Gangetic Delta. In *Handbook of Marine Macroalgae: Biotechnology and Applied Phycology*; Kim, S.K., Ed.; Wiley-Blackwell: Hoboken, NJ, USA, 2012.

24. Misurcová, L. Chemical composition of seaweeds. In *Handbook of Marine Macroalgae: Biotechnology and Applied Phycology*; Kim, S.-K., Ed.; John Wiley & Sons: Hoboken, NJ, USA, 2012; p. 567.

25. Al-Amoudi, O.A.; Mutawie, H.H.; Patel, A.V.; Blunden, G. Chemical composition and antioxidant activities of Jeddah corniche algae. *Saudi J. Biol. Sci.* **2009**, *16*, 23–29. [CrossRef]

26. Edwards, M.; Hanniffy, D.; Heesch, S.; Hernández-Kantún, J.; Moniz, M.; Queguineur, B.; Ratcliff, J.; Soler-Vila, A.; Wan, A. *Macroalgae Fact-Sheets*; Soler-Vila, A., Moniz, M., Eds.; Irish Seaweed Research Group, Ryan Institute, NUI Galway: Galway, Ireland, 2012; p. 40.

27. Shanura Fernando, I.P.; Asanka Sanjeewa, K.K.; Samarakoon, K.W.; Kim, H.S.; Gunasekara, U.K.D.S.S.; Park, Y.J.; Abeytungaa, D.T.U.; Lee, W.W.; Jeon, Y.-J. The potential of fucoidans from Chnoospora minima and Sargassum polycystum in cosmetics: Antioxidant, anti inflammatory, skin whitening, and antiwrinkle activities. *J. Appl. Phycol.* **2018**, *30*, 3223–3232. [CrossRef]

28. Hii, S.L.; Lim, J.; Ong, W.T.; Wong, C.L. Agar from Malaysian red seaweed as potential material for synthesis of bioplastic film. *J. Eng. Sci. Technol.* **2016**, *7*, 1–15.

29. Melo, M.R.S.; Feitosa, J.P.A.; Freitas, A.L.P.; De Paula, R.C.M. Isolation and characterization of soluble sulfated polysaccharide from the red seaweed Gracilaria cornea. *Carbohydr. Polym.* **2002**, *49*, 491. [CrossRef]

30. Hamed, I.; Ozogul, F.; Ozogul, Y.; Regenstein, J.M. Marine bioactive compounds and their health benefits: A review. *Compr. Rev. Food Sci. Food Saf.* **2015**, *14*, 446. [CrossRef]

31. Seedevi, P.; Moovendhan, M.; Viramani, S.; Shanmugam, A. A Bioactive potential and structural chracterization of sulfated polysaccharide from seaweed (*Gracilaria corticata*). *Carbohydr. Polym.* **2017**, *155*, 516–524. [CrossRef]

32. Hamouda, R.A.; Salman, A.S.; Alharbi, A.A.; Alhasani, R.H.; Elshamy, M.M. Assessment of the Antigenotoxic Effects of Alginate and ZnO/Alginate–Nanocomposites Extracted from Brown Alga *Fucus vesiculosus* in Mice. *Polymers* **2021**, *13*, 3839. [CrossRef]

33. Chen, X.; Song, L.; Wang, H.; Liu, S.; Yu, H.; Wang, X.; Li, R.; Liu, T.; Li, P. Partial characterization, the immune modulation and anticancer activities of sulfated polysaccharides from Filamentous microalgae *Tribonema* sp. *Molecules* **2019**, *24*, 322. [CrossRef]

34. He, D.; Wu, S.; Yan, L.; Zuo, J.; Cheng, Y.; Wang, H.; Liu, J.; Zhang, X.; Wu, M.; Choi, J.-I.; et al. Antitumor bioactivity of porphyran extracted from *Pyropia yezoensis* Chonsoo2 on human cancer cell lines. *J. Sci. Food Agr.* **2019**, *99*, 6722–6730. [CrossRef]

35. Nagamine, T.; Hayakawa, K.; Kusakabe, T.; Takada, H.; Nakazato, K.; Hisanaga, E.; Iha, M. Inhibitory effect of fucoidan on Huh7 hepatoma cells through downregulation of CXCL12. *Nutr. Cancer* **2009**, *61*, 340–347. [CrossRef]

36. Obluchinskaya, E.D.; Pozharitskaya, O.N.; Zakharov, D.V.; Flisyuk, E.V.; Terninko, I.I.; Generalova, Y.E.; Smekhova, I.E.; Shikov, A.N. The Biochemical Composition and Antioxidant Properties of *Fucus vesiculosus* from the Arctic Region. *Mar. Drugs* **2022**, *20*, 193. [CrossRef]

37. Xu, S.-Y.; Kan, J.; Hu, Z.; Liu, Y.; Du, H.; Pang, G.-C.; Cheong, K.-L. Quantification of Neoagaro-Oligosaccharide Production through Enzymatic Hydrolysis and Its Anti-Oxidant Activities. *Molecules* **2018**, *23*, 1354. [CrossRef] [PubMed]

38. Ozanne, H.; Toumi, H.; Roubinet, B.; Landemarre, L.; Lespessailles, E.; Daniellou, R.; Cesaro, A. Laminarin Effects, a β-(1,3)-Glucan, on Skin Cell Inflammation and Oxidation. *Cosmetics* **2020**, *7*, 66. [CrossRef]

39. Jiang, N.; Li, B.; Wang, X.; Xu, X.; Liu, X.; Li, W.; Chang, X.; Li, H.; Qi, H. The antioxidant and antihyperlipidemic activities of phosphorylated polysaccharide from *Ulva pertusa*. *Int. J. Biol. Macromol.* **2020**, *145*, 1059–1065. [CrossRef]

40. Li, B.; Xu, H.; Wang, X.; Wan, Y.; Jiang, N.; Qi, H.; Liu, X. Antioxidant and antihyperlipidemic activities of high sulfate content purified polysaccharide from Ulva pertusa. *Int. J. Biol. Macromol.* **2020**, *146*, 756–762. [CrossRef]

41. Pérez, M.J.; Falqué, E.; Domínguez, H. Antimicrobial action of compounds from marine seaweed. *Mar. Drugs* **2016**, *14*, 52. [CrossRef] [PubMed]

42. Damonte, E.; Matulewicz, M.; Cerezo, A. Sulfated Seaweed Polysaccharides as Antiviral Agents. *Curr. Med. Chem.* **2012**, *11*, 2399–2419. [CrossRef] [PubMed]

43. Cherry, P.; O'hara, C.; Magee, P.J.; Mcsorley, E.M.; Allsopp, P.J. Risks and benefits of consuming edible seaweeds. *Nutr. Rev.* **2019**, *77*, 307–329. [CrossRef]

44. Cheong, K.L.; Qiu, H.M.; Du, H.; Liu, Y.; Khan, B.M. Oligosaccharides derived from red seaweed: Production, properties, and potential health and cosmetic applications. *Molecules* **2018**, *23*, 2451. [CrossRef]

45. Mohamed, S.; Hashim, S.N.; Rahman, A. Seaweeds: A sustainable functional food for complementary and alternative therapy. *Trends Food Sci. Technol.* **2012**, *23*, 83–96. [CrossRef]

46. Venugopal, V. Sulfated and non-sulfated polysaccharides from seaweeds and their uses: An overview. *ECronicon Nutr.* **2019**, *2*, 126–141.

47. De Morais, M.G.; Vaz, B.D.S.; De Morais, E.G.; Costa, J.A.V. Biologically Active Metabolites Synthesized by Microalgae. *BioMed Res. Int.* **2015**, *2015*, 835761. [CrossRef] [PubMed]

48. Ouyang, Q.Q.; Hu, Z.; Li, S.D.; Quan, W.Y.; Wen, L.L.; Yang, Z.M.; Li, P.W. Thermal degradation of agar: Mechanism and toxicity of products. *Food Chem.* **2018**, *264*, 277–283. [CrossRef] [PubMed]

49. Mohsin, S.; Kurup, G.M. Mechanism underlying the anti-inflammatory effect of sulphated polysaccharide from *Padina tetrastromatica* against carrageenan induced paw edema in rats. *Biomed. Prev. Nutr.* **2011**, *1*, 294–301. [CrossRef]

50. Anastyuk, S.; Shervchenko, N.; Ermakova, S.; Vishchuk, O.; Nazarenko, E.; Dmitrenok, P.; Zvyagintseva, T. Anticancer activity in vitro of a fucoidan from the brown algae *Fucus evanescens* and its low-molecular fragments, structurally characterized by tandem mass-spectrometry. *Carbohydr. Polym.* **2012**, *87*, 186–194. [CrossRef] [PubMed]

51. Wang, Z.-J.; Xu, W.; Liang, J.-W.; Wang, C.-S.; Kang, Y. Effect of fucoidan on B16 murine melanoma cell melanin formation and apoptosis. *Afr. J. Tradit. Complement. Altern. Med.* **2017**, *14*, 149–155. [CrossRef]

52. Adrien, A.; Bonnet, A.; Dufour, D.; Baudouin, S.; Maugard, T.; Bridiau, N. Pilot production of ulvans from *Ulva* sp. and their effects on hyaluronan and collagen production in cultured dermal fibroblasts. *Carbohydr. Polym.* **2017**, *157*, 1306–1314. [CrossRef]

53. Fernando, I.S.; Sanjeewa, K.A.; Samarakoon, K.W.; Lee, W.W.; Kim, H.S.; Kang, N.; Ranasinghe, P.; Lee, H.S.; Jeon, Y.J. A fucoidan fraction purified from *Chnoospora minima*; a potential inhibitor of LPS-induced inflammatory responses. *Int. J. Boil. Macromol.* **2017**, *104*, 1185–1193. [CrossRef]

54. Zhang, Z.; Wang, F.; Wang, X.; Liu, X.; Hou, Y.; Zhang, Q. Extraction of the polysaccharides from five algae and their potential antioxidant activity in vitro. *Carbohydr. Polym.* **2010**, *82*, 118–121. [CrossRef]

55. Hwang, P.A.; Chien, S.Y.; Chan, Y.L.; Lu, M.K.; Wu, C.H.; Kong, Z.L.; Wu, C.J. Inhibition of lipopolysaccharide (LPS)-induced inflammatory responses by *Sargassum hemiphyllum* sulfated polysaccharide extract in RAW 264.7 macrophage cells. *J. Agric. Food Chem.* **2011**, *59*, 2062–2068. [CrossRef]

56. Ale, M.T.; Maruyama, H.; Tamauchi, H.; Mikkelsen, J.D.; Meyer, A.S. Fucose-containing sulfated polysaccharides from brown seaweeds inhibit proliferation of melanoma cells and induce apoptosis by activation of caspase-3 in vitro. *Mar. Drugs* **2011**, *9*, 2605–2621. [CrossRef]

57. Torres, M.D.; Flórez-Fernández, N.; Domínguez, H. Integral utilization of red seaweed for bioactive production. *Mar. Drugs* **2019**, *17*, 314. [CrossRef] [PubMed]

58. Hong, S.J.; Lee, J.H.; Kim, E.J.; Yang, H.J.; Park, J.S.; Hong, S.K. Toxicological evaluation of neoagarooligosaccharides prepared by enzymatic hydrolysis of agar. *Regul. Toxicol. Pharmacol.* **2017**, *90*, 9–21. [CrossRef] [PubMed]

59. Ellis, A.L.; Norton, A.B.; Mills, T.B.; Norton, I.T. Stabilisation of foams by agar gel particles. *Food Hydrocoll.* **2017**, *33*, 222–228. [CrossRef]

60. Hernandez-Carmona, G.; Freile-Pelegrín, Y.; Hernández-Garibay, E. Conventional and alternative technologies for the extraction of algal polysaccharides. In *Functional Ingredients from Algae for Foods and Nutraceuticals*; Woodhead Publishing: Cambridge, UK, 2013; pp. 475–516. [CrossRef]

61. Pegg, A.M. The application of natural hydrocolloids to foods and beverages. In *Natural Food Additives, Ingredients and Flavourings*; Woodhead Publishing: Cambridge, UK, 2012; pp. 175–196.

62. Scieszka, S.; Klewicka, E. Algae in food: A general review. *Crit. Rev. Food Sci. Nutr.* **2019**, *59*, 3538–3547. [CrossRef] [PubMed]

63. McHugh, D.J. *A Guide to the Seaweed Industry*; FAO Fisheries Technical Paper 441; Food and Agriculture Organization of the United Nations: Rome, Italy, 2003; Available online: https://www.fao.org/3/y4765e/y4765e00.htm (accessed on 15 July 2003).

64. Soukoulis, C.; Chandrinos, I.; Tzia, C. Study of the functionality of selected hydrocolloids and their blends with κ-carrageenan on storage quality of vanilla ice cream. *LWT* **2008**, *41*, 1816–1827. [CrossRef]

65. Pereira, L. *Carrageenans—Sources and Extraction Methods, Molecular Structure, Bioactive Properties and Health Effects*; Nova Science Publishers: Hauppauge, NY, USA, 2016; p. 293. ISBN 1634855035. Available online: https://novapublishers.com/shop/carrageenans-sources-and-extraction-methods-molecular-structure-bioactive-properties-and-health-effects/ (accessed on 1 September 2016).

66. Balboa, E.M.; Conde, E.; Soto, M.L.; Pérez-Armada, L.; Domínguez, H. Cosmetics from marine sources. In *Springer Handbook of Marine Biotechnology*; Kim, S.-K., Ed.; Springer: Berlin/Heidelberg, Germany, 2015; pp. 1015–1042. ISBN 978-3-642-53970-1. Available online: https://www.springerprofessional.de/en/cosmetics-from-marine-sources/4217512 (accessed on 1 February 2020).

67. Mafinowska, P. Algae extracts as active cosmetic ingredients. *Zesz. Nauk.* **2011**, *212*, 123–129.

68. Fabrowska, J.; Łęska, B.; Schroeder, G.; Messyasz, B.; Pikosz, M. Biomass and extracts of algae as material for cosmetics. In *Marine Algae Extracts*; Kim, S.-K., Chojnacka, K., Eds.; Wiley-VCH, Verlag GmbH & Co. KGaA: Weinheim, Germany, 2015; pp. 681–706. ISBN 9783527337088.

69. Hotchkiss, S.; Campbell, R.; Hepburn, C. Carrageenan: Sources and extraction methods. In *Carrageenans: Sources and Extraction Methods, Molecular Structure, Bioactive Properties and Health Effects*; Pereira, L., Ed.; Nova Science Publishers: New York, NY, USA, 2016; pp. 1–16. ISBN 978-1-63485-503-7.

70. Pereira, L.; Gheda, S.F.; Ribeiro-Claro, P.J. Analysis by vibrational spectroscopy of seaweed polysaccharides with potential use in food, pharmaceutical, and cosmetic industries. *Int. J. Carbohydr. Chem.* **2013**, *2013*, 537202. [CrossRef]

71. Fitton, J.H. Therapies from fucoidan; multifunctional marine polymers. *Mar. Drugs* **2011**, *9*, 1731–1760. [CrossRef]

72. Wu, L.; Sun, J.; Su, X.; Yu, Q.; Yu, Q.; Zhang, P. A review about the development of fucoidan in antitumor activity: Progress and challenges. *Carbohydr. Polym.* **2016**, *154*, 96–111. [CrossRef]

73. Saravana, P.S.; Cho, Y.-N.; Patil, M.P.; Cho, Y.-J.; Kim, G.-D.; Park, Y.B.; Woo, H.-C.; Chun, B.-S. Hydrothermal degradation of seaweed polysaccharide: Characterization and biological activities. *Food Chem.* **2018**, *268*, 179–187. [CrossRef]

74. Yaich, H.; Amira, A.B.; Abbes, F.; Bouaziz, M.; Besbes, S.; Richel, A.; Blecker, C.; Attia, H.; Garna, H. Effect of extraction procedures on structural, thermal and antioxidant properties of ulvan from *Ulva lactuca* collected in Monastir coast. *Int. J. Biol. Macromol.* **2017**, *105*, 1430–1439. [CrossRef] [PubMed]

75. Lahaye, M.; Robic, A. Structure and functional properties of ulvan, a polysaccharide from green seaweeds. *Biomacromolecules* **2007**, *8*, 1765–1774. [CrossRef] [PubMed]

76. Pereira, L. Biological and therapeutic properties of the seaweed polysaccharides. *Int. Biol. Rev.* **2018**, *2*, 1–50. [CrossRef]

77. Peñalver, R.; Lorenzo, J.M.; Ros, G.; Amarowicz, R.; Pateiro, M.; Nieto, G. Seaweeds as a Functional Ingredient for a Healthy Diet. *Mar. Drugs* **2020**, *18*, 301. [CrossRef]

78. Lordan, S.; Ross, R.P.; Stanton, C. Marine bioactives as functional food ingredients. Potential to reduce the incidence of chronic diseases. *Mar. Drugs* **2011**, *9*, 1056–1100. [CrossRef]

79. Pimentel, F.B.; Alves, R.C.; Rodrigues, F.; Oliveira, M.B.P.P. Macroalgae-Derived Ingredients for Cosmetic Industry—An Update. *Cosmetics* **2018**, *5*, 2. [CrossRef]

80. Admassu, H.; Abdalbasit, M.; Gasmalla, A.; Yang, R.; Zhao, W. Bioactive peptides derived from seaweed protein and their health benefits: Antihypertensive, antioxidant, and antidiabetic properties. *J. Food Sci.* **2018**, *83*, 6–16. [CrossRef]

81. Wijesekara, I.; Lang, M.; Marty, C.; Gemin, M.P.; Boulho, R.; Douzenel, P.; Wickramasinghe, I.; Bedoux, G.; Bourgougnon, N. Different extraction procedures and analysis of protein from *Ulva* Sp. In Brittany, France. *J. Appl. Phycol.* **2017**, *29*, 2503–2511. [CrossRef]

82. Abdel-fattah, A.F.; Sary, H.H. Glycoproteins from *Ulva lactuca*. *Phytochemistry* **1987**, *26*, 1447–1448. [CrossRef]

83. Kim, E.Y.; Kim, Y.R.; Nam, T.J.; Kong, I.S. Antioxidant and DNA protection activities of a glycoprotein isolated from a seaweed, *Saccharina japonica*. *Int. J. Food Sci. Technol.* **2012**, *47*, 1020–1027. [CrossRef]

84. Chaves, R.P.; Silva, S.R.D.; Nascimento Neto, L.G.; Carneiro, R.F.; Silva, A.L.C.D.; Sampaio, A.H.; Sousa, B.L.D.; Cabral, M.G.; Videira, P.A.; Teixeira, E.H.; et al. structural characterization of two isolectins from the marine red alga *Solieria Filiformis* (Kützing) P.W. Gabrielson and their anticancer effect on MCF-7 breast cancer cells. *Int. J. Biol. Macromol.* **2018**, *107*, 1320–1329. [CrossRef] [PubMed]

85. Abreu, T.M.; Monteiro, V.S.; Martins, A.B.S.; Teles, F.B.; Da Conceição Rivanor, R.L.; Mota, É.F.; Macedo, D.S.; de Vasconcelos, S.M.M.; Júnior, J.E.R.H.; Benevides, N.M.B. Involvement of the dopaminergic system in the antidepressant-like effect of the lectin isolated from the red marine alga *Solieria Filiformis* in mice. *Int. J. Biol. Macromol.* **2018**, *111*, 534–541. [CrossRef] [PubMed]

86. Oh, J.H.; Nam, T.J. Hydrophilic glycoproteins of an edible green alga *Capsosiphon fulvescens* prevent aging- induced spatial memory impairment by suppressing Gsk-3β-Mediated Er stress in *Dorsal hippocampus*. *Mar. Drugs.* **2019**, *17*, 168. [CrossRef] [PubMed]

87. Rafiquzzaman, S.M.; Kim, E.Y.; Lee, J.M.; Mohibbullah, M.; Alam, M.B.; Soo Moon, I.; Kim, J.M.; Kong, I.S. Anti-Alzheimers and anti-inflammatory activities of a glycoprotein purified from the edible brown alga *Undaria pinnatifida*. *Food Res. Int.* **2015**, *77*, 118–124. [CrossRef]

88. Ratana-arporn, P.; Chirapart, A. Nutritional Evaluation of Tropical Green Seaweeds Caulerpa Lentillifera and Ulva Reticulata. *Kasetsart J. Nat. Sci.* **2006**, *40*, 75–83.

89. Lumbessy, S.Y.; Andayani, S.; Nursyam, H.; Firdaus, M. Biochemical Study of Amino Acid Profile of *Kappaphycus alvarezii* and *Gracilaria salicornia* Seaweeds from Gerupuk Waters, West Nusa Tenggara (NTB). *Eur. Asian J. Biosci.* **2019**, *13*, 303–307.

90. Zubia, M.; Payri, C.E.; Deslandes, E.; Guezennec, J. Chemical Composition of Attached and Drift Specimens of Sargassum Mangarevense and Turbinaria Ornata (Phaeophyta: Fucales) from Tahiti, French Polynesia. *Bot. Mar.* **2003**, *46*, 562–571. [CrossRef]

91. Uribe, E.; Vega-Gálvez, A.; Vargas, N.; Pasten, A.; Rodríguez, K.; Ah-Hen, K.S. Phytochemical Components and Amino Acid Profile of Brown Seaweed Durvillaea Antarctica as Affected by Air Drying Temperature. *J. Food Sci. Technol.* **2018**, *55*, 4792–4801. [CrossRef]

92. Kadam, S.U.; Tiwari, B.K.; O'Donnell, C.P. Application of novel extraction technologies for bioactives from marine algae. *J. Agric. Food Chem.* **2013**, *61*, 4667–4675. [CrossRef]

93. Helmi, A.; Mohamed, H.I. Biochemical and ulturasturctural changes of some tomato cultivars to infestation with *Aphis gossypii* Glover (Hemiptera: Aphididae) at Qalyubiya, Egypt. *Gesunde Pflanzen.* **2016**, *68*, 41–50. [CrossRef]

94. Fleurence, J. Seaweed proteins. In *Proteins in Food Processing*; Yada, R.Y., Ed.; Woodhead Publishing: Cambridge, UK, 2004; pp. 197–213.

95. Galland-Irmouli, A.V.; Fleurence, J.; Lamghari, R.; Luçon, M.; Rouxel, C.; Barbaroux, O.; Bronowicki, J.P.; Villaume, C.; Guéant, J.L. Nutritional value of proteins from edible seaweed *Palmaria palmata* (dulse). *J. Nutr. Biochem.* **1999**, *10*, 353–359. [CrossRef]

96. Wu, G. (Ed.) *Amino Acids: Biochemistry and Nutrition*, 1st ed.; CRC Press: Boca Raton, FL, USA, 2013. [CrossRef]

97. Prabhasankar, P.; Ganesan, P.; Bhaskar, N.; Hirose, A.; Stephen, N.; Gowda, L.R. Edible Japanese seaweed, wakame (*Undaria pinnatifida*) as an ingredient in pasta: Chemical, functional and structural evaluation. *Food Chem.* **2009**, *115*, 501–508. [CrossRef]

98. Ramos-Romero, S.; Torrella, J.R.; Pagès, T.; Viscor, G.; Torres, J.L. Edible microalgae and their bioactive compounds in the prevention and treatment of metabolic alterations. *Nutrients.* **2021**, *13*, 563. [CrossRef] [PubMed]

99. Mabeau, S.; Fleurence, J. Seaweed in food products: Biochemical and nutritional aspects. *Trends Food Sci. Technol.* **1993**, *4*, 103–107. [CrossRef]

100. Lee, H.-A.; Kim, I.-H.; Nam, T.-J. Bioactive peptide from *Pyropia yezoensis* and its anti-inflammatory activities. *Int. J. Mol. Med.* **2015**, *36*, 1701–1706. [CrossRef]

101. Ryu, J.; Park, S.J.; Kim, I.H.; Choi, Y.H.; Nam, T.J. Protective effect of porphyra-334 on UVA-induced photoaging in human skin fibroblasts. *Int. J. Mol. Med.* **2014**, *34*, 796–803. [CrossRef]

102. Verdy, C.; Branka, J.E.; Mekideche, N. Quantitative assessment of lactate and progerin production in normal human cutaneous cells during normal ageing: Effect of an *Alaria esculenta* extract. *Int. J. Cosmet. Sci.* **2011**, *33*, 462–466. [CrossRef]

103. Mensi, F.; Nasraoui, S.; Bouguerra, S.; BenGhedifa, A.; Chalghaf, M. Effect of Lagoon and sea water depth on *Gracilaria gracilis* growth and biochemical composition in the Northeast of Tunisia. *Sci. Rep.* **2020**, *10*, 10014. [CrossRef]

104. Pliego-Cortés, H.; Bedoux, G.; Boulho, R.; Taupin, L.; Freile-Pelegrin, Y.; Bourgougnon, N.; Robledo, D. Stress tolerance and photoadaptation to solar radiation in *Rhodymenia pseudopalmata* (Rhodophyta) through mycosporine-like amino acids, phenolic compounds, and pigments in an Integrated Multi-Trophic Aquaculture System. *Algal Res.* **2019**, *41*, 101542. [CrossRef]

105. Athukorala, Y.; Trang, S.; Kwok, C.; Yuan, Y.V. Antiproliferative and antioxidant activities and mycosporine-Like amino acid profiles of wild-Harvested and cultivated edible Canadian marine red macroalgae. *Molecules* **2016**, *21*, 119. [CrossRef]

106. Barceló-Villalobos, M.; Figueroa, F.L.; Korbee, N.; Álvarez-Gómez, F.; Abreu, M.H. Production of Mycosporine-Like amino acids from *Gracilaria vermiculophylla* (Rhodophyta) cultured through one year in an integrated multi-trophic aquaculture (IMTA) system. *Mar. Biotechnol.* **2017**, *19*, 246–254. [CrossRef] [PubMed]

107. Holdt, S.L.; Kraan, S. Bioactive compounds in seaweed: Functional food applications and legislation. *J. Appl. Phycol.* **2011**, *23*, 543–597. [CrossRef]

108. Pereira, L. Seaweeds as Source of Bioactive Substances and Skin Care Therapy—Cosmeceuticals, Algotheraphy, and Thalassotherapy. *Cosmetics* **2018**, *5*, 68. [CrossRef]

109. Saadaoui, I.; Rasheed, R.; Abdulrahman, N.; Bounnit, T.; Cherif, M.; Al Jabri, H.; Mraiche, F. Algae-derived bioactive compounds with anti-lung cancer potential. *Mar. Drugs* **2020**, *18*, 197. [CrossRef] [PubMed]

110. Pangestutil, R.; Kim, S. *Seaweed Proteins, Peptides, and Amino Acids*; Elsevier Inc.: Amsterdam, The Netherlands, 2015; pp. 125–140. [CrossRef]

111. Cicero, A.F.; Fogacci, F.; Colletti, A. Potential role of bioactive peptides in prevention and treatment of chronic diseases: A narrative review. *Br. J. Pharmacol.* **2017**, *174*, 1378–1394. [CrossRef] [PubMed]

112. Chrapusta, E.; Kaminski, A.; Duchnik, K.; Bober, B.; Adamski, M.; Bialczyk, J. Mycosporine-like amino acids: Potential health and beauty ingredients. *Mar. Drugs* **2017**, *15*, 326. [CrossRef]

113. Morais, T.; Cotas, J.; Pacheco, D.; Pereira, L. Seaweeds Compounds: An Ecosustainable Source of Cosmetic Ingredients? *Cosmetics* **2021**, *8*, 8. [CrossRef]

114. Bedoux, G.; Hardouin, K.; Burlot, A.S.; Bourgougnon, N. Bioactive components from seaweeds: Cosmetic applications and future development. *Adv. Bot. Res.* **2014**, *71*, 345–378. [CrossRef]

115. Pereira, L. Chapter 6—Seaweed Flora of the European North Atlantic and Mediterranean. In *Springer Handbook of Marine Biotechnology*; Se-Kwon, K., Ed.; Springer: Berlin/Heidelberg, Germany, 2015; pp. 65–178. ISBN 978-3-642-53971-8. [CrossRef]

116. Notowidjojo, L. Seaweed as novel food for prevention and therapy for life style related disease. *World Nutr J.* **2021**, *5*, 1–5. [CrossRef]

117. Dhargalkar, V.K.; Verlecar, X.N. Southern Ocean seaweeds: A resource for exploration in food and drugs. *Aquaculture* **2009**, *287*, 229–242. [CrossRef]

118. Probst, Y. A review of the nutrient composition of selected rubus berries. *Nutr. Food Sci.* **2015**, *45*, 242–254. [CrossRef]

119. Conde, E.; Balboa, E.M.; Parada, M.; Falqué, E. Algal proteins, peptides and amino acids. In *Functional Ingredients from Algae for Foods and Nutraceuticals*; Domínguez, H., Ed.; Woodhead Publishing Limited: Cambridge, UK, 2013; pp. 135–180. ISBN 978-0-85709-512-1.

120. Quitral, V.; Morales, C.; Sepúlveda, M.; Schwartz, M. Propiedades nutritivas y saludables de algas marinas y su potencialidad como ingrediente funcional. *Rev. Chil. Neuropsiquiatr.* **2015**, *53*, 35–43. [CrossRef]

121. Ramadan, K.M.A.; El-Beltagi, H.S.; Shanab, S.M.M.; El-fayoumy, E.A.; Shalaby, E.A.; Bendary, E.S.A. Potential Antioxidant and Anticancer Activities of Secondary Metabolites of Nostoc linckia Cultivated under Zn and Cu Stress Conditions. *Processes* **2021**, *9*, 1972. [CrossRef]

122. Calder, P.C. Functional roles of fatty acids and their effects on human health. *J. Parenter. Enter. Nutr.* **2015**, *39*, 18S–32S. [CrossRef] [PubMed]

123. Menaa, F.; Wijesinghe, U.; Thiripuranathar, G.; Althobaiti, N.A.; Albalawi, A.E.; Khan, B.A.; Menaa, B. Marine Algae-Derived Bioactive Compounds: A New Wave of Nanodrugs? *Mar. Drugs* **2021**, *19*, 484. [CrossRef]

124. Gosch, B.J.; Magnusson, M.; Paul, N.A.; De Nys, R. Total lipid and fatty acid composition of seaweeds for the selection of species for oil-based biofuel and bioproducts. *GCB Bioenergy* **2012**, *4*, 919–930. [CrossRef]

125. Lopez-Huertas, E. Health effects of oleic acid and long chain omega-3 fatty acids (EPA and DHA) enriched milks. A review of intervention studies. *Pharmacol. Res.* **2010**, *61*, 200–207. [CrossRef]

126. Kumari, P.; Kumar, M.; Gupta, V.; Reddy, C.R.K.; Jha, B. Tropical marine macroalgae as potential sources of nutritionally important PUFAs. *Food Chem.* **2010**, *120*, 749–757. [CrossRef]

127. Matanjun, P.; Mohamed, S.; Mustapha, N.M.; Muhammad, K. Nutrient content of tropical edible seaweeds, *Eucheuma cottonii*, *Caulerpa lentillifera* and *Sargassum polycystum*. *J. Appl. Phycol.* **2009**, *21*, 75–80. [CrossRef]

128. Ortiz, J.; Uquiche, E.; Robert, P.; Romero, N.; Quitral, V.; Llantén, C. Functional and nutritional value of the Chilean seaweeds *Codium fragile*, *Gracilaria chilensis* and *Macrocystis pyrifera*. *Eur. J. Lipid Sci. Technol.* **2009**, *111*, 320–327. [CrossRef]

129. Ortiz, J.; Romero, N.; Robert, P.; Araya, J.; Lopez-Hernández, J.; Bozzo, C.; Navarrete, E.; Osorio, A.; Rios, A. Dietary fiber, amino acid, fatty acid and tocopherol contents of the edible seaweeds *Ulva lactuca* and *Durvillaea antarctica*. *Food Chem.* **2006**, *99*, 98–104. [CrossRef]

130. Lorenzo, J.M.; Agregán, R.; Munekata, P.E.S.; Franco, D.; Carballo, J.; Sahin, S.; Lacomba, R.; Barba, F.J. Proximate composition and nutritional value of three macroalgae: *Ascophyllum nodosum*, *Fucus vesiculosus* and *Bifurcaria bifurcata*. *Mar. Drugs* **2017**, *15*, 360. [CrossRef] [PubMed]

131. Cofrades, S.; Lopez-Lopez, I.; Bravo, L.; Ruiz-Capillas, C.; Bastida, S., Larrea, M.T., Jiménez-Colmenero, F. Nutritional and antioxidant properties of different brown and red spanish edible seaweeds. *Food Sci. Technol. Int.* **2010**, *16*, 361–370. [CrossRef] [PubMed]

132. Dawczynski, C.; Schubert, R.; Jahreis, G. Amino acids, fatty acids, and dietary fibre in edible seaweed products. *Food Chem.* **2007**, *103*, 891–899. [CrossRef]

133. Liu, B.; Kongstad, K.T.; Wiese, S.; Jager, A.K.; Staerk, D. Edible seaweed as future functional food: Identification of alpha-glucosidase inhibitors by combined use of high-resolution alpha-glucosidase inhibition profiling and HPLC-HRMS-SPE-NMR. *Food Chem.* **2016**, *203*, 16–22. [CrossRef]

134. Godfray, H.C.J.; Beddington, J.R.; Crute, I.R.; Haddad, L.; Lawrence, D.; Muir, J.F.; Pretty, J.; Robinson, S.; Thomas, S.M.; Toulmin, C. Food Security: The Challenge of Feeding 9 Billion People. *Science* **2010**, *327*, 812–818. [CrossRef]

135. Arao, T.; Yamada, M. Positional distribution of fatty acids in galactolipids of algae. *J. Phytochem.* **1989**, *28*, 805–810. [CrossRef]

136. Niaz, A.; Kashif, A. Chemical and Different Nutritional Characteristics of Brown Seaweed Lipids Advances in Science. *Technol. Eng. Syst. J.* **2016**, *1*, 23–25. [CrossRef]

137. Kanazawa, A. Sterols in marine invertebrates. *Fish. Sci.* **2001**, *67*, 997–1007. [CrossRef]

138. Francavilla, M.; Trotta, P.; Luque, R. Phytosterols from *Dunaliella tertiolecta* and *Dunaliella salina*: A potentially novel industrial application. *Bioresour. Technol.* **2010**, *101*, 4144–4150. [CrossRef]

139. da Vaz, B.S.; Moreira, J.B.; De Morais, M.G.; Costa, J.A.V. Microalgae as a new source of bioactive compounds in food supplements. *Curr. Opin. Food Sci.* **2016**, *7*, 73–77. [CrossRef]

140. Peng, Y.; Hu, J.; Yang, B.; Lin, X.P.; Zhou, X.F.; Yang, X.W.; Liu, Y. *Chemical Composition of Seaweeds*; Elsevier Inc.: Amsterdam, The Netherlands, 2015; pp. 79–124. ISBN 9780124199583.

141. Hamid, N.; Ma, Q.; Boulom, S.; Liu, T.; Zheng, Z.; Balbas, J.; Robertson, J. *Seaweed Minor Constituents*; Elsevier Inc.: Amsterdam, The Netherlands, 2015; pp. 193–242.

142. Aryee, A.N.; Agyei, D.; Akanbi, T.O. Recovery and utilization of seaweed pigments in food processing. *Curr. Opin. Food Sci.* **2018**, *19*, 113–119. [CrossRef]

143. Jia, X.; Yang, J.; Wang, Z.; Liu, R.; Xie, R. Polysaccharides from Laminaria japonica show hypoglycemic and hypolipidemic activities in mice with experimentally induced diabetes. *Exp. Biol. Med.* **2014**, *239*, 1663–1670. [CrossRef] [PubMed]

144. Bajpai, V.K.; Shukla, S.; Kang, S.M.; Hwang, S.K.; Song, X.; Huh, Y.S.; Han, Y.K. Developments of cyanobacteria for nano-marine drugs: Relevance of nanoformulations in cancer therapies. *Mar. Drugs* **2018**, *16*, 179. [CrossRef]

145. Camacho, F.; Macedo, A.; Malcata, F. Potential industrial applications and commercialization of microalgae in the functional food and feed industries: A short review. *Mar. Drugs* **2019**, *17*, 312. [CrossRef]

146. Maltsev, Y.; Maltseva, K. *Fatty Acids of Microalgae: Diversity and Applications*; Springer: Dordrecht, The Netherlands, 2021; Volume 3. ISBN 0123456789.

147. Da Silva, T.L.; Moniz, P.; Silva, C.; Reis, A. The dark side of microalgae biotechnology: A heterotrophic biorefinery platform directed to ω-3 rich lipid production. *Microorganisms* **2019**, *7*, 670. [CrossRef]

148. Molino, A.; Iovine, A.; Casella, P.; Mehariya, S.; Chianese, S.; Cerbone, A.; Rimauro, J.; Musmarra, D. Microalgae characterization for consolidated and new application in human food, animal feed and nutraceuticals. *Int. J. Environ. Res. Public Health* **2018**, *15*, 2436. [CrossRef]

149. Wynn, J.; Behrens, P.; Sundararajan, A.; Hansen, J.; Apt, K. Production of single cell oils from dinoflagellates. In *Single Cell Oils; Microbial and Algal Oils*; Cohen, Z., Ratledge, C., Eds.; AOCS Press: Champaign, IL, USA, 2010; pp. 115–129.

150. Ward, O.P.; Singh, A. Omega-3/6 fatty acids: Alternative sources of production. *Process Biochem.* **2005**, *40*, 3627–3652. [CrossRef]

151. Stengel, D.B.; Connan, S.; Popper, Z.A. Algal chemodiversity and bioactivity: Sources of natural variability and implications for commercial application. *Biotechnol. Adv.* **2011**, *29*, 483–501. [CrossRef]

152. Murphy, M.J.; Dow, A.A. Clinical studies of the safety and efficacy of macroalgae extracts in cosmeceuticals. *J. Clin. Aesthet. Dermatol.* **2021**, *14*, 37–41.

153. Yang, M.; Zhou, M.; Song, L. A review of fatty acids influencing skin condition. *J. Cosmet. Dermatol.* **2020**, *19*, 3199–3204. [CrossRef] [PubMed]

154. De Luca, M.; Pappalardo, I.; Limongi, A.R.; Viviano, E.; Radice, R.P.; Todisco, S.; Martelli, G.; Infantino, V.; Vassallo, A. Lipids from Microalgae for Cosmetic Applications. *Cosmetics* **2021**, *8*, 52. [CrossRef]

155. Yamada, K.; Nitta, T.; Atsuji, K.; Shiroyama, M.; Inoue, K.; Higuchi, C.; Nitta, N.; Oshiro, S.; Mochida, K.; Iwata, O.; et al. Characterization of sulfur-compound metabolism underlying wax-ester fermentation in Euglena gracilis. *Sci. Rep.* **2019**, *9*, 853. [CrossRef] [PubMed]

156. Huynh, A.; Maktabi, B.; Reddy, C.M.; O'Neil, G.W.; Chandler, M.; Baki, G. Evaluation of alkenones, a renewably sourced, plant-derived wax as a structuring agent for lipsticks. *Int. J. Cosmet. Sci.* **2020**, *42*, 146–155. [CrossRef] [PubMed]

157. Lee, H.J.; Dang, H.T.; Kang, G.J.; Yang, E.J.; Park, S.S.; Yoon, W.J.; Jung, J.H.; Kang, H.K.; Yoo, E.S. Two enone fatty acids isolated from Gracilaria verrucosa suppress the production of inflammatory mediators by down-regulating NF-êB and STAT1 activity in lipopolysaccharide-stimulated raw 264.7 cells. *Arch. Pharm. Res.* **2009**, *32*, 453–462. [CrossRef]

158. Patra, J.K.; Das, G.; Baek, K. Chemical composition and antioxidant and antibacterial activities of an essential oil extracted from an edible seaweed, *Laminaria japonica* L. *Molecules* **2015**, *20*, 12093–12113. [CrossRef]

159. Lee, Y.; Shin, K.; Jung, S.; Lee, S. Effects of the extracts from the marine algae *Pelvetia siliquosa* on hyperlipidemia in rats. *Korean J. Pharmacogn.* **2004**, *35*, 143–146.

160. Hwang, E.; Park, S.-Y.; Sun, Z.-W.; Shin, H.-S.; Lee, D.-G.; Yi, T.H. The protective effects of fucosterol against skin damage in UVB-Irradiated human dermal fibroblasts. *Mar. Biotechnol.* **2014**, *16*, 361–370. [CrossRef]

161. Neto, R.T.; Marçal, C.; Queirós, A.S.; Abreu, H.; Silva, A.M.S.; Cardoso, S.M. Screening of *Ulva rigida*, *Gracilaria* sp., *Fucus vesiculosus* and *Saccharina latissima* as Functional Ingredients. *Int. J. Mol. Sci.* **2018**, *19*, 2987. [CrossRef]

162. Udayan, A.; Arumugam, M.; Pandey, A. Nutraceuticals from algae and cyanobacteria. In *Algal Green Chemistry*; Elsevier: Amsterdam, The Netherlands, 2017; pp. 65–89. [CrossRef]

163. Kannaujiya, V.K.; Singh, P.R.; Kumar, D.; Sinha, R.P. Phycobiliproteins in microalgae: Occurrence, distribution, and biosynthesis. In *Pigments from Microalgae Handbook*; Springer: Berlin/Heidelberg, Germany, 2020; pp. 43–68. ISBN 978-3-030-50971-2.

164. Weill, P.; Plissonneau, C.; Legrand, P.; Rioux, V.; Thibault, R. May omega-3 fatty acid dietary supplementation help reduce severe complications in COVID-19 patients? *Biochimie* **2020**, *179*, 275–280. [CrossRef]

165. Shin, D.; Lee, S.; Huang, Y.-H.; Lim, H.-W.; Lee, Y.; Jang, K.; Cho, Y.; Park, J.S.; Kim, D.-D.; Lim, C.-J. Protective properties of geniposide against UV-B-induced photooxidative stress in human dermal fibroblasts. *Pharm. Biol.* **2018**, *56*, 176–182. [CrossRef] [PubMed]

166. Khan, M.N.A.; Yoon, S.J.; Choi, J.S.; Park, N.G.; Lee, H.H.; Cho, J.Y.; Hong, Y.K. Anti-edema effects of brown seaweed (*Undaria pinnatifida*) extract on phorbol 12-myristate 13-acetate-induced mouse ear inflammation. *Am. J. Chin. Med.* **2009**, *37*, 373–381. [CrossRef] [PubMed]

167. Richard, D.; Kefi, K.; Barbe, U.; Bausero, P.; Visioli, F. Polyunsaturated fatty acids as antioxidants. *Pharmacol. Res.* **2008**, *57*, 451–455. [CrossRef] [PubMed]

168. Gupta, S.; Abu-ghannam, N. Recent developments in the application of seaweeds or seaweed extracts as a means for enhancing the safety and quality attributes of foods. *Innov. Food Sci. Emerg. Technol.* **2011**, *12*, 600–609. [CrossRef]

169. Speranza, L.; Pesce, M.; Patruno, A.; Franceschelli, S.; DeLutiis, M.A. Astaxanthin treatment reduced oxidative induced pro-inflammatory cytokinessecretion in U937: SHP-1 as a novel biological target. *Mar. Drugs* **2012**, *10*, 890–899. [CrossRef]

170. Al-Amin, M.M.; Akhter, S.; Hasan, A.T.; Alam, T.; Nageeb Hasan, S.M.; Saifullah, A.R.; Shohel, C. The antioxidant effect of astaxanthin is higher in young mice than aged: A region specific study on brain. *Metab. Brain Dis.* **2015**, *27*, 15–25. [CrossRef]

171. Wang, J.-Y.; Lee, Y.-J.; Chou, M.-C.; Chang, R.; Chiu, C.-H.; Liang, Y.-J.; Wu, L.-S. Astaxanthin protects steroidogenesis from hydrogen peroxide-induced oxidative stress in mouse leydig cells. *Mar. Drugs* **2015**, *13*, 1375–1388. [CrossRef]

172. Sharoni, Y.; Agemy, L.; Giat, U.; Kirilov, E.; Danilenko, M.; Levy, J. Lycopene and astaxanthin inhibit human prostate cancer cell proliferation induced by androgens. In Proceedings of the 13th International Symposium on Carotenoids, Honolulu, HI, USA, 6–11 January 2002.

173. Jyonouchi, H.; Sun, S.; Iijima, K.; Gross, M.D. Antitumoractivity of astaxanthin and its mode of action. *Nutr. Cancer* **2000**, *36*, 59–65. [CrossRef]

174. Yoshida, H.; Yanai, H.; Ito, K.; Tomono, Y.; Koikeda, T.; Tsukahara, H.; Tada, N. Administration of natural astaxanthin increases serum HDL-cholesterol and adiponectin in subjects with mild hyperlipidemia. *Atherosclerosis* **2010**, *209*, 520–523. [CrossRef]

175. Hussein, G.; Nakamura, M.; Zhao, Q.; Iguchi, T.; Goto, H.; Sankawa, U.; Watanabe, H. Antihypertensive and neuroprotective effects of astaxanthin in experimental animals. *Biol. Pharm. Bull.* **2005**, *28*, 47–52. [CrossRef]

176. Heo, S.J.; Ko, S.C.; Kang, S.-M.; Kang, H.S.; Kim, J.P.; Kim, S.H.; Lee, K.W.; Cho, M.G.; Jeon, Y.J. Cytoprotective effect of fucoxanthin isolated from brown algae *Sargassum siliquastrum* against H_2O_2 induced cell damage. *Eur. Food Res. Technol.* **2008**, *228*, 145–151. [CrossRef]

177. Heo, S.J.; Jeon, Y.J. Protective effect of fucoxanthin isolated from Sargassum siliquastrum on UV-B induced cell damage. *J. Photochem. Photobiol. B Biol.* **2009**, *95*, 101–107. [CrossRef] [PubMed]

178. Sangeetha, R.K.; Bhaskar, N.; Baskaran, V. Comparative effects of β-carotene and fucoxanthin on retinol deficiency induced oxidative stress in rats. *Mol. Cell. Biochem.* **2009**, *331*, 59–67. [CrossRef] [PubMed]

179. Hosokawa, M.; Wanezaki, S.; Miyauchi, K.; Kurihara, H.; Kohno, H.; Kawabata, J.; Takahashi, K. Apoptosis-inducing effect of fucoxanthin on human leukemia cell HL-60. *Food Sci. Technol. Res.* **1999**, *5*, 243–246. [CrossRef]

180. Kotake-Nara, E.; Asai, A.; Nagao, A. Neoxanthin and fucoxanthin induce apoptosis in PC-3 human prostate cancer cells. *Cancer Lett.* **2005**, *220*, 75–84. [CrossRef]

181. Zhang, Z.; Zhang, P.; Hamada, M.; Takahashi, S.; Xing, G.; Liu, J.; Sugiura, N. Potential chemoprevention effect of dietary fucoxanthin on urinary bladder cancer EJ-1 cell line. *Oncol. Rep.* **2008**, *20*, 1099–1103. [CrossRef]

182. Gao, S.; Qin, T.; Liu, Z.; Caceres, M.A.; Ronchi, C.F.; Chen, C.-Y.O.; Shang, F. Lutein and zeaxanthin supplementation reduces H_2O_2 induced oxidative damage in human lens epithelial cells. *Mol. Vis.* **2011**, *17*, 3180–3190. Available online: http://www.molvis.org/molvis/v17/a343 (accessed on 7 December 2011).

183. Matsumoto, M.; Hosokawa, M.; Matsukawa, N.; Hagio, M.; Shinoki, A.; Nishimukai, M.; Hara, H. Suppressive effects of the marine carotenoids, fucoxanthin and fucoxanthinol on triglyceride absorption in lymph duct-cannulated rats. *Eur. J. Nutr.* **2010**, *49*, 243–249. [CrossRef]

184. Allard, J.P.; Royall, D.; Kurian, R.; Muggli, R.; Jeejeebhoy, K.N. Effects of beta-carotene supplementation on lipid peroxidation in humans. *Am. J. Clin. Nutr.* **1994**, *59*, 884–890. [CrossRef]

185. Lourenço-Lopes, C.; Fraga-Corral, M.; Jimenez-Lopez, C.; Carpena, M.; Pereira, A.G.; Garcia-Oliveira, P.; Prieto, M.A.; Simal-Gandara, J. Biological action mechanisms of fucoxanthin extracted from algae for application in food and cosmetic industries. *Trends Food Sci. Technol.* **2021**, *117*, 163–181. [CrossRef]

186. Rokkaku, T.; Kimura, R.; Ishikawa, C.; Yasumoto, T.; Senba, M.; Kanaya, F.; Mori, N. Anticancer effects of marine carotenoids, fucoxanthin and its deacetylated product, fucoxanthinol, on osteosarcoma. *Int. J. Oncol.* **2013**, *43*, 1176–1186. [CrossRef] [PubMed]

187. Di Tomo, P.; Canali, R.; Ciavardelli, D.; Di Silvestre, S.; De Marco, A.; Giardinelli, A.; Pipino, C.; Di Pietro, N.; Virgili, F.; Pandolfi, A. β-Carotene and lycopene affect endothelial response to TNF-a reducing nitro-oxidative stress and interaction with monocytes. *Mol. Nutr. Food Res.* **2012**, *56*, 217–227. [CrossRef] [PubMed]

188. Dwyer, J.H.; Navab, M.; Dwyer, K.M.; Hassan, K.; Sun, P.; Shircore, A.; Hama-Levy, S.; Hough, G.; Wang, X.; Drake, T.; et al. Oxygenated carotenoid lutein and progression of early atherosclerosis: The Los Angeles atherosclerosis study. *Circulation* **2001**, *103*, 2922–2927. [CrossRef] [PubMed]

189. Gullón, B.; Gagaoua, M.; Barba, F.J.; Gullón, P.; Zhang, W.; Lorenzo, J.M. Seaweeds as promising resource of bioactive compounds: Overview of novel extraction strategies and design of tailored meat products. *Trends Food Sci. Technol.* **2020**, *100*, 1–18. [CrossRef]

190. Afify, A.E.-M.M.R.; El-Beltagi, H.S.; Aly, A.A.; El-Ansary, A.E. Antioxidant enzyme activities and lipid peroxidation as biomarker for potato tuber stored by two essential oils from Caraway and Clove and its main component carvone and eugenol. *Asian Pac. J. Trop. Biomed.* **2012**, *2*, S772–S780. [CrossRef]

191. Kalasariya, H.S.; Pereira, L.; Patel, N.B. Pioneering role of marine macroalgae in cosmeceuticals. *Phycology* **2022**, *2*, 172–203. [CrossRef]
192. Farvin, K.H.S.; Jacobsen, C.; Sabeena Farvin, K.H.; Jacobsen, C. Phenolic compounds and antioxidant activities of selected species of seaweeds from Danish coast. *Food Chem.* **2013**, *138*, 1670–1681. [CrossRef]
193. Xu, T.; Sutour, S.; Casabianca, H.; Tomi, F.; Paoli, M.; Garrido, M.; Pasqualini, V.; Aiello, A.; Castola, V.; Bighelli, A. Rapid Screening of Chemical Compositions of *Gracilaria dura* and *Hypnea mucisformis* (Rhodophyta) from Corsican Lagoon. *Int. J. Phytocosmetics Nat. Ingred.* **2015**, *2*, 8. [CrossRef]
194. Lomartire, S.; Cotas, J.; Pacheco, D.; Marques, J.C.; Pereira, L.; Gonçalves, A.M.M. Environmental impact on seaweed phenolic production and activity: An important step for compound exploitation. *Mar. Drugs* **2021**, *19*, 245. [CrossRef]
195. Santos, S.A.O.; Félix, R.; Pais, A.C.S.; Rocha, S.M.; Silvestre, A.J.D. The quest for phenolic compounds from macroalgae: A review of extraction and identification methodologies. *Biomolecules* **2019**, *9*, 847. [CrossRef]
196. Klejdus, B.; Lojková, L.; Plaza, M.; Šnóblová, M.; Štěrbová, D. Hyphenated technique for the extraction and determination of isoflavones in algae: Ultrasound-assisted supercritical fluid extraction followed by fast chromatography with tandem mass spectrometry. *J. Chromatogr. A* **2010**, *1217*, 7956–7965. [CrossRef] [PubMed]
197. Reddy, P.; Urban, S. Meroditerpenoids from the southern Australian marine brown alga *Sargassum fallax*. *Phytochemistry* **2009**, *70*, 250–255. [CrossRef] [PubMed]
198. Stout, E.P.; Prudhomme, J.; Le Roch, K.; Fairchild, C.R.; Franzblau, S.G.; Aalbersberg, W.; Hay, M.E.; Kubanek, J. Unusual antimalarial meroditerpenes from tropical red macroalgae. *Bioorganic Med. Chem. Lett.* **2010**, *20*, 5662–5665. [CrossRef] [PubMed]
199. Blaustein, M.P.; Leenen, F.H.H.; Chen, L.; Golovina, V.A.; Hamlyn, J.M.; Pallone, T.L.; Van Huysse, J.W.; Zhang, J.; Wier, W.G. How NaCl raises blood pressure: A new paradigm for the pathogenesis of salt-dependent hypertension. *Am. J. Physiol. Heart Circ. Physiol.* **2012**, *302*, H1031–H1049. [CrossRef]
200. Bo, S.; Pisu, E. Role of dietary magnesium in cardiovascular disease prevention, insulin sensitivity and diabetes. *Curr. Opin. Lipidol.* **2008**, *19*, 50–56. [CrossRef]
201. Desideri, D.; Cantaluppi, C.; Ceccotto, F.; Meli, M.A.; Roselli, C.; Feduzi, L. Essential and toxic elements in seaweeds for human consumption. *J. Toxicol. Environ. Health Part A* **2016**, *79*, 112–122. [CrossRef]
202. Blaine, J.; Chonchol, M.; Levi, M. Renal control of calcium, phosphate, and magnesium homeostasis. *Clin. J. Am. Soci. Nephrol.* **2015**, *10*, 1257–1272. [CrossRef]
203. Schiener, P.; Black, K.D.; Stanley, M.S.; Green, D.H. The seasonal variation in the chemical composition of the kelp species *Laminaria digitata, Laminaria hyperborea, Saccharina latissima* and *Alaria esculenta*. *J. Appl. Phycol.* **2015**, *27*, 363–373. [CrossRef]
204. Parjikolaei, B.R.; Bruhn, A.; Eybye, K.L.; Larsen, M.M.; Rasmussen, M.B.; Christensen, K.V.; Fretté, X.C. Valuable biomolecules from nine north atlantic red macroalgae: Amino acids, fatty acids, carotenoids, minerals and metals. *Nat. Resour.* **2016**, *7*, 157–183. [CrossRef]
205. Dawczynski, C.; Schäfer, U.; Leiterer, M.; Jahreis, G. Nutritional and toxicological importance of macro, trace, and ultra-trace elements in algae food products. *J. Agric. Food Chem.* **2007**, *55*, 10470–10475. [CrossRef]
206. López-López, I.; Cofrades, S.; Cañeque, V.; Díaz, M.T.; López, O.; Jiménez-Colmenero, F. Effect of cooking on the chemical composition of low-salt, low-fat Wakame/olive oil added beef patties with special reference to fatty acid content. *Meat Sci.* **2011**, *89*, 27–34. [CrossRef] [PubMed]
207. López-López, I.; Bastida, S.; Ruiz-Capillas, C.; Bravo, L.; Larrea, M.T.; Sánchez-Muniz, F.; Cofrades, S.; Jiménez-Colmenero, F. Composition and antioxidant capacity of low-salt meat emulsion model systems containing edible seaweeds. *Meat Sci.* **2009**, *83*, 492–498. [CrossRef] [PubMed]
208. López-López, I.; Cofrades, S.; Yakan, A.; Solas, M.T.; Jiménez-Colmenero, F. Frozen storage characteristics of low-salt and low-fat beef patties as affected by Wakame addition and replacing pork backfat with olive oil-in-water emulsion. *Food Res. Int.* **2010**, *43*, 1244–1254. [CrossRef]
209. Circuncisão, A.R.; Catarino, M.D.; Cardoso, S.M.; Silva, A. Minerals from macroalgae origin: Health benefits and risks for consumers. *Mar. Drugs* **2018**, *16*, 400. [CrossRef]
210. Jacob, L.; Baker, C.; Farris, P. Vitamin-based cosmeceuticals. *Cosmet. Dermatol.* **2012**, *25*, 405.
211. Chakraborty, K.; Praveen, N.K.; Vijayan, K.K.; Rao, G.S. Evaluation of phenolic contents and antioxidant activities of brown seaweeds belonging to *Turbinaria* spp. (Phaeophyta, Sargassaceae) collected from Gulf of Mannar. *Asian Pac. J. Trop. Biomed.* **2013**, *3*, 8–16. [CrossRef]
212. Škrovánková, S. Seaweed vitamins as nutraceuticals. In *Advances in Food and Nutrition Research*; Elsevier: Amsterdam, The Netherlands, 2011; Volume 64, pp. 357–369. ISBN 9780123876690.
213. Searle, T.; Al-Niaimi, F.; Ali, F.R. The top 10 cosmeceuticals for facial hyperpigmentation. *Dermatol. Ther.* **2020**, *33*, 14095. [CrossRef]
214. Bissett, D.L.; Oblong, J.E.; Goodman, L.J. Topical Vitamins. In *Cosmetic Dermatology: Products and Procedures*; Draelos, Z.D., Ed.; Wiley & Sons, Ltd.: Hoboken, NJ, USA, 2015; pp. 336–345. [CrossRef]
215. Kilinç, B.; Semra, C.; Gamze, T.; Hatice, T.; Koru, E. Seaweeds for Food and Industrial Applications. In *Food Industry*; Muzzalupo, I., Ed.; InTech: Rijeka, Croatia, 2013; pp. 735–748. [CrossRef]

216. Campiche, R.; Curpen, S.J.; Lutchmanen-Kolanthan, V.; Gougeon, S.; Cherel, M.; Laurent, G.; Gempeler, M.; Schuetz, R. Pigmentation effects of blue light irradiation on skin and how to protect against them. *Int. J. Cosmet. Sci.* **2020**, *42*, 399–406. [CrossRef]

217. Watanabe, F.; Yabuta, Y.; Bito, T.; Teng, F. Vitamin B12-containing plant food sources for vegetarians. *Nutrients* **2014**, *6*, 1861–1873. [CrossRef]

218. Manela-Azulay, M.; Bagatin, E. Cosmeceuticals vitamins. *Clin. Dermatol.* **2009**, *27*, 469–474. [CrossRef]

219. Lorencini, M.; Brohem, C.A.; Dieamant, G.C.; Zanchin, N.I.; Maibach, H.I. Active ingredients against human epidermal aging. *Ageing Res. Rev.* **2014**, *15*, 100–115. [CrossRef] [PubMed]

220. Noriega-Fernández, E.; Sone, I.; Astráin-Redín, L.; Prabhu, L.; Sivertsvik, M.; Álvarez, I.; Cebrián, G. Innovative ultrasound-assisted approaches towards reduction of heavy metals and iodine in macroalgal biomass. *Foods* **2021**, *10*, 649. [CrossRef] [PubMed]

221. Cotas, J.; Leandro, A.; Monteiro, P.; Pacheco, D.; Figueirinha, A.; Gonçalves, A.M.M.; da Silva, G.J.; Pereira, L. Seaweed Phenolics: From Extraction to Applications. *Mar. Drugs* **2020**, *18*, 384. [CrossRef] [PubMed]

222. Falquet, J.; Hurni, J.P. The Nutritional Aspects of Spirulina. Antenna Foundation. 1997. Available online: https://www.antenna. ch/wp-content/uploads/2017/03/AspectNut_UK (accessed on 25 July 2017).

223. Kumar, C.S.; Ganesan, P.; Suresh, P.V.; Bhaskar, N. Seaweeds as a source of nutritionally beneficial compounds—A review. *J. Food Sci. Technol.* **2008**, *45*, 1.

224. Ganesan, A.R.; Tiwari, U.; Rajauria, G. Seaweed nutraceuticals and their therapeutic role in disease prevention. *Food Sci. Hum. Wellness* **2019**, *8*, 252–263. [CrossRef]

225. Jesumani, V.; Du, H.; Aslam, M.; Pei, P.; Huang, N. Potential Use of Seaweed Bioactive Compounds in Skincare—A Review. *Mar. Drugs* **2019**, *17*, 688. [CrossRef]

226. Chambial, S.; Dwivedi, S.; Shukla, K.K.; John, P.J.; Sharma, P. Vitamin C in disease prevention and cure: An overview. *Indian J. Clin. Biochem.* **2013**, *28*, 314–328. [CrossRef]

227. Mathew, S.; Ravishankar, C.N. *Seaweeds as a Source of Micro and Macro Nutrients*; ICAR-Central Institute of Fisheries Technology: Cochin, India, 2018. Available online: http://krishi.icar.gov.in/jspui/handle/123456789/20485 (accessed on 26 November 2018).

228. Vardi, M.; Levy, N.S.; Levy, A.P. Vitamin E in the prevention of cardiovascular disease: The importance of proper patient selection. *J. Lipid Res.* **2013**, *54*, 2307–2314. [CrossRef]

229. Ul-Haq, I.; Butt, M.S.; Amjad, N.; Yasmin, I.; Suleria, H.A.R. Marine-Algal Bioactive Compounds: A Comprehensive Appraisal. In *Handbook of Algal Technologies and Phytochemicals*; CRC Press: Boca Raton, FL, USA, 2019; pp. 71–80.

230. Romeilah, R.M.; El-Beltagi, H.S.; Shalaby, E.A.; Younes, K.M.; El Moll, H.; Rajendrasozhan, S.; Mohamed, H.I. Antioxidant and cytotoxic activities of Artemisia monosperma L. and Tamarix aphylla essential oils. *Not. Bot. Horti Agrobot. Cluj-Napoca* **2021**, *9*, 12233. [CrossRef]

231. Sellimi, S.; Kadri, N.; Barragan-Montero, V.; Laouer, H.; Hajji, M.; Nasri, M. Fucans from a Tunisian brown seaweed Cystoseira barbata: Structural characteristics and antioxidant activity. *Int. J. Biol. Macromol.* **2014**, *66*, 281–288. [CrossRef]

232. Sellimi, S.; Younes, I.; Ayed, H.B.; Maalej, H.; Montero, V.; Rinaudo, M.; Dahia, M.; Mechichi, T.; Hajji, M.; Nasri, M. Structural, physicochemical and antioxidant properties of sodium alginate isolated from a Tunisian brown seaweed. *Int. J. Biol. Macromol.* **2015**, *72*, 1358–1367. [CrossRef] [PubMed]

233. Hentati, F.; Tounsi, L.; Djomdi, D.; Pierre, G.; Delattre, C.; Ursu, A.V.; Fendri, I.; Abdelkafi, S.; Michaud, P. Bioactive polysaccharides from seaweeds. *Molecules* **2020**, *25*, 3152. [CrossRef] [PubMed]

234. Sofy, A.R.; Sofy, M.R.; Hmed, A.A.; Dawoud, R.A.; Refaey, E.E.; Mohamed, H.I.; El-Dougdoug, N.K. Molecular characterization of the Alfalfa mosaic virus infecting Solanum melongena in Egypt and control of its deleterious effects with melatonin and salicylic acid. *Plants* **2021**, *28*, 459. [CrossRef] [PubMed]

235. Abdel-Rahim, E.A.; El-Beltagi, H.S. Constituents of apple, parsley and lentil edible plants and their therapy treatments for blood picture as well as liver and kidney functions against lipidemic disease. *Elec. J. Environ. Agricult. Food Chem.* **2010**, *9*, 1117–1127.

236. Halliwell, B. Reactive Species and Antioxidants. Redox Biology Is a Fundamental Theme of Aerobic Life. *Plant Physiol.* **2006**, *141*, 312–322. [CrossRef] [PubMed]

237. Cornish, M.L.; Garbary, D.J. Antioxidants from macroalgae: Potential applications in human health and nutrition. *Algae* **2010**, *25*, 155–171. [CrossRef]

238. Fischbach, M.A.; Walsh, C.T. Antibiotics for Emerging Pathogens. *Science* **2009**, *325*, 1089–1093. [CrossRef]

239. Salama, H.M.H.; Marraiki, N. Antimicrobial activity and phytochemical analyses of *Polygonum aviculare* L. (Polygonaceae), naturally growing in Egypt. *Saudi J. Biol. Sci.* **2010**, *17*, 57–63. [CrossRef]

240. Tuney, I.; Cadirci, B.H.; Unal, D.; Sukatar, A. Antimicrobial activities of the extracts of marine algae from the coast of Urla (Izmir, Turkey). *Turkish J. Biol.* **2006**, *30*, 171–175.

241. Kandhasamy, M.; Arunachalam, K.D. Evaluation of in vitro antibacterial property of seaweeds of southeast coast of India. *Afr. J. Biotechnol.* **2008**, *7*, 1958–1961. [CrossRef]

242. Charway, G.N.A.; Yenumula, P.; Kim, Y.-M. Marine algae and their potential application as antimicrobial agents. *J. Food Hyg. Saf.* **2018**, *33*, 151–156. [CrossRef]

243. Lopez-Romero, J.C.; González-Ríos, H.; Borges, A.; Simõs, M. Antibacterial Effects and Mode of Action of Selected Essential Oils Components against *Escherichia coli* and *Staphylococcus aureus*. *Evid.-Based Complementary Altern. Med.* **2015**, *2015*, 795435. [CrossRef] [PubMed]

244. Lv, F.; Liang, H.; Yuan, Q.; Li, C. In Vitro Antimicrobial Effects and Mechanism of Action of Selected Plant Essential Oil Combinations against Four Food-Related Microorganisms. *Food Res. Int.* **2011**, *44*, 3057–3064. [CrossRef]

245. Sameeh, M.Y.; Mohamed, A.A.; Elazzazy, A.M. Polyphenolic contents and antimicrobial activity of different extracts of *Padina boryana Thivy* and *Enteromorpha* sp. marine algae. *J. Appl. Pharm. Sci.* **2016**, *6*, 87–92. [CrossRef]

246. El-Beltagi, H.S.; Mohamed, H.I.; Abdelazeem, A.S.; Youssef, R.; Safwat, G. GC-MS analysis, antioxidant, antimicrobial and anticancer activities of extracts from *Ficus sycomorus* fruits and leaves. *Not. Bot. Horti Agrobot. Cluj-Napoca* **2019**, *47*, 493–505. [CrossRef]

247. Hamed, M.M.; Abd El-Mobdy, M.A.; Kamel, M.T.; Mohamed, H.I.; Bayoumi, A.E. Phytochemical and biological activities of two asteraceae plants *Senecio vulgaris* and *Pluchea dioscoridis* L. *Pharmacol. Online* **2019**, *2*, 101–121.

248. Hussain, E.; Wang, L.J.; Jiang, B.; Riaz, S.; Butt, G.Y.; Shi, D.-Y. A review of the components of brown seaweeds as potential candidates in cancer therapy. *RSC Adv.* **2016**, *6*, 12592. [CrossRef]

249. Gutierrez-Rodriguez, A.G.; Juarez-Portilla, C.; Olivares-Banuelos, T.; Zepeda, R.C. Anticancer activity of seaweeds. *Drug Discov. Today* **2018**, *23*, 434–447. [CrossRef]

250. Algotiml, R.; Gab-Alla, A.; Seoudi, R.; Abulreesh, H.H.; El-Readi, M.Z.; Elbanna, K. Anticancer and antimicrobial activity of biosynthesized Red Sea marine algal silver nanoparticles. *Sci. Rep.* **2022**, *12*, 2421. [CrossRef]

251. Palanisamy, S.; Vinosha, M.; Marudhupandi, T.; Rajasekar, P.; Prabhu, N.M. Isolation of fucoidan from *Sargassum polycystum* brown algae: Structural characterization, in vitro antioxidant and anticancer activity. *Int. J. Biol. Macromol.* **2017**, *102*, 405–412. [CrossRef]

252. Usoltseva, R.V.; Anastyuk, S.D.; Surits, V.V.; Shevchenko, N.M.; Thinh, P.D.; Zadorozhny, P.A.; Ermakova, S.P. Comparison of structure and in vitro anticancer activity of native and modified fucoidans from *Sargassum feldmannii* and *S. duplicatum*. *Int. J. Biol. Macromol.* **2019**, *124*, 220–228. [CrossRef] [PubMed]

253. Narayani, S.S.; Saravanan, S.; Ravindran, J.; Ramasamy, M.S.; Chitra, J. In vitro anticancer activity of fucoidan extracted from *Sargassum cinereum* against Caco-2 cells. *Int. J. Biol. Macromol.* **2019**, *138*, 618–628. [CrossRef] [PubMed]

254. Athukorala, Y.; Jung, W.K.; Vasanthan, T.; Jeon, Y.J. An anticoagulative polysaccharide from an enzymatic hydrolysate of *Ecklonia cava*. *Carbohydr. Polym.* **2006**, *66*, 184–191. [CrossRef]

255. Souza, R.B.; Frota, A.F.; Silva, J.; Alves, C.; Neugebauer, A.Z.; Pinteus, S.; Rodrigues, J.A.G.; Cordeiro, E.M.S.; De Almeida, A.A.; Pedrosa, R.; et al. In vitro activities of kappa-carrageenan isolated from red marine alga *Hypnea musciformis*: Antimicrobial, anticancer and neuroprotective potential. *Int. J. Biol. Macromol.* **2018**, *112*, 1248–1256. [CrossRef]

256. Chen, H.; Zhang, L.; Long, X.; Li, P.; Chen, S.; Kuang, W.; Guo, J. Sargassum fusiforme polysaccharides inhibit VEGF-A-related angiogenesis and proliferation of lung cancer in vitro and in vivo. *Biomed. Pharmacother.* **2017**, *85*, 22–27. [CrossRef] [PubMed]

257. Ji, C.F.; Ji, Y.B. Laminarin-induced apoptosis in human colon cancer LoVo cells. *Oncol. Lett.* **2014**, *7*, 1728–1732. [CrossRef]

258. Synytsya, A.; Kim, W.J.; Kim, S.M.; Pohl, R.; Synytsya, A.; Kvasnička, F.; Čopíková, J.; Park, Y.I. Structure and antitumour activity of fucoidan isolated from sporophyll of Korean brown seaweed *Undaria pinnatifida*. *Carbohydras. Polym.* **2010**, *81*, 41–48. [CrossRef]

259. Yan, M.D.; Yao, C.J.; Chow, J.M.; Chang, C.L.; Hwang, P.A.; Chuang, S.E.; Whang-Peng, J.; Lai, G.M. Fucoidan elevates microRNA-29b to regulate DNMT3B-MTSS1 axis and inhibit EMT in human hepatocellular carcinoma cells. *Mar. Drugs* **2015**, *13*, 6099–6116. [CrossRef]

260. Lee, H.E.; Choi, E.S.; Shin, J.; Lee, S.O.; Park, K.S.; Cho, N.P.; Cho, S.D. Fucoidan induces caspase-dependent apoptosis in MC3 human mucoepidermoid carcinoma cells. *Exp. Ther. Med.* **2014**, *7*, 228–232. [CrossRef]

261. Elrggal, M.E.; Alamer, S.I.; Alkahtani, S.A.; Alshrahili, M.A.; Alharbi, A.; Alghamdi, B.A.; Zaitoun, M.F. Dispensing Practices for Weight Management Products in Eastern Saudi Arabia: A Survey of Community Pharmacists. *Int. J. Environ. Res. Public Health* **2021**, *18*, 13146. [CrossRef]

262. Krentz, A.J.; Bailey, C.J. Oral Antidiabetic Agents-Current Role in Type 2 Diabetes Mellitus. *Drugs* **2005**, *65*, 385–411. [CrossRef] [PubMed]

263. Garcimartín, A.; Benedí, J.; Bastida, S.; Sánchez-Muniz, F.J. Aqueous extracts and suspensions of restructured pork formulated with *Undaria pinnatifida*, Himanthaliaelongata and Porphyraumbilicalis distinctly affect the in vitro α-glucosidase activity and glucose diffusion. *LWT Food Sci. Technol.* **2015**, *64*, 720–726. [CrossRef]

264. Naveen, J.; Baskaran, R.; Baskaran, V. Profiling of bioactives and in vitro evaluation of antioxidant and antidiabetic property of polyphenols of marine algae *Padina tetrastromatica*. *Algal Res.* **2021**, *55*, 102250. [CrossRef]

265. Pacheco, L.V.; Parada, J.; Pérez-Correa, J.R.; Mariotti-Celis, M.S.; Erpel, F.; Zambrano, A.; Palacios, M. Bioactive polyphenols from southern chile seaweed as inhibitors of enzymes for starch digestion. *Mar. Drugs* **2020**, *18*, 353. [CrossRef]

266. Al-Araby, S.Q.; Rahman, M.A.; Chowdhury, M.A.; Das, R.R.; Chowdhury, T.A.; Hasan, C.M.M.; Afroze, M.; Hashem, M.A.; Hajjar, D.; Alelwani, W.; et al. *Padina tenuis* (marine alga) attenuates oxidative stress and streptozotocin-induced type 2 diabetic indices in Wistar albino rats. *S. Afr. J. Bot.* **2020**, *128*, 87–100. [CrossRef]

267. Abdel-Karim, O.H.; Abo-Shady, A.M.; Ismail, G.A.; Gheda, S.F. Potential effect of *Turbinaria decurrens* acetone extract on the biochemical and histological parameters of alloxan-induced diabetic rats. *Int. J. Environ. Health Res.* **2021**, *202*, 1–22. [CrossRef]

268. Abu, R.; Jiang, Z.; Ueno, M.; Isaka, S.; Nakazono, S.; Okimura, T.; Cho, K.; Yamaguchi, K.; Kim, D.; Oda, T. Anti-metastatic effects of the sulfated polysaccharide ascophyllan isolated from *Ascophyllum nodosum* on B16 melanoma. *Biochem. Biophys. Res. Commun.* **2015**, *458*, 727–732. [CrossRef]

269. Silva, J.; Alves, C.; Freitas, R.; Martins, A.; Pinteus, S.; Ribeiro, J.; Gaspar, H.; Alfonso, A.; Pedrosa, R. Antioxidant and Neuroprotective Potential of the Brown Seaweed *Bifurcaria bifurcata* in an in vitro Parkinson's Disease Model. *Mar. Drugs* **2019**, *17*, 85. [CrossRef]

270. Muñoz-Ochoa, M.; Murillo-Álvarez, J.I.; Zermeño-Cervantes, L.A.; Martínez-Díaz, S.; Rodríguez-Riosmena, R. Screening of extracts of algae from Baja California Sur, Mexico as reversers of the antibiotic resistance of some pathogenic bacteria. *Eur. Rev. Med. Pharmacol. Sci.* **2010**, *14*, 739–747.

271. Mise, T.; Ueda, M.; Yasumoto, T. Production of fucoxanthin-rich powder from *Cladosiphon okamuranus*. *Adv. J. Food Sci. Technol.* **2011**, *3*, 73–76.

272. Panayotova, V.; Merzdhanova, A.; Dobreva, D.A.; Zlatanov, M.; Makedonski, L. Lipids of black sea algae: Unveiling their potential for pharmaceutical and cosmetic applications. *J. IMAB Ann. Proc. Sci. Pap.* **2017**, *23*, 1747–1751. [CrossRef]

273. Kosani´c, M.; Rankovi´c, B.; Stanojkovi´c, T. Brown macroalgae from the Adriatic Sea as a promising source of bioactive nutrients. *J. Food Meas. Charact.* **2019**, *13*, 330–338. [CrossRef]

274. Sugiura, Y.; Takeuchi, Y.; Kakinuma, M.; Amano, H. Inhibitory effects of seaweeds on histamine release from rat basophile leukemia cells (RBL-2H3). *Fish. Sci.* **2006**, *72*, 1286–1291. [CrossRef]

275. Campos, A.M.; Matos, J.; Afonso, C.; Gomes, R.; Bandarra, N.M.; Cardoso, C. Azorean macroalgae (*Petalonia binghamiae, Halopteris scoparia* and *Osmundea pinnatifida*) bioprospection: A study of fatty acid profiles and bioactivity. *Int. J. Food Sci. Technol.* **2018**, *54*, 880–890. [CrossRef]

276. Shimoda, H.; Tanaka, J.; Shan, S.J.; Maoka, T. Anti-pigmentary activity of fucoxanthin and its influence on skin mRNA expression of melanogenic molecules. *J. Pharm. Pharm.* **2010**, *62*, 1137–1145. [CrossRef]

277. Sappati, P.K.; Nayak, B.; VanWalsum, G.P.; Mulrey, O.T. Combined effects of seasonal variation and drying methods on the physicochemical properties and antioxidant activity of sugar kelp (*Saccharina latissima*). *J. Appl. Phycol.* **2019**, *31*, 1311–1332. [CrossRef]

278. Rhimou, B.; Hassane, R.; José, M.; Nathalie, B. The antibacterial potential of the seaweeds (Rhodophyceae) of the Strait of Gibraltar and the Mediterranean Coast of Morocco. *Afr. J. Biotechnol.* **2010**, *9*, 6365–6372.

279. SpecialChem—The Universal Selection Source: Cosmetics Ingredients. Available online: https://cosmetics.specialchem.com/ (accessed on 5 May 2020).

280. Thomas, N.V.; Kim, S.K. Beneficial e_ects of marine algal compounds in cosmeceuticals. *Mar. Drugs* **2013**, *11*, 146–164. [CrossRef]

281. Santos, J.P.; Torres, P.B.; dos Santos, D.Y.; Motta, L.B.; Chow, F. Seasonal effects on antioxidant and anti-HIV activities of Brazilian seaweeds. *J. Appl. Phycol.* **2018**, *31*, 1333–1341. [CrossRef]

282. De Jesus Raposo, M.; de Morais, A.; de Morais, R. Marine polysaccharides from algae with potential biomedical applications. *Mar. Drugs* **2015**, *13*, 2967–3028. [CrossRef]

283. Azam, M.S.; Choi, J.; Lee, M.S.; Kim, H.R. Hypopigmenting effects of brown algae-derived phytochemicals: A review on molecular mechanisms. *Mar. Drugs* **2017**, *15*, 297. [CrossRef] [PubMed]

284. Pezeshk, F.; Babaei, S.; Abedian Kenari, A.; Hedayati, M.; Naseri, M. The effect of supplementing diets with extracts derived from three different species of macroalgae on growth, thermal stress resistance, antioxidant enzyme activities and skin colour of electric yellow cichlid (*Labidochromis caeruleus*). *Aquac. Nutr.* **2019**, *25*, 436–443. [CrossRef]

285. Kelman, D.; Posner, E.K.; McDermid, K.J.; Tabandera, N.K.; Wright, P.R.; Wright, A.D. Antioxidant activity of Hawaiian marine algae. *Mar. Drugs* **2012**, *10*, 403–416. [CrossRef] [PubMed]

286. Premalatha, M.; Dhasarathan, P.; Theriappan, P. Phytochemical characterization and antimicrobial effciency of seaweed samples, *Ulva fasciata* and *Chaetomorpha antennina*. *Int. J. Pharm. Biol. Sci.* **2011**, *2*, 288–293.

287. Mourelle, M.L.; Gómez, C.P.; Legido, J.L. The potential use of marine microalgae and cyanobacteria in cosmetics and thalassotherapy. *Cosmetics* **2017**, *4*, 46. [CrossRef]

288. José de Andrade, C.; Maria de Andrade, L. An overview on the application of genus Chlorella in biotechnological processes. *J. Adv. Res. Biotechnol.* **2017**, *2*, 1–9. [CrossRef]

289. Berthon, J.Y.; Nachat-Kappes, R.; Bey, M.; Cadoret, J.P.; Renimel, I.; Filaire, E. Marine algae as attractive source to skin care. *Free Radic. Res.* **2017**, *51*, 555–567. [CrossRef]

290. Makpol, S.; Yeoh, T.W.; Ruslam, F.A.C.; Arifin, K.T.; Yusof, Y.A.M. Comparative effect of Piper betle, *Chlorella vulgaris* and tocotrienol-rich fraction on antioxidant enzymes activity in cellular ageing of human diploid fibroblasts. *BMC Complement. Altern. Med.* **2013**, *13*, 210. [CrossRef]

291. Kang, H.; Lee, C.H.; Kim, J.R.; Kwon, J.Y.; Seo, S.G.; Han, J.G.; Kim, B.; Kim, J.; Lee, K.W. *Chlorella vulgaris* attenuates dermatophagoides farinae-induced atopic dermatitis-like symptoms in NC/Nga mice. *Int. J. Mol. Sci.* **2015**, *16*, 21021–21034. [CrossRef]

292. Murthy, K.; Vanitha, A.; Rajesha, J.; Swamy, M.; Sowmya, P.; Ravishankar, G. In vivo antioxidant activity of carotenoids from *Dunaliella salina*—A green microalga. *Life Sci.* **2005**, *76*, 1381–1390. [CrossRef]

293. Yang, D.J.; Lin, J.T.; Chen, Y.C.; Liu, S.C.; Lu, F.J.; Chang, T.J.; Wang, M.; Lin, H.W.; Chang, Y.Y. Suppressive effect of carotenoid extract of *Dunaliella salina* alga on production of LPS-stimulated pro-inflammatory mediators in RAW264. 7 cells via NF-B and JNK inactivation. *J. Funct. Foods* **2013**, *5*, 607–615. [CrossRef]

294. Shin, J.; Kim, J.E.; Pak, K.J.; Kang, J.I.; Kim, T.S.; Lee, S.Y.; Yeo, I.H.; Park, J.H.Y.; Kim, J.H.; Kang, N.J.; et al. A Combination of soybean and Haematococcus extract alleviates ultraviolet B-induced photoaging. *Int. J. Mol. Sci.* **2017**, *18*, 682. [CrossRef] [PubMed]

295. Rao, A.R.; Sindhuja, H.N.; Dharmesh, S.M.; Sankar, K.U.; Sarada, R.; Ravishankar, G.A. Effective inhibition of skin cancer, tyrosinase, and antioxidative properties by astaxanthin and astaxanthin esters from the green alga *Haematococcus pluvialis*. *J. Agric. Food Chem.* **2013**, *61*, 3842–3851. [CrossRef]

296. Banskota, A.H.; Sperker, S.; Stefanova, R.; McGinn, P.J.; O'Leary, S.J. Antioxidant properties and lipid composition of selected microalgae. *J. Appl. Phycol.* **2019**, *31*, 309–318. [CrossRef]

297. Shen, C.T.; Chen, P.Y.; Wu, J.J.; Lee, T.M.; Hsu, S.L.; Chang, C.M.J.; Young, C.C.; Shieh, C.J. Purification of algal anti-tyrosinase zeaxanthin from Nannochloropsis oculate using supercritical anti-solvent precipitation. *J. Supercrit. Fluids* **2011**, *55*, 955–962. [CrossRef]

298. Wu, H.L.; Fu, X.Y.; Cao, W.Q.; Xiang, W.Z.; Hou, Y.J.; Ma, J.K.; Wang, Y.; Fan, C.D. Induction of apoptosis in human glioma cells by fucoxanthin via triggering of ROS-mediated oxidative damage and regulation of MAPKs and PI3K-AKT pathways. *J. Agric. Food Chem.* **2019**, *67*, 2212. [CrossRef] [PubMed]

299. Rastogi, R.P.; Sonani, R.R.; Madamwar, D.; Incharoensakdi, A. Characterization and antioxidant functions of mycosporine-like amino acids in the cyanobacterium *Nostoc* sp. R76DM. *Algal Res.* **2016**, *16*, 110–118. [CrossRef]

300. Haimeur, A.; Ulmann, L.; Mimouni, V.; Guéno, F.; Pineau-Vincent, F.; Meskini, N.; Tremblin, G. The role of *Odontella aurita*, a marine diatom rich in EPA, as a dietary supplement in dyslipidemia, platelet function and oxidative stress in high-fat fed rats. *Lipids Health Dis.* **2012**, *11*, 147. [CrossRef]

301. Shannon, E.; Abu-Ghannam, N. Antibacterial derivatives of marine algae: An overview of pharmacological mechanisms and applications. *Mar. Drugs* **2016**, *14*, 81. [CrossRef]

302. Lauritano, C.; Andersen, J.H.; Hansen, E.; Albrigtsen, M.; Escalera, L.; Esposito, F.; Helland, K.; Hanssen, K.Ø.; Romano, G.; Ianora, A. Bioactivity screening of microalgae for antioxidant, anti-inflammatory, anticancer, anti-diabetes, and antibacterial activities. *Front. Mar. Sci.* **2016**, *3*, 68. [CrossRef]

303. Wu, Q.; Liu, L.; Miron, A.; Klímová, B.; Wan, D.; Kuča, K. The antioxidant, immunomodulatory, and anti-inflammatory activities of Spirulina: An overview. *Arch. Toxicol.* **2016**, *90*, 1817–1840. [CrossRef]

304. El-Sheekh, M.M.; Daboor, S.M.; Swelim, M.A.; Mohamed, S. Production and characterization of antimicrobial active substance from *Spirulina platensis*. *Iran. J. Microbiol.* **2014**, *6*, 112–119.

305. Plaza, M.; Santoyo, S.; Jaime, L.; Reina, G.G.B.; Herrero, M.; Señoráns, F.J.; Ibáñez, E. Screening for bioactive compounds from algae. *J. Pharm. Biomed. Anal.* **2010**, *51*, 450–455. [CrossRef]

306. Jae-Llane, D.; Carlos Braisv, C. Versatility of the Humble Seaweed in Biomanufacturing. *Procedia Manuf.* **2019**, *32*, 87–94. [CrossRef]

307. Abu-Shahba, M.S.; Mansour, M.M.; Mohamed, H.I.; Sofy, M.R. Comparative cultivation and biochemical analysis of iceberg lettuce grown in sand soil and hydroponics with or without microbubble and microbubble. *J. Soil Sci. Plant Nutr.* **2021**, *21*, 389–403. [CrossRef]

308. Eissa, M.A.; Nasralla, N.N.; Gomah, N.H.; Osman, D.M.; El-Derwy, Y.M. Evaluation of natural fertilizer extracted from expired dairy products as a soil amendment. *J. Soil Sci. Plant Nutr.* **2018**, *18*, 694–704. [CrossRef]

309. Bixler, H.J.; Porse, H. A decade of change in the seaweed hydrocolloids industry. *J. Appl. Phycol.* **2011**, *23*, 321–335. [CrossRef]

310. Nkemka, V.N.; Murto, M. Exploring strategies for seaweed hydrolysis: Effect on methane potential and heavy metal mobilisation. *Process Biochem.* **2012**, *47*, 2523–2526. [CrossRef]

311. Garcia-Vaquero, M.; Hayes, M. Red and green macroalgae for fish and animal feed and human functional food development. *Food Rev. Int.* **2016**, *32*, 15–45. [CrossRef]

312. Abdel Khalik, K.; Osman, G. Genetic analysis of *Plectranthus* L. (Lamiaceae) in Saudi Arabia based on RAPD and ISSR markers. *Pak. J. Bot.* **2017**, *49*, 1073–1084.

313. Anisimov, M.; Chaikina, E.; Klykov, A.; Rasskazov, V. Effect of seaweeds extracts on the growth of seedling roots of buckwheat (*Fagopyrum esculentum* Moench) is depended on the season of algae collection. *Agric. Sci. Dev.* **2013**, *2*, 67–75.

314. Mukherjee, A.; Patel, J.S. Seaweed extract: Biostimulator of plant defense and plant productivity. *Int. J. Environ. Sci. Technol.* **2020**, *17*, 553–558. [CrossRef]

315. EL Boukhari, M.E.; Barakate, M.; Bouhia, Y.; Lyamlouli, K. Trends in seaweed extract based biostimulants: Manufacturing process and beneficial effect on soil-plant systems. *Plants* **2020**, *9*, 359. [CrossRef]

316. Lomartire, S.; Marques, J.C.; Gonçalves, A.M.M. An Overview to the Health Benefits of Seaweeds Consumption. *Mar. Drugs* **2021**, *19*, 341. [CrossRef]

317. Myers, S.P.; O'Connor, J.; Fitton, J.H.; Brooks, L.; Rolfe, M.; Connellan, P.; Wohlmuth, H.; Cheras, P.A.; Morris, C. A combined Phase I and II open-label study on the Immunomodulatory effects of seaweed extract nutrient complex. *Biol. Targets Ther.* **2011**, *5*, 45–60. [CrossRef]

318. Houghton, P.J.; Hylands, P.J.; Mensah, A.Y.; Hensel, A.; Deters, A.M. In vitro tests and ethnopharmacological investigations: Wound healing as an example. *J. Ethnopharmacol.* **2005**, *100*, 100–107. [CrossRef]

319. EMA. *Community Herbal Monograph on Fucus vesiculosus L., Thallus*; EMA: Amsterdam, The Netherlands, 2012.
320. Yoon, S.J.; Pyun, Y.R.; Hwang, J.K.; Mourão, P.A.S. A sulfated fucan from the brown alga *Laminaria cichorioides* has mainly heparin cofactor II-dependent anticoagulant activity. *Carbohydr. Res.* **2007**, *342*, 2326–2330. [CrossRef]
321. Drozd, N.N.; Tolstenkov, A.S.; Makarov, V.A.; Kuznetsova, T.A.; Besednova, N.N.; Shevchenko, N.M.; Zvyagintseva, T.N. Pharmacodynamic parameters of anticoagulants based on sulfated polysaccharides from marine algae. *Bull. Exp. Biol. Med.* **2006**, *142*, 591–593. [CrossRef]
322. Mansour, A.T.; Alsaqufi, A.S.; Omar, E.A.; El-Beltagi, H.S.; Srour, T.M.; Yousef, M.I. Ginseng, Tribulus extracts and pollen grains supplementation improves sexual state, testes redox status, and testicular histology in *Nile Tilapia* Males. *Antioxidants* **2022**, *11*, 875. [CrossRef]
323. Millet, J.K.; Séron, K.; Labitt, R.N.; Danneels, A.; Palmer, K.E.; Whittaker, G.R.; Dubuisson, J.; Belouzard, S. Middle East respiratory syndrome coronavirus infection is inhibited by griffithsin. *Antivir. Res.* **2016**, *133*, 1–8. [CrossRef]
324. Celikler, S.; Tas, S.; Vatan, O.; Ziyanok-Ayvalik, S.; Yildiz, G.; Bilaloglu, R. Anti-hyperglycemic and antigenotoxic potential of *Ulva rigida* ethanolic extract in the experimental diabetes mellitus. *Food Chem. Toxicol.* **2009**, *47*, 1837–1840. [CrossRef]
325. Kang, J.Y.; Khan, M.N.A.; Park, N.H.; Cho, J.Y.; Lee, M.C.; Fujii, H.; Hong, Y.K. Antipyretic, analgesic, and anti-inflammatory activities of the seaweed *Sargassum fulvellum* and *Sargassum thunbergii* in mice. *J. Ethnopharmacol.* **2008**, *116*, 187–190. [CrossRef]
326. Mukherjee, P.K.; Maity, N.; Nema, N.K.; Sarkar, B.K. Bioactive compounds from natural resources against skin aging. *Phytomedicine* **2011**, *19*, 64–73. [CrossRef]
327. Hong, D.D.; Hien, H.M.; Son, P.N. Seaweeds from Vietnam used for functional food, medicine and biofertilizer. *J. Appl. Phycol.* **2007**, *19*, 817–826. [CrossRef]
328. Khotimchenko, M.; Tiasto, V.; Kalitnik, A.; Begun, M.; Khotimchenko, R.; Leonteva, E.; Bryukhovetskiy, I.; Khotimchenko, Y. Antitumor potential of carrageenans from marine red algae. *Carbohydr. Polym.* **2020**, *246*, 116568. [CrossRef]
329. Yuan, H.; Song, J. Preparation, structural characterization and in vitro antitumor activity of kappa-carrageenan oligosaccharide fraction from *Kappaphycus striatum*. *J. Appl. Phycol.* **2005**, *17*, 7–13. [CrossRef]
330. Tannoury, M.Y.; Saab, A.M.; Elia, J.M.; Harb, N.N.; Makhlouf, H.Y.; Diab-Assaf, M. In vitro cytotoxic activity of *Laurencia papillosa*, marine red algae from the Lebanese coast. *J. Appl. Pharm. Sci.* **2017**, *7*, 175–179. [CrossRef]
331. Patra, S.; Muthuraman, M.S. *Gracilaria edulis* extract induces apoptosis and inhibits tumor in Ehrlich Ascites tumor cells in vivo. *BMC Complement. Altern. Med.* **2013**, *13*, 331. [CrossRef]
332. Alarif, W.M.; Al-Lihaibi, S.S.; Ayyad, S.E.N.; Abdel-Rhman, M.H.; Badria, F.A. Laurene-type sesquiterpenes from the Red Sea red alga *Laurencia obtusa* as potential antitumor-antimicrobial agents. *Eur. J. Med. Chem.* **2012**, *55*, 462–466. [CrossRef]
333. Celikler, S.; Yildiz, G.; Vatan, O.; Bilaloglu, R. In vitro antigenotoxicity of *Ulva rigida* C. Agardh (Chlorophyceae) extract against induction of chromosome aberration, sister chromatid exchange and micronuclei by mutagenic agent MMC. *Biomed. Environ. Sci.* **2008**, *21*, 492–498. [CrossRef]
334. Cho, K.S.; Shin, M.; Kim, S.; Lee, S.B. Recent advances in studies on the therapeutic potential of dietary carotenoids in neurodegenerative diseases. *Oxid. Med. Cell. Longev.* **2018**, *2018*, 4120458. [CrossRef]
335. Bauer, S.; Jin, W.; Zhang, F.; Linhardt, R.J. The application of seaweed polysaccharides and their derived products with potential for the treatment of Alzheimer's disease. *Mar. Drugs* **2021**, *19*, 89. [CrossRef]
336. Park, S.K.; Kang, J.Y.; Kim, J.M.; Yoo, S.K.; Han, H.J.; Chung, D.H.; Kim, D.O.; Kim, G.H.; Heo, H.J. Fucoidan-rich substances from *Ecklonia cava* improve trimethyltin-induced cognitive dysfunction via down-regulation of amyloid_production/Tau Hyperphosphorylation. *Mar. Drugs* **2019**, *17*, 591. [CrossRef]
337. Bogie, J.; Hoeks, C.; Schepers, M.; Tiane, A.; Cuypers, A.; Leijten, F.; Chintapakorn, Y.; Suttiyut, T.; Pornpakakul, S.; Struik, D.; et al. Dietary Sargassum fusiforme improves memory and reduces amyloid plaque load in an Alzheimer's disease mouse model. *Sci. Rep.* **2019**, *9*, 4908. [CrossRef]
338. Myung, C.S.; Shin, H.C.; Hai, Y.B.; Soo, J.Y.; Bong, H.L.; Jong, S.K. Improvement of memory by dieckol and phlorofucofuroeckol in ethanol-treated mice: Possible involvement of the inhibition of acetylcholinesterase. *Arch. Pharm. Res.* **2005**, *28*, 691–698. [CrossRef]
339. Ahn, B.R.; Moon, H.E.; Kim, H.R.; Jung, H.A.; Choi, J.S. Neuroprotective effect of edible brown alga *Eisenia bicyclis* on amyloid beta peptide-induced toxicity in PC12 cells. *Arch. Pharm. Res.* **2012**, *35*, 1989–1998. [CrossRef]
340. Cumashi, A.; Ushakova, N.A.; Preobrazhenskaya, M.E.; D'Incecco, A.; Piccoli, A.; Totani, L.; Tinari, N.; Morozevich, G.E.; Berman, A.E.; Bilan, M.I.; et al. A comparative study of the anti-inflammatory, anticoagulant, antiangiogenic, and antiadhesive activities of nine different fucoidans from brown seaweeds. *Glycobiology* **2007**, *17*, 541–552. [CrossRef]
341. Mei, C.H.; Zhou, S.C.; Zhu, L.; Ming, J.X.; Zeng, F.D.; Xu, R. Antitumor effects of laminaria extract fucoxanthin on lung cancer. *Mar. Drugs* **2017**, *15*, 39. [CrossRef]
342. Atya, M.E.; El-Hawiet, A.; Alyeldeen, M.A.; Ghareeb, D.A.; Abdel-Daim, M.M.; El-Sadek, M.M. In vitro biological activities and in vivo hepatoprotective role of brown algae isolated fucoidans. *Environ. Sci. Pollut. Res.* **2021**, *28*, 19664–19676. [CrossRef]
343. Wang, S.; Li, Y.; White, W.; Lu, J. Extracts from New Zealand *Undaria pinnatifida* containing fucoxanthin as potential functional biomaterials against cancer in vitro. *J. Funct. Biomater.* **2014**, *5*, 29–42. [CrossRef]
344. Shibata, H.; Iimuro, M.; Uchiya, N.; Kawamori, T.; Nagaoka, M.; Ueyama, S.; Hashimoto, S.; Yokokura, T.; Sugimura, T.; Wakabayashi, K. Preventive effects of Cladosiphon fucoidan against Helicobacter pylori infection in *Mongolian gerbils*. *Helicobacter* **2003**, *8*, 59–65. [CrossRef] [PubMed]

345. Liu, M.; Liu, Y.; Cao, M.J.; Liu, G.M.; Chen, Q.; Sun, L.; Chen, H. Antibacterial activity and mechanisms of depolymerized fucoidans isolated from *Laminaria japonica*. *Carbohydr. Polym.* **2017**, *172*, 294–305. [CrossRef] [PubMed]

346. Ayrapetyan, O.N.; Obluchinskaya, E.D.; Zhurishkina, E.V.; Skorik, Y.A.; Lebedev, D.V.; Kulminskaya, A.A.; Lapina, I.M. Antibacterial properties of fucoidans from the brown algae *Fucus vesiculosus* L. of the barents sea. *Biology* **2021**, *10*, 67. [CrossRef] [PubMed]

347. Krylova, N.V.; Ermakova, S.P.; Lavrov, V.F.; Leneva, I.A.; Kompanets, G.G.; Iunikhina, O.V.; Nosik, M.N.; Ebralidze, L.K.; Falynskova, I.N.; Silchenko, A.S.; et al. The comparative analysis of antiviral activity of native and modified fucoidans from brown algae *Fucus evanescens* In Vitro and In Vivo. *Mar. Drugs* **2020**, *18*, 224. [CrossRef]

348. Zhu, W.; Chiu, L.C.M.; Ooi, V.E.C.; Chan, P.K.S.; Ang, P.O. Antiviral property and mode of action of a sulphated polysaccharide from Sargassum patens against Herpes simplex virus type 2. *Int. J. Antimicrob. Agents* **2004**, *24*, 279–283. [CrossRef]

349. Chan, P.T.; Matanjun, P.; Yasir, S.M.; Tan, T.S. Histopathological studies on liver, kidney and heart of normal and dietary induced hyperlipidaemic rats fed with tropical red seaweed *Gracilaria changii*. *J. Funct. Foods* **2015**, *17*, 202–213. [CrossRef]

350. Kim, M.M.; Kim, S.K. Effect of phloroglucinol on oxidative stress and inflammation. *Food Chem. Toxicol.* **2010**, *48*, 2925–2933. [CrossRef]

351. Liu, X.; Wang, S.; Cao, S.; He, X.; Qin, L.; He, M.; Yang, Y.; Hao, J.; Mao, W. Structural characteristics and anticoagulant property in vitro and in vivo of a seaweed sulfated Rhamnan. *Mar. Drugs* **2018**, *16*, 243. [CrossRef]

352. Adrien, A.; Bonnet, A.; Dufour, D.; Baudouin, S.; Maugard, T.; Bridiau, N. Anticoagulant Activity of Sulfated Ulvan Isolated from the Green Macroalga Ulva rigida. *Mar. Drugs* **2019**, *17*, 291. [CrossRef]

353. Pozharitskaya, O.N.; Obluchinskaya, E.D.; Shikov, A.N. Mechanisms of Bioactivities of Fucoidan from the Brown Seaweed *Fucus vesiculosus* L. of the Barents Sea. *Mar. Drugs* **2020**, *18*, 275. [CrossRef]

354. De Zoysa, M.; Nikapitiya, C.; Jeon, Y.J.; Jee, Y.; Lee, J. Anticoagulant activity of sulfated polysaccharide isolated from fermented brown seaweed Sargassum fulvellum. *J. Appl. Phycol.* **2008**, *20*, 67–74. [CrossRef]

355. Gwon, W.G.; Lee, M.S.; Kim, J.S.; Kim, J.I.; Lim, C.W.; Kim, N.G.; Kim, H.R. Hexane fraction from Sargassum fulvellum inhibits lipopolysaccharide- induced inducible nitric oxide synthase expression in RAW 264.7 cells via NF-_B pathways. *Am. J. Chin. Med.* **2013**, *41*, 565–584. [CrossRef] [PubMed]

356. Pal, A.; Kamthania, M.C.; Kumar, A. Bioactive Compounds and Properties of Seaweeds—A Review. *Open Access Libr. J.* **2014**, *1*, 1–17. [CrossRef]

357. de Almeida, C.L.F.; Falcão, D.S.H.; Lima, D.M.G.R.; Montenegro, D.A.C.; Lira, N.S.; de Athayde-Filho, P.F.; Rodrigues, L.C.; de Souza, M.F.V.; Barbosa-Filho, J.M.; Batista, L.M. Bioactivities from marine algae of the genus Gracilaria. *Int. J. Mol. Sci.* **2011**, *12*, 4550–4573. [CrossRef] [PubMed]

358. Gunathilaka, T.L.; Samarakoon, K.W.; Ranasinghe, P.; Peiris, L.C.D. *In-Vitro* Antioxidant, Hypoglycemic Activity, and Identification of Bioactive Compounds in Phenol-Rich Extract from the Marine Red Algae Gracilaria edulis (Gmelin) Silva. *Molecules* **2019**, *24*, 3708. [CrossRef] [PubMed]

359. El-Beltagi, H.S.; El-Mogy, M.M.; Parmar, A.; Mansour, A.T.; Shalaby, T.A.; Ali, M.R. Phytochemical characterization and utilization of dried red beetroot (*Beta vulgaris*) peel extract in maintaining the quality of *Nile Tilapia* fish fillet. *Antioxidants* **2022**, *11*, 906. [CrossRef]

360. Shi, Q.; Wang, A.; Lu, Z.; Qin, C.; Hu, J.; Yin, J. Overview on the antiviral activities and mechanisms of marine polysaccharides from seaweeds. *Carbohydr. Res.* **2017**, *453–454*, 1–9. [CrossRef]

361. Panzella, L.; Napolitano, A. Natural phenol polymers: Recent advances in food and health applications. *Antioxidants* **2017**, *6*, 30. [CrossRef]

362. Gheda, S.F.; El-Adawi, H.I.; El-Deeb, N.M. Antiviral Profile of Brown and Red Seaweed Polysaccharides against Hepatitis C Virus. *Iran. J. Pharm. Res. IJPR* **2016**, *15*, 483–491.

363. Soares, A.R.; Robaina, M.C.S.; Mendes, G.S.; Silva, T.S.L.; Gestinari, L.M.S.; Pamplona, O.S.; Yoneshigue-Valentin, Y.; Kaiser, C.R.; Romanos, M.T.V. Antiviral activity of extracts from Brazilian seaweeds against herpes simplex virus. *Braz. J. Pharmacogn.* **2012**, *22*, 714–723. [CrossRef]

364. Lakshmi, V.; Goel, A.K.; Srivastava, M.N.; Raghubir, R. Bioactivity of marine organisms: Part X-Screening of some marine fauna from the Indian coasts. *Indian J. Exp. Biol.* **2006**, *44*, 754–756. [CrossRef] [PubMed]

365. Mendes, G.D.S.; Soares, A.R.; Martins, F.O.; De Albuquerque, M.C.M.; Costa, S.S.; Yoneshigue-Valentin, Y.; Gestinari, L.M.D.S.; Santos, N.; Romanos, M.T.V. Antiviral activity of the green marine alga *Ulva fasciata* on the replication of human metapneumovirus. *Rev. Inst. Med. Trop. Sao Paulo* **2010**, *52*, 3–10. [CrossRef] [PubMed]

366. Mohamed, M.E.; Kandeel, M.; Abd El-Lateef, H.M.; El-Beltagi, H.S.; Younis, N.S. The Protective effect of Anethole against Renal Ischemia/Reperfusion: The role of the TLR2,4/MYD88/NF_B pathway. *Antioxidants* **2022**, *11*, 535. [CrossRef] [PubMed]

367. Aslam, A.; Bahadar, A.; Liaquat, R.; Saleem, M.; Waqas, A.; Zwawi, M. Algae as an attractive source for cosmetics to counter environmental stress. *Sci. Total Environ.* **2021**, *772*, 144905. [CrossRef]

368. Gellenbeck, K.W. Utilization of algal materials for nutraceutical and cosmeceutical applications—What do manufacturers need to know? *J. Appl. Phycol.* **2012**, *24*, 309–313. [CrossRef]

369. Mansour, A.T.; Hamed, H.S.; El-Beltagi, H.S.; Mohamed, W.F. Modulatory effect of papaya extract against chlorpyrifos-induced oxidative stress, immune suppression, endocrine disruption, and dna damage in female *Clarias gariepinus*. *Int. J. Environ. Res. Public Health* **2022**, *19*, 4640. [CrossRef]

370. Mansour, A.T.; Alprol, A.E.; Abualnaja, K.M.; El-Beltagi, H.S.; Ramadan, K.M.A.; Ashour, M. Dried brown seaweed's phytoremediation potential for methylene blue dye removal from aquatic environments. *Polymers* **2022**, *14*, 1375. [CrossRef]

371. El-Beltagi, H.S.; Mohamed, H.I.; Abou El-Enain, M.M. Role of secondary metabolites from seaweeds in the context of plant development and crop production. In *Seaweeds as Plant Fertilizer, Agricultural Biostimulants and Animal Fodder*; Pereira, L., Bahcevandziev, K., Joshi, N.H., Eds.; CRC Press: Boca Raton, FL, USA, 2019; pp. 64–79.

372. Afify, A.E.M.M.; El-Beltagi, H.S. Effect of insecticide cyanophos on liver function in adult male rats. *Fresen. Environ. Bull.* **2011**, *20*, 1084–1088.

373. El-desoky, A.H.; Abdel-Rahman, A.H.; Rehab, F.; Ahmed, O.K.; El-Beltagi, H.S.; Hattori, M. Anti-inflammatory and antioxidant activities of naringin isolated from *Carissa carandas* L.: In vitro and in vivo evidence. *Phytomedicine* **2018**, *42*, 126–134. [CrossRef]

374. Riani Mansauda, K.L.; Anwar, E.; Nurhayati, T. Antioxidant and anti-collagenase activity of *Sargassum plagyophyllum* extract as an anti-wrinkle cosmetic ingredient. *Pharmacogn. Mag.* **2018**, *10*, 932–936. [CrossRef]

375. Mohamed, A.A.; El-Beltagi, H.S.; Rashed, M.M. Cadmium stress induced change in some hydrolytic enzymes, free radical formation and ultrastructural disorders in radish plant. *Electron. J. Environ. Agric. Food Chem.* **2009**, *8*, 969–983.

376. Unnikrishnan, P.S.; Jayasri, M.A. Marine algae as a prospective source for antidiabetic compounds—A Brief Review. *Curr. Diabetes Rev.* **2018**, *14*, 237–245. [CrossRef] [PubMed]

377. El-Beltagi, H.S.; Mohamed, H.I.; Aldaej, M.I.; Al-Khayri, J.M.; Rezk, A.A.; Al-Mssallem, M.Q.; Sattar, M.N.; Ramadan, K.M.A. Production and antioxidant activity of secondary metabolites in Hassawi rice (*Oryza sativa* L.) cell suspension under salicylic acid, yeast extract, and pectin elicitation. *In Vitro Cell. Dev. Biol. Plant.* **2022**. [CrossRef]

378. Wang, L.; Je, J.-G.; Yang, H.-W.; Jeon, Y.-J.; Lee, S. Dieckol, an algae-derived phenolic compound, suppresses UVB-induced skin damage in human dermal fibroblasts and its underlying mechanisms. *Antioxidants* **2021**, *10*, 352. [CrossRef]

379. Li, Y.; Fu, X.; Duan, D.; Liu, X.; Xu, J.; Gao, X. Extraction and identification of phlorotannins from the brown alga, *Sargassum fusiforme* (Harvey) Setchell. *Mar. Drugs* **2017**, *15*, 49. [CrossRef] [PubMed]

380. Le Lann, K.; Surget, G.; Couteau, C.; Coiffard, L.; Cérantola, S.; Gaillard, F.; Larnicol, M.; Zubia, M.; Guérard, F.; Poupart, N.; et al. Sunscreen, antioxidant, and bactericide capacities of phlorotannins from the brown macroalga Halidrys siliquosa. *J. Appl. Phycol.* **2016**, *28*, 3547–3559. [CrossRef]

381. Thiyagarasaiyar, K.; Mahendra, C.K.; Goh, B.-H.; Gew, L.T.; Yow, Y.-Y. UVB radiation protective effect of brown Alga *Padina australis*: A potential cosmeceutical application of Malaysian Seaweed. *Cosmetics* **2021**, *8*, 58. [CrossRef]

382. Fernando, I.P.S.; Dias, M.K.H.M.; Madusanka, D.M.D.; Han, E.J.; Kim, M.J.; Jeon, Y.-J.; Ahn, G. Fucoidan refined by *Sargassum confusum* indicate protective effects suppressing photo-oxidative stress and skin barrier perturbation in UVB-induced human keratinocytes. *Int. J. Biol. Macromol.* **2020**, *164*, 149–161. [CrossRef]

383. Soleimani, S.; Yousefzadi, M.; Nezhad, S.B.M.; Pozharitskaya, O.N.; Shikov, A.N. Evaluation of fractions extracted from *Polycladia myrica*: Biological activities, UVR protective effect, and stability of cream formulation based on it. *J. Appl. Phycol.* **2022**. [CrossRef]

384. Echave, J.; Otero, P.; Garcia-Oliveira, P.; Munekata, P.E.S.; Pateiro, M.; Lorenzo, J.M.; Simal-Gandara, J.; Prieto, M.A. Seaweed-Derived Proteins and Peptides: Promising Marine Bioactives. *Antioxidants* **2022**, *11*, 176. [CrossRef]